Innovative Drug Development for Headache Disorders

Frontiers in Headache Research
Volume 16

FRONTIERS IN HEADACHE RESEARCH SERIES

Published by Lippincott-Raven

Volume 1: *Migraine and Other Headaches: The Vascular Mechanisms*
J. Olesen, editor; 1991

Volume 2: *5-Hydroxytryptamine Mechanisms in Primary Headaches*
J. Olesen and P.R. Saxena, editors; 1992

Volume 3: *Tension-Type headache: Classification, Mechanisms and Treatment*
J. Olesen and J. Schoenen, editors; 1993

Volume 4: *Headache Classification and Epidemiology*
J. Olesen, editor; 1994

Volume 5: *Experimental Headache Models*
J. Olesen and M.A. Moskowitz, editors; 1995

Volume 6: *Headache Treatment: Trial Methodology and New Drugs*
J. Olesen and P. Tfelt-Hansen, editors; 1995

Volume 7: *Headache Pathogenesis: Monoamines, Neuropeptides, Purines and Nitric Oxide*
J. Olesen and L. Edvinsson, editors; 1997

Volume 8: *Genetics of Headache Disorders*
J. Olesen, editors; 1998

Published by Oxford University Press

Volume 9: *Cluster Headache and Related Conditions*
J. Olesen and P. Goadsby, editors; 1999

Volume 10: *The Triptans: Novel Drugs for Migraine*
P. Humphrey, M Ferrari, and J. Olesen, editors; 2001

Volume 11: *Reducing the Burden of Headache*
J. Olesen, T.J. Steiner, and R. Lipton, editors; 2003

Volume 12: *Preventive Pharmacotherapy of Headache Disorders*
J. Olesen, S.D. Silberstein, and P. Tfelt-Hansen, editors; 2004

Volume 13: *The Classification and Diagnosis of Headache Disorders*
J. Olesen, editor; 2005

Volume 14: *From Basic Pain Mechanisms to Headache*
J. Olesen and T.S. Jensen, editors; 2006

Volume 15: *Headache Clinics: Organization, Patients and Treatment*
R. Jensen, H-C. Diener, and J. Olesen, editors; 2007

Volume 16: *Innovative Drug Development for Headache Disorders*
J. Olesen and N. Ramadan, editors; 2008

Innovative Drug Development for Headache Disorders

Frontiers in Headache Research
Volume 16

Edited by

Jes Olesen
Department of Neurology and
Danish Headache Centre, Glostrup Hospital,
University of Copenhagen,
Denmark

Nabih Ramadan
Diamond Headache Clinic
Chicago, Illinois, USA

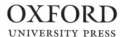

OXFORD
UNIVERSITY PRESS

OXFORD

UNIVERSITY PRESS

Great Clarendon Street, Oxford OX2 6DP

Oxford University Press is a department of the University of Oxford.
It furthers the University's objective of excellence in research, scholarship,
and education by publishing worldwide in

Oxford New York

Auckland Cape Town Dar es Salaam Hong Kong Karachi
Kuala Lumpur Madrid Melbourne Mexico City Nairobi
New Delhi Shanghai Taipei Toronto

With offices in

Argentina Austria Brazil Chile Czech Republic France Greece
Guatemala Hungary Italy Japan Poland Portugal Singapore
South Korea Switzerland Thailand Turkey Ukraine Vietnam

Oxford is a registered trade mark of Oxford University Press
in the UK and in certain other countries

Published in the United States
by Oxford University Press Inc., New York

A catalog record for this title is available from the British Library

Data available

Library of Congress Cataloging in Publication Data

Data available

Typeset by Cepha Imaging Private Ltd., Bangalore, India
Printed in Great Britain
on acid-free paper by
Biddles Ltd., King's Lynn, Norfolk

ISBN 978–0–19–955276–4

10 9 8 7 6 5 4 3 2 1

While every effort has been made to ensure that the contents of this book are as
complete, accurate and up-to-date as possible at the date of writing, Oxford
University Press is not able to give any guarantee or assurance that such is the case.
Readers are urged to take appropriately qualified medical advice in all cases. The
information in this book is intended to be useful to the general reader, but should
not be used as a means of self-diagnosis or for the prescription of medication.

Contents

Preface

Migraine treatment was very much improved with the advent of the triptans in the 1990s. While previous drugs have had efficacy, compounds such as ergotamine, had bothersome side-effects and their overuse could lead to severe complications. The triptans were the first class of drugs with high receptor specificity and disease specificity. In the early days of the triptans, it was widely presumed that migraine was no longer a treatment problem. However, it has gradually been recognized that a significant proportion of patients are not responsive to triptans or do not tolerate them. Furthermore, the success criteria in the triptan trials were quite relaxed. With more strict success criteria, particularly the sustained pain-free response, one-third of the patients or lower respond. It is now clear that, even with effective attack treatment, patients with frequent attacks are not treated well exclusively with acute medications. This is partly because patients are still bothered by the attacks and partly because frequent intake of acute medication may result in medication overuse headache. These problems have led to a renewed interest in preventive migraine drugs. In relation to the other major primary headache disorder, chronic tension-type headache, there has not been much progress. Amitriptyline is still the mainstay of treatment but recently mirtazapine has also proven to be of value. There is a great need for preventive drugs for chronic tension-type headache.

Recent European data have shown that research funding of the migraine in Europe is the lowest of all of 12 major brain disorders studied. Research support to other types of headache could not be identified at all. The combined headache field probably receives less than 10% of the funding of epilepsy or movement disorders but costs society four times more. How can therapeutic progress then be expected? The happy message is that despite the gloomy figures on research support, there have been significant advances in migraine research over recent years. As demonstrated in this volume, there are several promising new avenues for the development of future drugs for migraine. The main principles with proof of concept, but not yet in full clinical development, are cortical spreading depression inhibition, nitric oxide synthase inhibition, and calcitonin gene-related peptide receptor antagonism. The present book presents frontline knowledge as far as it is available in the public domain. Hopefully, readers and their patients will find it exciting to learn about all the novel possibilities, and hopefully the impressive research advances in migraine will lead to increased funding, not only of migraine but also of other types of headache. Only then can we fully exploit all the academic advances for the benefit of our patients.

Contributors

Ashina, Messoud
Danish Headache Center and Department
of Neurology, Glostrup Hospital,
University of Copenhagen,
Glostrup, Denmark

Bleakman, David
Lilly Research Laboratories, Lilly
Corporate Center,
Indianapolis, USA

Blower, Peter R.
Minster Pharmaceuticals plc.,
Audley End Business Centre,
The Old Forge, Saffron Walden,
Essex, UK

Bräuner-Osborne, Hans
Department of Medical Chemistry,
Faculty of Pharmaceutical Sciences,
University of Copenhagen,
Copenhagen, Denmark

Brennan, Kevin C.
Headache Research and Treatment
Program, Department of Neurology,
David Geffen School of Medicine at
UCLA, Los Angeles, California, USA

Buscone, Simona
University Centre for the Study of
Adaptive Disorder and Headache,
University of Pavia, Italy

Charles, Andrew C.
Headache Research and Treatment
Program, Department of Neurology,
David Geffen School of Medicine at
UCLA, Los Angeles, USA

Chizh, Boris A.
GlaxoSmithKline, Addenbrooke's
Centre for Clinical Investigation,
Addenbrooke's Hospital,
Cambridge, UK

Christiansen, Bolette
Department of Medical Chemistry,
Faculty of Pharmaceutical Sciences,
University of Copenhagen,
Copenhagen, Denmark

Clemens-Smith, Amy
Lilly Research Laboratories, Lilly
Corporate Center,
Indianapolis, USA

Colnaghi, S.
Laboratory of Ocular Movements,
Foundation IRCCS 'C. Mondino',
Pavia, Italy

Dahlöf, Carl G.H.
Institute of Neuroscience and Physiology,
Department of Clinical Neuroscience
and Rehabilitation,
Sahlgrenska University Hospital,
Göteborg, Sweden

Dehlinger, Veronique
Eli Lilly and Co. Ltd., Lilly Research
Centre, Erl Wood Manor,
Windlesham,
Surrey, UK

Dell, Colin P.
Eli Lilly and Co. Ltd., Lilly Research
Centre, Erl Wood Manor,
Windlesham
Surrey, UK

Dieckman, Donna K.
Lilly Research Laboratories,
Lilly Corporate Center,
Indianapolis, USA

Edvinsson, Lars
Clinical Experimental Research,
Glostrup Research Institute,
Glostrup Hospital,
Glostrup, Denmark

Ferrari, Michel D.
Leiden University Medical Centre,
Leiden, The Netherlands

Filla, Sandra A.
Lilly Research Laboratories,
Lilly Corporate Center,
Indianapolis, USA

Fioravanti, Beatriz
Department of Pharmacology,
College of Medicine, University of
Arizona, Tucson, Arizona, USA

Greco, Rosaria
IRCCS Neurological Institute
'C. Mondino Foundation', Pavia, Italy

Hansen, Jakob Møller
Danish Headache Center and
Department of Neurology,
Glostrup Hospital, Faculty of
Health Sciences, University of
Copenhagen, Glostrup,
Denmark

Hudziak, Kevin J.
Lilly Research Laboratories,
Lilly Corporate Center,
Indianapolis, USA

Jansen-Olesen, Inger
Department of Neurology and Danish
Headache Center,
Glostrup Research Institute, Glostrup
Hospital, University of Copenhagen,
Glostrup, Denmark

Jensen, Anders A.
Department of Medical Chemistry,
Faculty of Pharmaceutical Sciences,
University of Copenhagen,
Copenhagen, Denmark

Jensen, Rigmor
Danish Headache Center and
Department of Neurology,
Glostrup Hospital, University of
Copenhagen, Glostrup, Denmark

Johnson, Kirk W.
Lilly Research Laboratories,
Lilly Corporate Center,
Indianapolis, USA

Johnson, Michael P.
Lilly Research Laboratories,
Lilly Corporate Center,
Indianapolis, USA

Juhl, Louise
Department of Neurology,
Glostrup Research Institute,
Glostrup Hospital,
Glostrup, Denmark

Kvist, Trine
Department of Medical Chemistry,
Faculty of Pharmaceutical Sciences,
University of Copenhagen,
Copenhagen, Denmark

Marchioni, E.
Department of Clinical Neurology,
IRCCS Foundation 'C. Mondino',
Pavia, Italy

Nappi, Giuseppe
Scientific Direction, IRCCS Foundation
'C. Mondino', Pavia, Italy, and Department
of Neurology and ORL, University 'La
Sapienza', Rome, Italy, and Headache Unit
and University Centre for Adaptive
Disorders and Headache (UCADH),
University of Pavia, Italy

Nisenbaum, Eric S.
Eli Lilly and Co. Ltd., Lilly Research
Centre Erl Wood Manor, Windlesham,
Surrey, UK

Olesen, Jes
Department of Neurology and
Danish Headache Centre, Glostrup
Hospital, University of Copenhagen,
Glostrup, Denmark

Ornstein, Paul L.
Lilly Research Laboratories,
Lilly Corporate Center,
Indianapolis, USA

Perrotta, Armando
University Centre for the Study of
Adaptive Disorder and Headache
(UCADH), University of Pavia,
Italy

Pichiecchio, A.
Neuroradiology Department,
Foundation IRCCS 'C. Mondino',
Pavia, Italy

Ploug, Kenneth Beri
Department of Neurology
and Danish Headache Centre,
Glostrup Research Institute, Glostrup
Hospital, University of Copenhagen,
Glostrup, Denmark

Rahmann, Alexandra Maria
Department of Neurology,
University Hospital Münster,
Münster, Germany

Ramadan, Nabih M.
Rosalind Franklin University of
Medicine and Science,
North Chicago, USA

Rogawski, Michael A.
Department of Neurology, School of
Medicine, University of California,
Sacramento, California, USA

Sandrini, Giorgio
University Centre for the Study of
Adaptive Disorder and Headache
(UCADH), University of Pavia,
Italy and IRCCS Neurological
Institute 'C. Mondino Foundation',
Pavia, Italy

Saxena, Pramod R.
Department of Pharmacology,
Erasmus MC, University Medical Center,
Rotterdam, The Netherlands

Sharpe, Paul C.
Minster Pharmaceuticals plc.,
Saffron Walden,
Essex, UK

Siuda, Edward R.
Lilly Research Laboratories,
Lilly Corporate Center,
Indianapolis, USA

Tassorelli, Cristina
University Centre for the Study of
Adaptive Disorder and Headache
(UCADH), University of Pavia,
Italy and IRCCS Neurological Institute
'C. Mondino Foundation',
Pavia, Italy

Tavazzi, E.
Department of Clinical Neurology, IRCCS
Foundation 'C. Mondino', Pavia, Italy

Tfelt-Hansen, Peer
Department of Neurology,
Glostrup Hospital,
University of Copenhagen,
Glostrup, Denmark

Van den Maagdenberg, Arn M.J.M.
Department of Neurology, Leiden
University Medical Center, Leiden,
The Netherlands, and Department of
Human Genetics, Leiden University
Medical Center, The Netherlands

Vanderah, Todd W.
Department of Pharmacology, College of
Medicine, University of Arizona, Tucson,
Arizona, USA

Versino, M.
Laboratory of Ocular Movements,
Foundation IRCCS 'C. Mondino',
Pavia, Italy

Waeber, Christian
Department of Radiology,
Massachusetts General Hospital,
Charlestown, Massachusetts, USA

Wienecke, Troels
Danish Headache Center
and Department of Neurology,
Glostrup Hospital,
Faculty of Health Sciences,
University of Copenhagen,
Glostrup, Denmark

Session I

Screening models

The human γ-aminobutyric acid transporter GAT-2: from cloning to high throughput screening

Bolette Christiansen,* Trine Kvist,*
Anders A. Jensen, and Hans Bräuner-Osborne

γ-Aminobutyric acid (GABA) is the major inhibitory neurotransmitter in the mammalian central nervous system (CNS). In the GABAergic synapse, GABA is released from presynaptic nerve terminals and it exerts its physiological effects through the ionotropic $GABA_A$ and $GABA_C$ receptors and the metabotropic $GABA_B$ receptors. The GABAergic neurotransmission is terminated by rapid uptake of the neurotransmitter from the synaptic cleft into neurones and glial cells by specific high-affinity GABA transporters. To date, four different plasma membrane GABA transporter (GAT) subtypes have been identified in the CNS and some peripheral tissues in several mammalian species. Unless otherwise specified, we will use the nomenclature introduced by Guastella et al.[1] and Borden et al.[2] for human and rat GATs and refer to the transporters as GAT-1, betaine/GABA transporter-1 (BGT-1), GAT-2, and GAT-3. A different nomenclature, originally suggested by Liu et al.,[3] names the corresponding homologous transporters in mouse GAT1–GAT4 (without hyphen), respectively.

The GABA transporters belong to the family of Na^+/Cl^--dependent transporters (SLC6 gene family), which also includes transporters for the neurotransmitters dopamine, serotonin, noradrenaline, and glycine.[4] The topologies of these membrane-bound proteins are composed of 12 transmembrane domains connected by intracellular and extracellular loops, and intracellular amino and carboxy termini. Recently, crystal structures of a bacterial homologue of the transporters have been resolved, and they have contributed with considerable information about the structure and function of the Na^+/Cl^--dependent transporters.[5–7]

Neurotransmitter transporters are drug targets for several neurological and psychiatric disorders.[4] Diseases such as epilepsy, anxiety disorders, schizophrenia, drug addiction, and various pain states are related to the GABA system, and pharmacological inhibition of GABA transport constitutes an attractive approach to increase overall GABA neurotransmission. So far, this concept has been exploited in the treatment of epilepsy where

* These authors contributed equally to this work.

the GAT-1 selective inhibitor tiagabine is administered clinically as adjunctive therapy for partial seizures. In contrast to the availability of GAT-1 selective inhibitors, selective ligands for the three other GABA transporter subtypes have so far not been published.

In contrast to the four identified plasma membrane GABA transporter subtypes in mouse and rat, only three orthologue subtypes, hGAT-1, hBGT-1, and hGAT-3, have been characterized in humans. The human orthologue of mouse (m) GAT3 and rat (r) GAT-2 has remained enigmatic and is typically referred to as 'not cloned' in the literature.[8] In 2001, the cDNA supposedly encoding for the hGAT-2 was reported cloned but functional uptake of [³H]GABA in mammalian cells transiently transfected with this cDNA could not be demonstrated.[9] Bioinformatic analysis of this putative hGAT-2 sequence revealed that it was likely to be an incomplete cDNA sequence with several truncations. Here we describe the cloning of the full-length hGAT-2 and the pharmacological characterization of the transporter using a number of standard GABA transporter substrates and inhibitors. Furthermore, we have performed a screening of a small commercial compound library with the objective of identifying subtype-selective ligands for GAT-2.

Experimental procedures

Materials

GlutaMAX-I Dulbecco's modified Eagle medium, Ham's F12 with L-glutamine, dialysed foetal bovine serum, penicillin, streptomycin, zeocin, hygromycin B, Hanks' balanced salt solution, and bovine serum albumin were purchased from Invitrogen (Paisley, UK). Plasmocin was purchased from InvivoGen (San Diego, CA, USA). Dimethyl sulphoxide and buffer reagents were obtained from Sigma-Aldrich (St Louis, MO, USA). [2,3-³H(N)]GABA (specific radioactivity either 27.6 Ci/mmol or 40.0 Ci/mmol) and D-[2,3-³H]Aspartate (specific radioactivity 40.0 Ci/mmol) were purchased from Perkin Elmer (Waltham, MA, USA).

β-Alanine, taurine, L-2,4-diamino-n-butyric acid (L-DABA), quinidine, NNC-711, and (S)-SNAP-5114 were purchased from Sigma-Aldrich. GABA was obtained from Fluka Chemie AG, Buchs SG (Dübendorf, Switzerland), betaine from B.A.S. Synteselaboratorium (Denmark), nipecotic acid from Aldrich Chemical Company Inc. (Milwaukee, WI, USA), and DL-2,3-diaminopropionic acid (DAPA) from TCI Europe nv (Zwijndrecht, Belgium). The following compounds were synthesized in house: 4,5,6, 7-tetrahydroisoxazolo(4,5-c)pyridin-3-ol (THPO), guvacine, and N-[4,4-bis(3-methyl-2-thienyl)-3-butenyl]-3-hydroxy-4-(methylamino)-4,5,6,7-tetrahydrobenzo[d]isoxazol-3-ol (EF1502) (see reference 10 for references).

Cloning of hGAT-2

The IMAGE cDNA clone 4612245 was purchased and subsequent sequencing revealed the presence of the full-length nucleotide sequence encoding for the open reading frame of hGAT-2. The cDNA of hGAT-2 was amplified by polymerase chain reaction (PCR) using the forward primer 5´-gggatggatagcagggtctc-3´ and the reverse primer

5′-ctagcagtgagactctagctc-3′, and subcloned into the mammalian pcDNA5 vector according to the protocol of the manufacturer (pcDNA5/FRT/V5-His TOPO® TA Expression Kit, Invitrogen). The sequence of the cDNA and the absence of mutations were confirmed by automated DNA sequencing.

Bioinformatic analysis of the protein sequence of hGAT-2

An alignment of the amino acid sequence of hGAT-2 with the previous reported sequences of hGAT-2[9] and of the mouse orthologue mGAT3[3] was performed using the ClustalW alignment program available at the home page maintained by The European Bioinformatics Institute (http://www.ebi.ac.uk/Tools/clustalw/index.html). Transmembrane segments in the hGAT-2 protein were identified by the hidden Markov model for prediction of transmembrane helices. The algorithm is publicly accessible at the Center for Biological Sequence Analysis, Technical University of Denmark through internet services (http://www.cbs.dtu.dk/services/TMHMM/). Furthermore, a hydrophobicity analysis using the TMpred program was performed. This algorithm is based on the statistical analysis of TMbase, a database of naturally occurring transmembrane proteins, and is available at the home page maintained by Swiss EMBnet (http://www.ch.embnet.org/software/TMPRED_form.html).

Cell culture and transfections

tsA201 cells (a transformed HEK293 cell line) were cultured in GlutaMAX-I Dulbecco's modified Eagle medium supplemented with 10% dialysed foetal bovine serum, penicillin (100 U/ml), and streptomycin (100 µg/ml) at 37°C in a humidified atmosphere of 95% air and 5% CO_2. The constructs encoding the hGAT-2 and the human excitatory amino acid transporter hEAAT3 were transiently transfected into cells using PolyFect according to the protocol of the manufacturer (Qiagen, West Sussex, UK), and the functional assays were performed 36–48 h later.

Construction of a stable cell line expressing hGAT-2

Flp-In™-CHO cells (Invitrogen) were cultured in Ham's F12 medium with L-glutamine supplemented with 10% foetal bovine serum, penicillin (100 U/ml), streptomycin (100 µg/ml), plasmocin (5 µg/ml), and zeocin (100 µg/ml) at 37°C in a humidified atmosphere of 95% air and 5% CO_2. The cells were co-transfected with pOG44 (Invitrogen) and hGAT-2-pcDNA5/FRT using PolyFect, and the stable cell line was generated according to the protocol of the manufacturer (Invitrogen). After transfection, the cells were cultured under selection pressure due to the presence of hygromycin B (200 µg/ml) in Ham's F12 with L-glutamine supplemented with 10% foetal bovine serum, penicillin (100 U/ml), streptomycin (100 µg/ml), and plasmocin (5 µg/ml).

Validation of integration of hGAT-2 into the Flp-In™-CHO cells

Genomic DNA was prepared by solubilizing CHO cells stably expressing hGAT-2 in a buffer containing 50 mM KCl, 10 mM Tris–HCl, 2 mM MgCl2, 0.1 mg/ml gelatin, 0.45% Nonidet P40, 0.45% TWEEN 20, pH 8.3. Proteinase K was added and the mixture was incubated at 56°C for 2 h. Next, the mixture was placed at 95°C for 10 min and subsequently stored at 4°C. The genomic DNA was amplified by PCR using the forward hGAT-2 primer 5′-gggatggatagcagggtctc-3′ and the reverse hGAT-2 primer 5′-ctagcagtgagactctagctc-3′. PCR was performed using Advantage polymerase as described by the manufacturer (Clontech, Mountain View, CA, USA). The reactions were heated to 94°C for 1 min and then cycled 35 times at 94°C for 30 s and 68°C for 2 min. The final elongation step was performed at 68°C for 10 min. Untransfected Flp-In™-CHO cells were used as negative control. The reactions were run on a 1% agarose gel containing SYBR Safe™ (Invitrogen) to visualize the PCR products.

[³H]GABA and D-[³H]Asp uptake assays

tsA201 cells transfected with hGAT-2-pcDNA5, tsA201 cells transfected with hEAAT3-pcDNA3, or Flp-In™-CHO cells stably expressing hGAT-2 were split into poly-D-lysine-coated white 96-well plates (Perkin Elmer, Boston, MA, USA). The next day, the medium was removed and cells were washed with 100 µl assay buffer (Hanks' balanced salt solution supplemented with 20 mM HEPES, 1 mM $CaCl_2$, and 1 mM $MgCl_2$, pH 7.4). Then assay buffer supplemented with [³H]GABA or D-[³H]Asp and various test compounds was added on to the cells, and the plate was incubated at 37°C for 3 min. Then the cells were washed with 3 × 100 µl ice-cold assay buffer and 150 µl Microscint™20 scintillation fluid (Perkin Elmer, Boston, MA, USA) was added. The plate was shaken for at least 1 h and counted in a Packard TopCount microplate scintillation counter.

In the saturation experiments, 75 µl assay buffer supplemented with [³H]GABA in concentration up to 100 nM was used and in order to measure transport at higher concentrations the radioligand (100 nM [³H]GABA) was diluted with various concentrations of 'cold' GABA. Non-specific transport was determined in the presence of 3 mM GABA.

In the competition transport experiments, 75 µl of assay buffer supplemented with either 30 nM [³H]GABA (in the experiments with hGAT-2) or 30 nM D-[³H]Asp (in the experiments with hEAAT3) was used. The [³H]GABA competition curves were constructed based on measurements obtained typically for eight different concentrations of the test compounds. The following maximum concentrations of the test compounds were applied: GABA, 3 mM; DAPA, 1 mM; β-alanine, 3 mM; (S)-SNAP-5114, 500 µM; EF1502, 250 µM; nipecotic acid, 10 mM; L-DABA, 3 mM; quinidine, 1 mM; guvacine, 10 mM; NNC-711, 1.6 mM; THPO, 10 mM; taurine, 10 mM; betaine, 10 mM. These maximum concentrations were also applied to cells expressing hEAAT3.

In the high throughput screening experiments, 50 µl assay buffer supplemented with 30 nM [³H]GABA was used. The compounds were transferred from each well on the duplex plate to the respective well on the cell plate. When estimating the Z' factor, 75 µl assay buffer supplemented with 30 nM [³H]GABA was used as negative control and 1 mM GABA was used as positive control.

High throughput screening

A compound library (ChemBridge Inc, San Diego, CA, USA) was screened at CHO cells stably expressing hGAT-2 in the search for inhibitors of [³H]GABA uptake through this transporter. The compound library contained 3040 compounds distributed into the wells of a total of 38 96-well plates. Each 96-well plate was composed of 16 empty wells and 80 wells containing 0.1 mg of solid compound with a molecular weight of 230–500 g/mol. The 16 empty wells were placed diagonally across the plate with two empty wells in each row (Figure 1.4A).

Preparation of a 'daughter library'

To each well of all 38 mother plates was added 20 µl dimethyl sulphoxide. The plates were shaken for 1 h followed by centrifugation at 2000 rpm for 1 min. 2 µl from each well on the mother plate was transferred to a 'daughter plate', the 'mother library' giving rise to a total of seven 'daughter libraries'. The 38 plates representing a complete 'daughter library' were sealed and stored at -18°C until the day of testing.

Preparation of duplex plates

On the day of testing, a duplex plate was produced by pooling two daughter plates. A 130 µl assay buffer supplemented with 30 nM [^{3}H]GABA was added to each well on the daughter plate. From an odd numbered plate, plate no. X, 120 µl was transferred to an even numbered plate, plate number X+1, giving a total amount of 250 µl in each well of this duplex plate. A final concentration of 2 mM GABA was added as positive control to eight of the 16 wells without compound. Each duplex plate was screened at hGAT-2 at a concentration of 80–170 µM of each single compound using the [^{3}H]GABA uptake assay.

Data analysis

Data was analysed using Prism 4.0b (GraphPad Software, San Diego, CA, USA). The saturation curves and the inhibition curves were all fitted by non-linear regression (see reference 10 for further details).

Z' and Z were calculated using the formulas $Z' = 1 - ((3\sigma_{c+} + 3\sigma_{c-})/|\mu_{c+} - \mu_{c-}|)$ and $Z = 1 - ((3\sigma_s + 3\sigma_{c+})/|\mu_s - \mu_{c+}|)$ where σ_{c+}, σ_{c-}, and σ_s are the standard deviation of the positive control, the negative control, and the sample, respectively, and μ_{c+}, μ_{c-}, and μ_s are the mean of the positive control, the negative control, and the sample, respectively.

Results

Cloning of the hGAT-2

Initially we performed a multiple alignment of the amino acid sequence of the previously cloned non-functional hGAT-2 (GenBank accession number U76343[9]) with the mouse and rat orthologues. This comparison revealed that the previously reported hGAT-2 cDNA clone contained four truncations and a fairly different C-terminal sequence compared with the murine sequences. Owing to these differences we next performed a tBLASTn search of the human genome and expressed sequence tag (EST) databases at the NCBI website using the mGAT3 amino acid sequence as query. Results from both of these databases suggested that the truncations and deviating C-terminal sequence of the previously reported hGAT-2 cDNA clone was erroneous and that a full-length human orthologue does exist. Further searches of GenBank at NCBI revealed a full-length cDNA clone identified by the Mammalian Gene Collection Program Team (accession number BC022392) that could be obtained from the I.M.A.G.E. Consortium. We then used PCR to amplify a nucleotide sequence from the I.M.A.G.E. clone which is identical to the GenBank entry BC022392. The cDNA has a predicted amino acid sequence containing an open reading frame of 602 amino acids, which is in good agreement with the lengths of the rat and mouse orthologues.[2,3] Alignment analysis demonstrates that the sequence is different from the truncated hGAT-2 of 569 amino acids previously reported by Gong et al.,[9] and that the amino acid sequence of the full-length hGAT-2, described here, displays high similarity to mGAT3 (Figure 1.1).

Analysis of sequence

A search in the gene database maintained by NCBI demonstrated that the gene for hGAT-2 (SLC6A13) is localized to human chromosome 12p13.3. The presence of 14 exons in the gene was found by comparison between the amino acid sequence of hGAT-2 and the genomic DNA. These findings are similar to what has recently been reported for hGAT-2 in a description of the complete repertoire of the SLC6 family.[11]

The topology of the predicted protein was analysed using two different analysis tools for prediction of transmembrane helices. Analysis by the hidden Markov model predicted the presence of 12 transmembrane α-helices. Hydrophobicity analysis using the TMpred program identified two possible models for transmembrane topology with 11 and 12 transmembrane α-helices, respectively, depending on the predicted orientation of the membrane spanning segments. Collectively, the two algorithms demonstrate that hGAT-2 contains 12 putative transmembrane α-helices, which is expected for a member of the Na^+/Cl^--dependent neurotransmitter transporter superfamily.[12]

Pharmacological characterization of hGAT-2 in the [³H]GABA uptake assay

In order to determine whether the cloned hGAT-2 cDNA encodes for a functional GABA transporter, we expressed the hGAT-2 construct in tsA201 cells. Using a [³H]GABA uptake assay, we could demonstrate transporter-specific uptake of GABA, and in saturation experiments, a dose-dependent increase in [³H]GABA uptake reaching saturation levels at higher concentrations was observed. The saturable transport of GABA was characterized by a Km value of 8.24 ± 0.38 μM ($n = 4$) (Figure 1.2A).

The pharmacological properties of 13 standard GABA transporter ligands were characterized at the hGAT-2 in the [³H]GABA uptake assay using a tracer concentration of 30 nM [³H]GABA. In this assay, all test compounds displayed dose-dependent inhibition curves, with the exception of betaine, which only displayed minor inhibitory activity at concentrations up to 10 mM. GABA, DAPA, and β-alanine displayed the most potent inhibition of GABA-transport at hGAT-2 (IC_{50} values in the 10–100 μM range). The compounds (S)-SNAP-5114, EF1502, nipecotic acid, L-DABA, and quinidine displayed some inhibition of [³H]GABA-transport (IC_{50} values 100–800 μM), whereas guvacine,

```
hGAT-2    MDSRVSGTTSNGETKPVYPVMEKKEEDGTLERGHWNNKMEFVLSVAGEIIGLGNVWRFPY 60
mGAT3     MENRASGTTSNGETKPVCPAMEKVEEDGTLEREHWNNKMEFVLSVAGEIIGLGNVWRFPY 60
U76343    MDSRVSGTTSNGETKP------------------YHKMEFVLSVAGEIIGLGNVWRFPY 41
          *:.*.**********                   :*********************

hGAT-2    LCYKNGGGAFFIPYLVFLFTCGIPVFLLETALGQYTSQGGVTAWRRICPIFEGIGYASQM 120
mGAT3     LCYKNGGGAFFIPYLIFLFTCGIPVFFLETALGQYTNQGGITAWRRICPIFEGIGYASQM 120
U76343    LCYKNGGGAFFIPYLVFLFTCGIPVFLLETALGQYTSQGGVTAWRKICPIFEGIGYASQM 101
          ***************:**********:*********.*** ***:**** :*************

hGAT-2    IVILLNVYYIIVLAWALFYLFSSFTIDLPWGGCYHEWNTEHCMEFQKTNGSLNGTSENAT 180
mGAT3     IVSLLNVYYIVVLAWALFYLFSSFTTDLPWGSCSHEWNTENCVEFQKANDSMNVTSENAT 180
U76343    IVILLNVYYIIVLAWALFYLFSSFTIDLPWGGCYHEWNTEHCMEFQKTNGSLNGTSENAT 161
          ** *******:************** *****.* ******:*:****:*.*:* ******

hGAT-2    SPVIEFWERRVLKISDGIQHLGALRWELALCLLLAWVICYFCIWKGVKSTGKVVYFTATF 240
mGAT3     SPVIEFWERRVLKLSDGIQHLGSLRWELVLCLLLAWIICYFCIWKGVKSTGKVVYFTATF 240
U76343    SPVIEFWERRVLKISDGIQHLGALRWELALCLLLAWVICYFCIWKGVKSTGKVVYFTATF 221
          *************:********:*****.*******:***********************

hGAT-2    PYLMLVVLLIRGVTLPGAAQGIQFYLYPNLTRLWDPQVWMDAGTQIFFSFATCLGCLTAL 300
mGAT3     PYLMLVVLLIRGVTLPGAAQGIQFYLYPNITRLWDPQVWMDAGTQIFFSFAICLGCLTAL 300
U76343    PYLMLVVLLIRGVTLPGAAQGIQFYLYPNLTRLWDPQVWMDAGTQIFFSFAICLGCLTAL 281
          *****************************:********************:***********

hGAT-2    GSYNKYHNNCYRDCIALFGLNSGTSFVAGFAIFSILGFMSQEQGVPISEVAESGPGLAFI 360
mGAT3     GSYNKYHNNCYRDCIALCILNSSTSFMAGFAIFSILGFMSQEQGVPISEVAESGPGLAFI 360
U76343    GSYNKYHNNCY----------SGTSFVAGFAIFSILGFMSQEQGVPISEVAESGPGLAFI 331
          ***********          *.***.*********************************

hGAT-2    AYPRAVVMLPFSPLWACCFFFMVVLLGLDSQFVCVESLVTALVDMYPHVFRKKNRREVLI 420
mGAT3     AYPRAVVMLPFSPLWACCFFFMVVLLGLDSQFVCVESLVTALVDMYPRVFRKKNRREVLI 420
U76343    AYPRAVVMLPFSPLWACCFFFMVVLLGLDSQFVCVESLVTALVDMYPHVFRKKNRREVLI 391
          ***********************************************:.************

hGAT-2    LGVSVVSFLVGLIMLTEGGMYVFQLFDYYAASGMCLLFVAIFESLCVAWVYGAKRFYDNI 480
mGAT3     LIVSVISFFIGLIMLTEGGMYVFQLFDYYAASGMCLLFVAIFESLCVAWVYGAGRFYDNI 480
U76343    LGVSVVSFPVGLIMLTEGGMYVFQLFDYYAASGMCLLFVAIFESLCVAWVYGAKRFYDNI 451
          * ***:** :***************************************** ******

hGAT-2    EDMIGYRPWPLIKYCWLFLTPAVCTATFLFSLIKYTPLTYNKKYTYPWWGDALGWLLALS 540
mGAT3     EDMIGYKPWPLIKYCWLFFTPAVCLATFLFSLIKYTPLTYNKKYTYPWWGDALGWLLALS 540
U76343    EDMIGYRPWPLIKYCWLFLTPAVCTATFLFSLIKYTPLTYNKKYTYPWWGDALGWLLALS 511
          ******:***********:*****.***** ****************************

hGAT-2    SMVCIPAWSLYRLGTLKGPFRERIRQLMCPAEDLPQRNPAGPSAPATPRTSLLRLTELES 600
mGAT3     SMICIPAWSIYKLRTLKGPLRERLRQLVCPAEDLPQKNQPEPTAPATPMTSLLRLTELES 600
U76343    SWSAFLPGASTDSEPSRAPSERESVSSCAQPRTCPSGTQQDPRLPPPPGP---HCSDSQS 568
          *  .: .:     . :.*  ...  . ...  *. .    *  *..*

hGAT-2    HC 602
mGAT3     NC 602
U76343    --
```

Fig. 1.1 Alignment analysis. Shown are the amino acid sequence of hGAT-2 described in this study (accession number NP_057699), and the deduced amino acid sequence of the previously reported non-functional hGAT-2 (accession number U76343).[9] The amino acid sequence of mGAT3 (accession number NP_653095) is shown for comparison. The alignment was made using the ClustalW alignment tool provided by the European Molecular Biology Laboratory: star (*) indicates that a residue in a certain position is identical in all three sequences in the alignment, colon (:) indicates a conserved substitution, period (.) indicates a semi-conserved substitution. Reproduced from *The Journal of Biological Chemistry*, 282 (27), Christiansen B, Meinild AK, Jensen AA, Bräuner-Osborne H, Cloning and characterization of a functional human γ-aminobutyric acid (GABA) transporter, human GAT-2 (2007), pp.19331–41 with permission from the American Society for Biochemistry and Molecular Biology.

NNC-711, THPO, taurine, and betaine were weak or very weak inhibitors of the transporter activity (IC$_{50}$ values ≥ 1000 μM) (Table 1.1 and Figure 1.2B). As a control for nonspecific inhibition of [^{3}H]GABA uptake, the test compounds were also characterized at hEAAT3-expressing tsA201 cells. None of the compounds inhibited the uptake of D-[^{3}H]Asp by hEAAT3 in the maximum concentrations used for hGAT-2 (data not shown).

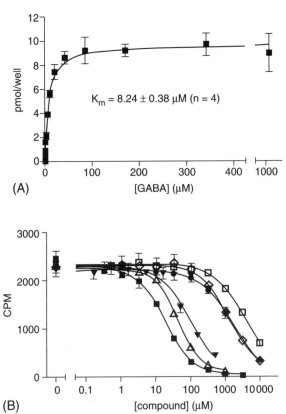

(A)

(B)

Fig. 1.2 Pharmacological characterization of hGAT-2 in the [^{3}H]GABA uptake assay using tsA201 cells transiently transfected with hGAT-2. (A) Saturation curve for GABA transport where specific uptake of increasing concentrations of GABA was measured. The uptake assay was performed as described in Experimental procedures. Data are given as pmol/well and are mean ± SD of triplicate determinations of a single representative experiment. The K$_m$ for GABA was determined to be 8.24 ± 0.38 μM ($n = 4$). Reproduced from *The Journal of Biological Chemistry*, 282 (27), Christiansen B, Meinild AK, Jensen AA, Bräuner-Osborne H, Cloning and characterization of a functional human Á-aminobutyric acid (GABA) transporter, human GAT-2 (2007), pp.19331–41, with permission from the American Society for Biochemistry and Molecular Biology. (B) Concentration–inhibition curves for standard substrates and inhibitors of hGAT-2 transport. Inhibition of the uptake of 30 nM [^{3}H]GABA by hGAT-2 by the indicated standard ligands was performed as described in Experimental procedures. Results are given as counts per minute (CPM) and are mean ± SD of triplicate determinations of single representative experiments. At least two additional experiments performed on different days gave similar results. Modified from reference 10. ■ GABA; △ DAPA; ▼ (*S*)-SNAP-5114; ◇ Guvacine; ● THPO; ☐ Taurine.

Table 1.1 IC_{50} values for standard GAT substrates and inhibitors at hGAT-2 expressed transiently in tsA201 cells. The test compounds were examined for their ability to inhibit uptake of 30 nM [^{3}H]GABA as described in Experimental procedures. All experiments were performed in triplicate in at least three independent experiments.

Compound	hGAT-2 IC_{50} ($pIC_{50} \pm$ SEM) μM
GABA	10.9 (4.99 ± 0.07)
DAPA	28.2 (4.58 ± 0.13)
β-alanine	41.9 (4.41 ± 0.12)
(S)-SNAP-5114	126 (3.91 ± 0.06)[a]
EF1502	286 (3.55 ± 0.02)[a]
Nipecotic acid	530 (3.28 ± 0.05)
L-DABA	633 (3.20 ± 0.05)[a]
Quinidine	716 (3.15 ± 0.05)[a]
Guvacine	1000 (3.01 ± 0.08)
NNC-711	1210 (2.93 ± 0.07)[a]
THPO	1450 (2.84 ± 0.01)[a]
Taurine	>3000[a]
Betaine	>3000[a]

[a] The concentration–inhibition curves for compounds that displayed <90% inhibition of hGAT-2 at the maximal tested concentration were fitted to the value of 100% inhibition (1 mM GABA). These compounds exhibited the following maximal inhibition (in %): (S)-SNAP-5114 (500 μM), 80.3 ± 1.3; EF1502 (250 μM), 47.4 ± 2.1; L-DABA (3 mM), 77.9 ± 1.9; quinidine (1 mM), 61.6 ± 4.2; NNC-711 (1.6 mM), 58.9 ± 3.9; THPO (10 mM), 87.6 ± 1.0; taurine (10 mM), 74.1 ± 0.2; betaine (10 mM), 21.3 ± 1.6.

Setting up a high throughput screening assay

In the search for novel inhibitors of GAT-2 we decided to perform a screening of a compound library at the transporter. We first used the Flp-In™ system to establish a stable CHO cell line expressing the hGAT-2. Stable integration of the transporter into the genome was confirmed by PCR. A single PCR product was amplified from the genomic DNA using specific hGAT-2 primers. The band corresponds to the predicted size of 1812 nucleotides (data not shown). No visible PCR products were amplified from genomic DNA from untransfected Flp-In™-CHO cells (data not shown).

The [^{3}H]GABA uptake assay was used to confirm functional uptake of GABA in the cell line. Furthermore, the applicability of the screening assay was validated by calculating the Z'-factor, a statistical parameter used as a measure of the suitability of an assay for high throughput screening.[13] The Z'-factor for hGAT-2 was $Z' = 0.70$ ($n = 1$, Figure 1.3). In the range $0.5 \leq Z < 1$ the Z' factor is indicating a large separation between the positive and the negative controls. The assay is therefore categorized as an excellent assay with adequate sensitivity, reproducibility, and accuracy.[13]

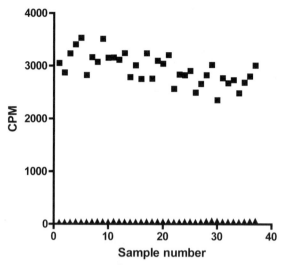

Fig. 1.3 Evaluation of the suitability of the [³H]GABA uptake assay for high throughput screening. The response to assay buffer containing 30 nM [³H]GABA (buffer) and assay buffer containing 30 nM [³H]GABA and 1 mM GABA (1 mM GABA) was measured at CHO cells stably expressing hGAT-2 (n = 1). Results are given as counts per minute (CPM). The Z'-factor was calculated to be $Z' = 0.70$. ■, Buffer; ▲, 1 mM GABA.

High throughput screening of a small compound library at GAT-2

We screened a compound library consisting of 3040 compounds at hGAT-2 using the [³H]GABA uptake assay. A hit was defined as a compound able to inhibit [³H]GABA uptake by 50% or more. The response from the compounds was compared with the positive GABA control (2 mM GABA) and the negative buffer control on the same row on the 96-well plate (Figure 1.4A,B). From the preliminary screening we identified compounds from ten wells as hits at hGAT-2. With two compounds in each well of the duplex plate, this gave a total of 20 compounds that were tested individually to identify the hit compounds. From this second testing we confirmed eight of the potential ten hits from the preliminary screening at hGAT-2. This gives a total hit rate of 0.26% at hGAT-2.

The Z-factor is the screening window coefficient, which reflects the quality of a configured assay for a particular high throughput screening.[13] For hGAT-2 the estimated Z-factor was $Z = 0.70$ (data not shown). At the defined screening conditions, the Z-factor defines a characteristic parameter of the capability of hit identification for a given assay, contrary to the Z'-factor that is a characteristic parameter for the suitability and quality of the assay itself. The Z-factor is sensitive to the composition of the small compound library as well as the compound concentration at which the screening is performed and not only sensitive to the assay procedure.[13]

Discussion

Since the cloning of the rat, mouse, and human GABA transporters in the early 1990s, the possible existence of hGAT-2 remained enigmatic until a non-functional clone was

(A)

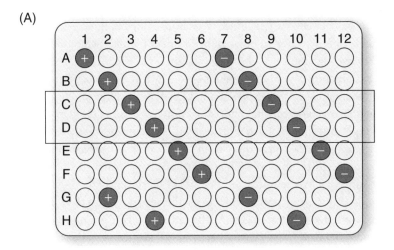

(B)

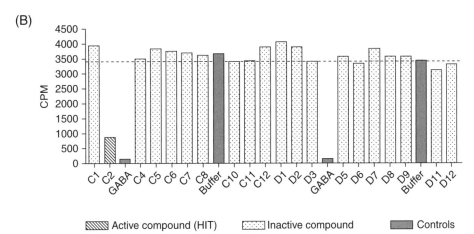

▨ Active compound (HIT)   ⬚ Inactive compound   ■ Controls

Fig. 1.4 High throughput screening of a small compound library at hGAT-2. (A) Plate design for the screening of the compound library. The position of the positive controls (+) and the negative controls (−) is indicated. (B) Illustration of hit identification in the screening of the compound library at CHO cells stably expressing hGAT-2. Each compound was tested for inhibition of uptake of 30 nM [³H]GABA as described in Experimental procedures. Results are given as counts per minute (CPM). Assay buffer (containing 30 nM [³H]GABA) was used as negative control while assay buffer supplemented with 2 mM GABA was used as positive control. All compounds were tested in a concentration of 80–170 µM. Shown are compounds C1–D12 on a selected duplex plate. Compound C2 (▨) was identified as a hit at hGAT-2.

reported in 2001.[9] Our analysis of this sequence revealed that it contains several truncations and a C-terminal deviating considerably from those of the rat and mouse orthologues, which was puzzling considering the close sequence relationship shared by the orthologues of the other three GABA transporter subtypes. This observation led us to use bioinformatic tools to identify the full-length open reading frame of hGAT-2 containing a C-terminal similar to the rat and mouse orthologues. Here we describe the cDNA cloning of the human GABA transporter, hGAT-2, which is functional and displays pharmacological characteristics similar to its murine orthologues rGAT-2 and mGAT3. The protein is closely related to other cloned human plasma membrane GABA transporters and displays high amino acid sequence similarity to mGAT3 (91% amino acid identity). Our examination of mRNA levels of hGAT-2 by reverse transcription–PCR in tissues from adult individuals reveals expression in kidney, brain, lung, and testis.[10]

We examined the pharmacological characteristics of hGAT-2 transiently expressed in tsA201 cells using a number of both synthesized and commercially available compounds. These compounds have previously been tested as substrates or inhibitors of GABA transport and found to possess different selectivity profiles at the cloned GABA transporter subtypes. We demonstrate that hGAT-2, similarly to hGAT-1 and hGAT-3, displays high-affinity transport of GABA. Furthermore, we find the following order of affinities for the tested substrates: GABA ≥ β-alanine > L-DABA = nipecotic acid ≥guvacine > taurine = betaine. These results are overall similar to what has been described for the rat and mouse orthologues rGAT-2 and mGAT3 (described in further detail in reference 10).

To date, no selective inhibitors of hGAT-2 have been published, and we therefore decided to use a high throughput screening assay to search for such compounds. Initial testing revealed a Z'-factor of 0.70, which indicates that the assay is well suited for screening purposes. We therefore performed a screening of a small compound library of 3040 diverse compounds randomly selected to be representative of a larger compound library consisting of a total of 430 000 compounds. All compounds in the library are in compliance with the Lipinski 'rule of fives'[14] and are likely to be reasonably good leads for future drug design. Eight hits with inhibitory activities at GAT-2 were identified, and this number represents a hit rate of 0.26%. Furthermore, the estimated Z-factor of the screening was 0.70 (i.e. $0.5 \leq Z < 1$) reflecting the excellent suitability of the assay for high throughput screening.[13]

The therapeutic potential of targeting the hGAT-2 remains to be clarified. It has previously been suggested to be unlikely that GAT-2 is involved in regulation of GABA inside and outside intracerebral synapses.[8] However, it may be noted that BGT-1, which, similarly to GAT-2, is expressed in non-neural tissues, only recently has been suggested to have a functional role in the CNS.[15] This finding was based on the discovery of the novel GABA transport inhibitor EF1502, which acts at both GAT-1 and BGT-1.[16]

Selective GAT inhibitors can provide essential information about the physiological function and therapeutic potential of the individual human GABA transporter subtypes. The finding of the new inhibitors of hGAT-2 will hopefully reveal more about the function of GAT-2 both in the central nervous system and in the periphery. Furthermore, the hits from the screening are considered potential candidates for further lead structure optimization.

Acknowledgements

The authors wish to thank Dr Susan Amara for the hEAAT3 cDNA. Bente Frølund is acknowledged for providing THPO and guvacine, Rasmus P. Clausen for EF1502, and

Christian A. Olsen for DAPA. This work was supported by the Lundbeck Foundation, the Augustinus Foundation, the Direktør Ib Henriksen Foundation, the Novo Nordisk PhD Plus Prize (BC), and the Drug Research Academy (TK).

References

1. Guastella J, Nelson N, Nelson H, *et al.* (1990) Cloning and expression of a rat brain GABA transporter. *Science* 249, 1303–6.

2. Borden LA, Smith KE, Hartig PR, Branchek TA, Weinshank RL (1992) Molecular heterogeneity of the γ-aminobutyric acid (GABA) transport system. Cloning of two novel high affinity GABA transporters from rat brain. *J Biol Chem* 267, 21098–104.

3. Liu QR, López-Corcuera B, Mandiyan S, Nelson H, Nelson N (1993) Molecular characterization of four pharmacologically distinct γ-aminobutyric acid transporters in mouse brain [corrected]. *J Biol Chem* 268, 2106–12.

4. Gether U, Andersen PH, Larsson OM, Schousboe A (2006) Neurotransmitter transporters: molecular function of important drug targets. *Trends Pharmacol Sci* 27, 375–83.

5. Yamashita A, Singh SK, Kawate T, Jin Y, Gouaux E (2007) Crystal structure of a bacterial homologue of Na^+/Cl^--dependent neurotransmitter transporters. *Nature* 437, 215–23.

6. Zhou Z, Zhen J, Karpowich NK, *et al.* (2007) LeuT-desipramine structure reveals how antidepressants block neurotransmitter reuptake. *Science* 317, 1390–3.

7. Singh SK, Yamashita A, Gouaux E (2007) Antidepressant binding site in a bacterial homologue of neurotransmitter transporters. *Nature* 448, 952–6.

8. Dalby NO (2003) Inhibition of γ-aminobutyric acid uptake: anatomy, physiology and effects against epileptic seizures. *Eur J Pharmacol* 479, 127–37.

9. Gong Y, Zhang M, Cui L, Minuk GY (2001) Sequence and chromosomal assignment of a human novel cDNA: similarity to gamma-aminobutyric acid transporter. *Can J Physiol Pharmacol* 79, 977–84.

10. Christiansen B, Meinild AK, Jensen AA, Bräuner-Osborne H (2007) Cloning and characterization of a functional human γ-aminobutyric acid (GABA) transporter, human GAT-2. *J Biol Chem* 282, 19331–41.

11. Höglund PJ, Adzic D, Scicluna SJ, Lindblom J, Fredriksson R (2005) The repertoire of solute carriers of family 6: identification of new human and rodent genes. *Biochem Biophys Res Commun* 336, 175–89.

12. Nelson N (1998) The family of Na^+/Cl^- neurotransmitter transporters. *J Neurochem* 71, 1785–803.

13. Zhang JH, Chung TD, Oldenburg KR (1999) A simple statistical parameter for use in evaluation and validation of high throughput screening assays. *J Biomol Screen* 4, 67–73.

14. Lipinski CA, Lombardo F, Dominy BW, Feeney PJ (2001) Experimental and computational approaches to estimate solubility and permeability in drug discovery and development settings. *Adv Drug Deliv Rev* 46, 3–26.

15. Clausen RP, Frølund B, Larsson OM, Schousboe A, Krogsgaard-Larsen P, White HS (2006) A novel selective γ-aminobutyric acid transport inhibitor demonstrates a functional role for GABA transporter subtype GAT2/BGT-1 in the CNS. *Neurochem Int* 48, 637–42.

16. Clausen RP, Moltzen EK, Perregaard J, *et al.* (2005) Selective inhibitors of GABA uptake: synthesis and molecular pharmacology of 4-*N*-methylamino-4,5,6,7-tetrahydrobenzo[*d*]isoxazol-3-ol analogues. *Bioorg Med Chem* 13, 895–908.

Low throughput preclinical models for headache*

Peter J. Goadsby

Migraine is an episodic brain disorder that affects about 15% of the population,[4,5] can be highly disabling,[6] and has been estimated to be the most costly neurological disorder in the European Community at more than €27 billion per year.[7] Patients with the highest frequency of attacks are the most disabled.[8] In clinical practice one sees far too many patients fitting this description and thus in need of better treatments. Against this background migraine is complex, involves brain systems that are just now being understood,[9] and thus offers many targets for the development of new medicines.[2] In this setting the difficult and rewarding challenge of selecting new medicines must be made.

   Preclinically, candidate compound selection must be done by model systems that may be 'high' or 'low' throughput. The former are addressed in the previous chapter, whose authors and I arbitrarily divided these models by complexity. To a novice to high-throughput screening, this author included, robotic screening seems *complex* so the designation of complexity is not pejorative; rather a clumsy attempt to draw lines between a continuum. Moreover, modelling is an iterative process that seeks to dissect the disorder at hand, i.e. headache, into component parts, to simplify the process of its study. Modelling is essentially hypothesis generation that is tested in patients with headache. It is an iterative process that should loop from bench to bedside, ideally learning from both. Modelling hopefully teaches something about the disorder, should generate some interest in the problem, and at its best drives forward new prospects for medicines. Below I will set out some models as examples, which are not meant to be exhaustive. Interested readers are directed to texts[10,11] and more complete reviews.[12,13] Migraine aura as modelled by cortical spreading depression is covered elsewhere in this volume (see Chapter 10).

Modelling the peripheral trigeminovascular system *in vivo*: intravital microscopy

Intravital microscopy permits the direct study of the peripheral branch of the trigeminovascular system. The model was developed by Williamson and colleagues and is well

---

* Some aspects of this text have been derived from the author's previous work.[1–3]

suited to pharmacological studies as within animal comparisons and dose ranging is possible.[14] This approach uses a thinned closed cranial window and video microscopy to visualize cranial, dural, and pial blood vessels and allows measurement of changes to their diameter.[14,15] Electrical stimulation of the cranial window causes a reproducible dural and pial blood vessel dilation via activation of the trigeminal nerve that is thought to be via the release of calcitonin gene-related peptide (CGRP) from presynaptic trigeminal nerve endings.[14,16,17] Inhibition of neurogenic dural vasodilation has proved historically successful in predicting antimigraine efficacy.

Triptans, 5-hydroxytryptamine 1B/1D receptor agonists,[18] dihydroergotamine, and CGRP receptor antagonists are each able to inhibit neurogenic dural vasodilation.[14,17,19,20] In contrast, neurokinin 1 receptor antagonists were unable to inhibit neurogenic dural vasodilation,[14] similar to results found in clinical trials.[21–26] Other compounds inhibiting neurogenic dural vasodilation and useful, or potentially useful, as antimigraine therapies are μ-opioid receptor antagonists,[27] neuronal nitric oxide synthase inhibitors,[16] and the non-steroidal anti-inflammatory, indomethacin.[28]

A number of novel targets for antimigraine medicine development have been suggested by studies demonstrating they inhibit neurogenic dural vasodilation. Cannabinoid CB_1 receptor agonists,[29] P/Q-, N-, and L-type voltage-dependent calcium channel blockers,[30] nociceptin,[31] and adenosine A_1 receptor agonists[32] each inhibit neurogenic dural vasodilation. TRPV1 receptor antagonists, although present in the human trigeminal gangli in a small percentage of cell bodies,[33] do not seem a potent target in this model.[34] Clinical results with the potent TRPV1 receptor antagonist SB-705498[35] will be very informative in terms of the utility of this model system that effectively predicts a poor clinical outcome. Neurogenic dural vasodilation also highlights that certain migraine preventives do not have potential to exert their action in the trigeminovascular system. Propranolol, α_1 and α_2 adrenoceptor agonists, sodium valproate, and flunarizine were all unsuccessful at inhibiting neurogenic dural vasodilation,[28,36,37] thus it appears their action is not at the level of the peripheral side of the trigeminal nerve.

CGRP and nitric oxide potent vasodilators are both able to cause a headache and a delayed migraine in patients.[38–41] When used in intravital microscopy they are able to cause reproducible dural blood vessel dilation,[16,29] and are thus used to model acute migraine. CGRP-induced dilation is attenuated by CGRP antagonists, nitric oxide synthase inhibitors, and cannabinoid CB_1 receptor agonists.[14,16,17,29] Nitric oxide-induced dilation is attenuated by triptans, CGRP antagonists, cannabinoid CB_1 receptor agonist, and indomethacin.[28,42] Therefore these models are able to predict anti migraine efficacy and may highlight potential new targets.

Modelling central trigeminovascular activation using Fos immunohistochemistry

Fos protein immunoreactivity was first shown to be a marker of nociception after peripheral noxious stimulation.[43] Fos protein expression within the trigeminal nucleus can be induced by applying mechanical, electrical, or chemical stimuli in either extracranial or intracranial tissues innervated by the trigeminal nerve. A range of studies have employed this method to map trigeminovascular nociceptive afferents and to quantify interventions.[44–48] One important property of Fos is its ability to respond to polysynaptic activation. This property has been utilized to map neuronal pathways involved in the modulatory control of pathways potentially involved in migraine, including the periaqueductal grey[49–51] and hypothalamus.[52,53]

Trigeminal ganglion stimulation

Typically electrodes are placed into both trigeminal ganglia, after which a single ganglion is stimulated for several minutes using paired rectangular pulses. This technique induces expression of c-*fos* mRNA and Fos immunoreactivity[54] within the ipsilateral trigeminal nucleus caudalis. A limitation is that trigeminal ganglion electrical stimulation may cause widespread Fos expression by discharging many more afferents than those innervating the meninges.

Chemical stimulation of the meninges

A small catheter is placed into the cisterna magna through the atlanto-occipital membrane of anaesthetized rats,[55] mice,[56] or guinea pigs.[57] An irritant substance, such as autologous blood,[58] capsaicin,[55] or carrageenin[59] is injected via the catheter, activating the primary sensory fibres supplying the meninges. Capsaicin induces Fos protein expression in a dose-dependent manner.[55] An important limitation of this model is that the stimulus is not restricted in its area, and that in effect, it is a model of meningitis.

Superior sagittal sinus stimulation

Stimulation of the superior sagittal sinus in humans produces pain referred to the head.[60–63] This model has been applied in rat, cat,[44] and non-human primate[46,48,49] to study trigeminovascular nociceptive afferents. Electrical stimulation of the pain-producing structures of the head including the superior sagittal sinus and direct stimulation of the trigeminal ganglion, both established methods of trigeminovascular activation, have been utilized to investigate the effect of a variety of compounds on Fos expression. The 5-hydroxytryptamine 1B/1D receptor agonists zolmitriptan[64] and eletriptan[65,66] have both been shown to reduce Fos immunoreactivity in the trigeminocervical complex, whereas the less lipophilic sumatriptan was unable to reduce Fos expression[66] unless the blood–brain barrier was disrupted.[67] Taken together, the evidence suggested a peripheral as well as central site of action for the triptans.[18] The NMDA receptor (MK-801) and the iGluR5 kainate receptor ([3S,4aR,6S,8aR]-6-[4-carboxyimidazol-1-ylmethyl] decahydroisoquinoline-3-carboxylic acid) antagonists both inhibit Fos expression in this model of trigeminovascular activation[68,69] implicating their receptor systems in the pathophysiology of migraine.

Conclusions

There is no preclinical model of migraine, rather many ways to examine portions of the putative pathways and systems that may be involved in the disorder. Despite increased complexity low throughput models do not model the disorder itself. Having said this, central trigeminovascular nociceptive models are emerging to provide a good correlation with clinical results, as well as increased understanding of the disorder. No doubt these and other models discussed in this monograph will facilitate the development of new treatments for migraine.

References

1. Bergerot A, Storer RJ, Goadsby PJ (2007) Dopamine inhibits trigeminovascular transmission in the rat. *Ann Neurol* 61, 251–62.
2. Goadsby PJ (2005) Can we develop neurally-acting drugs for the treatment of migraine? *Nat Rev Drug Disc* 4, 741–50.
3. Goadsby PJ (2006) Migraine: nonvascular/neurally acting drugs as novel treatment strategies. *Drug Future* 31, 969–77.
4. Lipton RB, Stewart WF, Diamond S, Diamond ML, Reed M (2001) Prevalence and burden of migraine in the United States: data from the American Migraine Study II. *Headache* 41, 646–57.
5. Steiner TJ, Scher AI, Stewart WF, Kolodner K, Liberman J, Lipton RB (2003) The prevalence and disability burden of adult migraine in England and their relationships to age, gender and ethnicity. *Cephalalgia* 23, 519–27.
6. Menken M, Munsat TL, Toole JF (2000) The global burden of disease study—implications for neurology. *Arch Neurol* 57, 418–20.
7. Andlin-Sobocki P, Jonsson B, Wittchen HU, Olesen J (2005) Cost of disorders of the brain in Europe. *Eur J Neurol* 12(Suppl 1), 1–27.
8. Lipton RB, Stewart WF, Sawyer J, Edmeads JG (2001) Clinical utility of an instrument assessing migraine disability: the migraine disability assessment (MIDAS) questionnaire. *Headache* 41, 854–61.
9. Goadsby PJ, Oshinsky M (2007) The pathophysiology of migraine. In: Silberstein SD, Lipton RB, Dodick D (eds) *Wolff's Headache and Other Head Pain*, 8th edn. Oxford University Press, New York.
10. Olesen J, Tfelt-Hansen P, Ramadan N, Goadsby PJ, Welch KMA (2005) *The Headaches*. Lippincott, Williams & Wilkins, Philadelphia, PA.
11. Edvinsson L (1999) *Experimental Headache Models in Animals and Man*. Martin Dunitz, London.
12. Bergerot A, Holland PR, Akerman S, *et al.* (2006) Animal models of migraine. Looking at the component parts of a complex disorder. *Eur J Neurosci* 24, 1517–34.
13. De Vries P, Villalon CM, Saxena PR (1999) Pharmacological aspects of experimental headache models in relation to acute antimigraine therapy. *Eur J Pharmacol* 375, 61–74.
14. Williamson DJ, Hargreaves RJ, Hill RG, Shepheard SL (1997) Intravital microscope studies on the effects of neurokinin agonists and calcitonin gene-related peptide on dural blood vessel diameter in the anaesthetized rat. *Cephalalgia* 17, 518–24.
15. Williamson DJ, Hargreaves RJ, Hill RG, Shepheard SL (1997) Sumatriptan inhibits neurogenic vasodilation of dural blood vessels in the anaesthetized rat—intravital microscope studies. *Cephalalgia* 17, 525–31.
16. Akerman S, Williamson DJ, Kaube H, Goadsby PJ (2002) Nitric oxide synthase inhibitors can antagonise neurogenic and calcitonin gene-related peptide induced dilation of dural meningeal vessels. *Br J Pharmacol* 137, 62–8.
17. Petersen KA, Birk S, Doods H, Edvinsson L, Olesen J (2004) Inhibitory effect of BIBN4096BS on cephalic vasodilatation induced by CGRP or transcranial electrical stimulation in the rat. *Br J Pharmacol* 143, 697–704.

18. Goadsby PJ (2000) The pharmacology of headache. *Prog Neurobiol* 62, 509–25.

19. Williamson DJ, Hill RG, Shepheard SL, Hargreaves RJ (2001) The anti-migraine 5-HT$_{1B/1D}$ agonist rizatriptan inhibits neurogenic dural vasodilation in anaesthetized guinea-pigs. *Br J Pharmacol* 133, 1029–34.

20. Williamson DJ, Shepheard SL, Hill RG, Hargreaves RJ (1997) The novel anti-migraine agent rizatriptan inhibits neurogenic dural vasodilation and extravasation. *Eur J Pharmacol* 328, 61–4.

21. Connor HE, Bertin L, Gillies S, Beattie DT, Ward P, The GR205171 Clinical Study Group (1998) Clinical evaluation of a novel, potent, CNS penetrating NK$_1$ receptor antagonist in the acute treatment of migraine. *Cephalalgia* 18, 392.

22. Norman B, Panebianco D, Block GA (1998) A placebo-controlled, in-clinic study to explore the preliminary safety and efficacy of intravenous L-758,298 (a prodrug of the NK1 receptor antagonist L-754,030) in the acute treatment of migraine. *Cephalalgia* 18, 407.

23. Goldstein DJ, Wang O, Saper JR, Stoltz R, Silberstein SD, Mathew NT (1997) Ineffectiveness of neurokinin-1 antagonist in acute migraine: a crossover study. *Cephalalgia* 17, 785–90.

24. Goldstein DJ, Offen WW, Klein EG, *et al.* (2001) Lanepitant, an NK-1 antagonist, in migraine prevention. *Cephalalgia* 21, 102–6.

25. Diener H-C, The RPR100893 Study Group (2003) RPR100893, a substance-P antagonist, is not effective in the treatment of migraine attacks. *Cephalalgia* 23, 183–5.

26. May A, Goadsby PJ (2001) Substance P receptor antagonists in the therapy of migraine. *Expert Opin Invest Drugs* 10, 1–6.

27. Williamson DJ, Shepheard SL, Cook DA, Hargreaves RJ, Hill RG, Cumberbatch MJ (2001) Role of opioid receptors in neurogenic dural vasodilation and sensitization of trigeminal neurones in anaesthetized rats. *Br J Pharmacol* 133, 807–14.

28. Akerman S, Kaube H, Goadsby PJ (2002) The effect of anti-migraine compounds on nitric oxide induced dilation of dural meningeal vessels. *Eur J Pharmacol* 452, 223–8.

29. Akerman S, Kaube H, Goadsby PJ (2004) Anandamide acts as a vasodilator of dural blood vessels in vivo by activating TRPV1 receptors. *Br J Pharmacol* 142, 1354–60.

30. Akerman S, Williamson D, Goadsby PJ (2003) Voltage-dependent calcium channels are involved in neurogenic dural vasodilation via a pre-synaptic transmitter release mechanism. *Br J Pharmacol* 140, 558–66.

31. Bartsch T, Akerman S, Goadsby PJ (2002) The ORL-1 (NOP$_1$) receptor ligand nociceptin/orphanin FQ (N/OFQ) inhibits neurogenic vasodilatation in the rat. *Neuropharmacology* 43, 991–8.

32. Honey AC, Bland-Ward PA, Connor HE, Feniuk W, Humphrey PPA (2000) Study of an adenosine A1 receptor agonist on trigeminally evoked dural blood vessel dilation in the anaesthetized rat. *Cephalalgia* 22, 260–4.

33. Hou M, Uddman R, Tajti J, Kanje M, Edvinsson L (2002) Capsaicin receptor immunoreactivity in the human trigeminal ganglion. *Neurosci Lett* 330, 223–6.

34. Akerman S, Kaube H, Goadsby PJ (2003) Vanilloid type 1 receptor (VR1) evoked CGRP release plays a minor role in causing dural vessel dilation via the trigeminovascular system. *Br J Pharmacol* 140, 718–24.

35. Rami HK, Thompson M, Stemp G, *et al.* (2006) Discovery of SB-705498: A potent, selective and orally bioavailable TRPV1 antagonist suitable for clinical development. *Bioorg Med Chem Lett* 16, 3287–91.

36. Akerman S, Williamson D, Hill RG, Goadsby PJ (2001) The effect of adrenergic compounds on neurogenic dural vasodilatation. *Eur J Pharmacol* 424, 53–8.

37. Williamson DJ, Hargreaves RJ (2001) Neurogenic inflammation in the context of migraine. *Microsc Res Tech* 53, 167–78.

38. Lassen LH, Haderslev PA, Jacobsen VB, Iversen HK, Sperling B, Olesen J (2002) CGRP may play a causative role in migraine. *Cephalalgia* 22, 54–61.
39. Olesen J, Iversen HK, Thomsen LL (1993) Nitric oxide supersensitivity, a possible molecular mechanism of migraine pain. *Neuroreport* 4, 1027–30.
40. Olesen J, Thomsen LL, Iversen HK (1994) Nitric oxide is a key molecule in migraine and other vascular headaches. *Trends Pharmacol Sci* 15, 149–53.
41. Iversen HK, Olesen J, Tfelt-Hansen P (1989) Intravenous nitroglycerin as an experimental headache model. Basic characteristics. *Pain* 38, 17–24.
42. Akerman S, Kaube H, Goadsby PJ (2004) Anandamide is able to inhibit trigeminal neurons using an *in vivo* model of trigeminovascular-mediated nociception. *J Pharmacol Exp Ther* 309, 56–63.
43. Hunt SP, Pini A, Evan G (1987) Induction of c-fos like protein in spinal cord neurons following sensory stimulation. *Nature* 328, 1686–704.
44. Kaube H, Keay KA, Hoskin KL, Bandler R, Goadsby PJ (1993) Expression of c-*Fos*-like immunore-activity in the caudal medulla and upper cervical cord following stimulation of the superior sagittal sinus in the cat. *Brain Res* 629, 95–102.
45. Strassman AM, Mineta Y, Vos BP (1994) Distribution of fos-like immunoreactivity in the medullary and upper cervical dorsal horn produced by stimulation of dural blood vessels in the rat. *J Neurosci* 14, 3725–35.
46. Goadsby PJ, Hoskin KL (1997) The distribution of trigeminovascular afferents in the nonhuman primate brain *Macaca nemestrina*: a c-fos immunocytochemical study. *J Anat* 190, 367–75.
47. Sugimoto T, He YF, Xiao C, Ichikawa H (1998) c-Fos induction in the subnucleus oralis following trigeminal nerve stimulation. *Brain Res* 783, 158–62.
48. Hoskin KL, Zagami A, Goadsby PJ (1999) Stimulation of the middle meningeal artery leads to Fos expression in the trigeminocervical nucleus: a comparative study of monkey and cat. *J Anat* 194, 579–88.
49. Hoskin KL, Bulmer DCE, Lasalandra M, Jonkman A, Goadsby PJ (2001) Fos expression in the midbrain periaqueductal grey after trigeminovascular stimulation. *J Anat* 197, 29–35.
50. Keay KA, Bandler R (1998) Vascular head pain selectively activates ventrolateral periaqueductal gray in the cat. *Neurosci Lett* 245, 58–60.
51. Keay KA, Bandler R (2002) Distinct central representations of inescapable and escapable pain: observations and speculation. *Exp Physiol* 87, 275–9.
52. Malick A, Burstein R (2001) A neurohistochemical blueprint for pain-induced loss of appetite. *Proc Natl Acad Sci USA* 98, 9930–5.
53. Benjamin L, Levy MJ, Lasalandra MP, *et al.* (2004) Hypothalamic activation after stimulation of the superior sagittal sinus in the cat: a Fos study. *Neurobiol Dis* 16, 500–5.
54. Clayton JS, Gaskin PJ, Beattie DT (1997) Attenuation of Fos-like immunoreactivity in the trigeminal nucleus caudalis following trigeminovascular activation in the anaesthetised guinea-pig. *Brain Res* 775, 74–80.
55. Mitsikostas DD, Sanchez del Rio M, Waeber C, Moskowitz MA, Cutrer FM (1998) The NMDA receptor antagonist MK-801 reduces capsaicin-induced *c-fos* expression within rat trigeminal nucleus caudalis. *Pain* 76, 239–48.
56. Mitsikostas DD, Sanchez del Rio M, Waeber C (2002) 5-Hydroxytryptamine(1B/1D) and 5-hydroxytryptamine1F receptors inhibit capsaicin-induced c-fos immunoreactivity within mouse trigeminal nucleus caudalis. *Cephalalgia* 22, 384–94.
57. Cutrer FM, Mitsikostas DD, Ayata G, Sanchez del Rio M (1999) Attenuation by butalbital of capsaicin-induced c-fos-like immunoreactivity in trigeminal nucleus caudalis. *Headache* 39, 697–704.
58. Nozaki K, Boccalini P, Moskowitz MA (1992) Expression of c-fos-like immunoreactivity in brain-stem after meningeal irritation by blood in the subarachnoid space. *Neuroscience* 49, 669–80.

59. Nozaki K, Moskowitz MA, Boccalini P (1992) CP-93,129, sumatriptan, dihydroergotamine block c-fos expression within the rat trigeminal nucleus caudalis caused by chemical stimulation of the meninges. *Br J Pharmacol* 106, 409–15.

60. Wolff HG (1948) *Headache and Other Head Pain*. Oxford University Press, New York.

61. Ray BS, Wolff HG (1940) Experimental studies on headache. Pain sensitive structures of the head and their significance in headache. *Arch Surg* 41, 813–56.

62. Feindel W, Penfield W, McNaughton F (1960) The tentorial nerves and localization of intracranial pain in man. *Neurology* 10, 555–63.

63. McNaughton FL, Feindel WH (1997) Innervation of intracranial structures: a reappraisal. In: Rose FC (ed.) *Physiological aspects of Clinical Neurology*, pp. 279–93. Blackwell Scientific Publications, Oxford.

64. Hoskin KL, Goadsby PJ (1998) Comparison of a more and less lipophilic serotonin ($5HT_{1B/1D}$) agonist in a model of trigeminovascular nociception in cat. *Exp Neurol* 150, 45–51.

65. Knyihar-Csillik E, Tajti J, Csillik AE, Chadaide Z, Mihaly A, Vecsei L (2000) Effects of eletriptan on the peptidergic innervation of the cerebral dura mater and trigeminal ganglion, and on the expression of c-fos and c-jun in the trigeminal complex of the rat in an experimental migraine model. *Eur J Neurosci* 12, 3991–4002.

66. Goadsby PJ, Hoskin KL (1999) Differential effects of low dose CP122,288 and eletriptan on fos expression due to stimulation of the superior sagittal sinus in cat. *Pain* 82, 15–22.

67. Kaube H, Hoskin KL, Goadsby PJ (1993) Inhibition by sumatriptan of central trigeminal neurones only after blood-brain barrier disruption. *Br J Pharmacol* 109, 788–92.

68. Classey JD, Knight YE, Goadsby PJ (2001) The NMDA receptor antagonist MK-801 reduces Fos-like immunoreactivity within the trigeminocervical complex following superior sagittal sinus stimulation in the cat. *Brain Res* 907, 117–24.

69. Filla SA, Winter MA, Johnson KW, *et al.* (2002) Ethyl (3S,4aR,6S,8aR)-6-(4-ethoxycar-bonylimidazol-1-ylmethyl)decahydroiso-quinoline-3-carboxylic ester: a prodrug of a GluR5 kainate receptor antagonist active in two animal models of acute migraine. *J Med Chem* 45, 4383–6.

Human models: screening models

Messoud Ashina

Introduction

Animal migraine models have a substantial impact on development and early screening of novel antimigraine drugs. However, an animal model that is identical or almost identical to human migraine has not yet been developed. It is, therefore, difficult to predict the antimigraine action of drugs, and early and cost-effective proof of concept studies in humans are important.

A fundamental feature of migraine is that attacks are triggered by various things such as missed sleep, menstruation, and drugs. The clinical phenotype of glyceryl trinitrate (GTN) induced migraine, including premonitory symptoms,[1] is indistinguishable from spontaneous migraine.[2] Given that the GTN model is the best studied model to trigger migraine attack I shall discuss its possible use as a screening model to test antimigraine drugs.

Acute antimigraine drugs

The effect of sumatriptan on a GTN-induced headache has been examined in two studies.[3,4] In a double-blind crossover study Iversen and Olesen[4] injected subcutaneously sumatriptan 6 mg or placebo in ten healthy subjects, followed by a 20-min infusion of GTN (0.12 mg/kg per min). This study demonstrated that sumatriptan significantly reduced the GTN-induced immediate headache and the temporal and radial artery diameter.[4] Another study by Schmetterer et al.[3] confirmed the efficacy of sumatriptan in GTN-induced headache and in addition demonstrated that sumatriptan also prevents GTN-induced dilatation of the MCA.

Prophylactic antimigraine drugs

No migraine-specific prophylactic drugs have so far been developed. One of the problems in prophylactic drug development for migraine is that there are no animal models with reasonable sensitivity and validity in predicting prophylactic antimigraine activity. The GTN model of migraine could be sensitive and valid in predicting prophylactic antimigraine activity. Tvedskov et al.[5,6] introduced for the first time the GTN model of migraine to validate the use of the model by testing the effect of recognized prophylactic drugs, sodium valproate and propranolol.

The major outcome of the valproate study was that a prophylactic effect of valproate might be demonstrated using the GTN human migraine model[5] (Figure 3.1). Other major outcomes were that the authors gained valuable information concerning study methodology, in particular end-points applied and suggestions to improve study design in the future studies. Tvedskov *et al.*[5] used the difference between placebo and GTN in the reduction of incidence of migraine attack as a primary end-point. Using very strict International Headache Society (IHS) criteria the authors failed to show a statistical difference between valproate and placebo. The authors discovered that some patients reported probable migraine and took rescue medication during onset of attack, i.e. when the attack did not fulfil the IHS criteria for migraine. In fact, adding these patients in statistical analysis resulted in a statistical difference in reported migraine attacks.[5]

Given the prophylactic drugs usually reduce the intensity of spontaneous attacks one would expect effect on the area under the (headache) curve (AUC) and median peak intensity during the GTN-induced migraine attack. The latter is more specific and should obviously be considered to test the effect of prophylactic drugs on attack severity. Tvedskov *et al.*[5] reported that peak headache showed a numerical but non-significant efficacy of valproate (Figure 3.1). The authors suggested that if a patient on placebo develops severe headache or migraine after GTN, the patient would take rescue medication very early and abort the headache. On the valproate arm the same patient may get a much less pronounced headache not requiring rescue medication. In addition, anticipation of attack reduces patients' threshold to take a medication. In support, it was reported that most migraine patients took their rescue medication very early to abort their attacks.[5] In future studies, patients could be asked to refrain from abortive medication until they fulfilled migraine criteria or patient reported migraine rather than IHS migraine could be chosen as an outcome parameter.

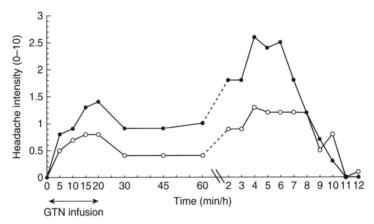

Fig. 3.1 Mean headache intensity over time, immediate (0–60 min) and delayed (up to 12 h). ●, Placebo; ○, valproate. Reproduced from *Cephalalgia*, 24, Tvedskov JF, Thomsen LL, Iverson HK, *et al.* The prophylactic effect of valproate on glyceryltrinitrate induced migraine (2004a), pp. 576–585, with permission from Blackwell Publishing.

In studies by Tvedskov *et al.*[5] valproate was given daily, each for a minimum of 13 days. In clinical practice the onset of prophylactic migraine activity after prophylactic drugs may not occur until after 1–2 months of treatment. Therefore, it would be better to pretreat patients for 2 months before challenging with GTN. However, it would require active and washout periods, and the long-lasting placebo arm. This crossover design might be considered ethically unacceptable and it would also eliminate many of the advantages of using the GTN model such as the testing of drugs with only 2 weeks toxicology.

The results of a propranolol study[6] showed no sign of efficacy for propranolol in the GTN migraine model on any of several outcome parameters, such as number with IHS migraine, immediate or delayed peak headache. These data suggested that the efficacy of future prophylactic drugs in the GTN model depends on their mechanism of action. There may also be different mechanisms involved in different patients, so new drugs may not be effective in all patients or all attacks depending on the causative mechanism. The ineffectiveness of a well-proven migraine prophylaxis in this study limits the usefulness of the model, and must be considered in future testing of new migraine prophylactic drugs.

Future perspectives

The results of drug testing in human models of migraine show the major advantage of the GTN model. Thus, a potential prophylactic migraine agent can be tested at a very early stage of development with approximately 2 weeks toxicology testing available. Furthermore, the model allows extensive testing of safety parameters such as blood pressure, heart rate, and effects of drugs on cerebral circulation.[5,6] The GTN studies have also shown that the sensitivity of models could be improved with some changes in experimental design. Thus, it would be desirable to increase sample size to 30 to achieve statistical relevant difference between two experimental conditions. Furthermore, the clinical difference could be increased by adapting less conservative IHS criteria such as probable or migraine like headache.

One limitation of the model is that lack of efficacy is no proof that the drug does not work in spontaneous migraine. Thus, spontaneous migraine may be induced via a number of different mechanisms, whereas GTN induces migraine via one particular pathway (nitric oxide–cGMP). The efficacy on the other hand would imply a high likelihood of clinical efficacy. Future studies may reveal whether all prophylactic migraine drugs work in the GTN model, whether the model can be used for dose finding in prophylactic studies, and how such a dose-finding study should best be designed.

References

1. Afridi SK, Kaube H, Goadsby PJ (2004) Glyceryl trinitrate triggers premonitory symptoms in migraineurs. *Pain* 110, 675–80.
2. Thomsen LL, Kruuse C, Iversen HK, Olesen J (1994) A nitric oxide donor (nitroglycerin) triggers genuine migraine attacks. *Eur Neurol* 1, 73–80.

3. Schmetterer L, Wolzt M, Krejcy K, *et al.* (1996) Cerebral and ocular hemodynamic effects of suma-triptan in the nitroglycerin headache model. *Clin Pharmacol Ther* 60, 199–205.

4. Iversen HK, Olesen J (1996) Headache induced by a nitric oxide donor (nitroglycerin) responds to sumatriptan. A human model for development of migraine drugs. *Cephalalgia* 16, 412–18.

5. Tvedskov JF, Thomsen LL, Iversen HK, Gibson A, Wiliams P, Olesen J (2004) The prophylactic effect of valproate on glyceryltrinitrate induced migraine. *Cephalalgia* 24, 576–85.

6. Tvedskov JF, Thomsen LL, Thomsen LL, *et al.* (2004) The effect of propranolol on glyceryltrinitrate-induced headache and arterial response. *Cephalalgia* 24, 1076–87.

Session II

Trials methodology

4

Stricter success criteria, qualitative and quantitative end-points: acute versus prevention trials

Peer Tfelt-Hansen

Introduction

Migraine can be regarded as an episodic-chronic disorder[1] and in the treatment of migraine one should consider treatment of the migraine attacks and in many cases also preventive treatment.

In acute migraine treatment patients want to be pain free within a reasonable time.[2] In 30–40% of the cases the migraine attack relapses after a primary successful treatment with triptans[3–5] and this is of course disliked by the patients. In addition, the patients want consistency of effect from attacks to attacks. During migraine attacks the general well-being of the patients is decreased[6] and quite naturally patients want treatment that can normalize their general well-being. In the following an overview will be given of the current status of success criteria with the specific acute antimigraine drugs, the 5-HT$_{1B/1D}$ receptor agonists, the triptans. Possible improvements for future medicines with more strict and more clinically relevant success criteria, including measurement of general well-being,[6] will be discussed. Current acute migraine treatment is not without *adverse events* (AEs) and measurement of general well-being[6] after acute treatment will also cover the aspect of tolerability.

The triptans are usually regarded as very effective acute migraine drugs. This fact, however, is not always evident in current randomized clinical trials (RCTs). One could argue that this is so because only the most severely afflicted patients participate in these RCTs. In migraine patients with infrequent attacks recruited by general practitioners and by advertisement the results are, however, quite similar.[7]

In preventive treatment of migraine the primary efficacy measure has been a decrease in attack frequency.[8] Tolerability has also been registered. In clinical practice lack of tolerability, most often due to non-serious AEs, is a major problem in migraine prophylaxis and the current way of reporting AEs in migraine prophylactic trials is unsatisfactory because it does not reflect this clinical experience.[9] A task force of the International Headache Society has suggested a better way to evaluate and report AEs in migraine trials (Tfelt-Hansen, personal communication).

Qualitative measures in acute migraine trials (see Table 4.1)

In 1991 the clinical drug trial committee of the International Headache Society made the following recommendation: the number of migraine attacks that resolved within 2 h, before any escape medication, should usually be the primary parameter of efficacy. Whenever an attack remits within 2 h, and relapses within 24 h, it is a treatment failure by this criterion.[10] This ideal efficacy parameter has, however, never been used in RCTs in migraine. It is most likely a too strict efficacy parameter. Instead Glaxo introduced headache relief[11] (see below).

Pain free after 2 h is the currently suggested primary efficacy parameter.[8] When the headaches are moderate or severe treatment with an oral triptan results in pain-free responses from 30% to 40%.[3,12] When the migraine attacks are treated in the mild phase in RCTs the 2-h pain-free responder rate increases considerably. Thus the pain-free response was 43% after zolmitriptan 2.5 mg,[13] 51–66% after sumatriptan 50–100 mg,[14,15] and 70% after rizatriptan 10 mg.[16] In the mild phase of a migraine attack some patients can have difficulties in distinguishing a migraine attack from episodic tension-type headache. Owing to this diagnostic uncertainty I do not recommend to use treatment in the mild phase of migraine in phase II and early phase III RCTs. Pain free after established moderate or severe migraine headache[8] should remain the primary efficacy measure in these phases of drug development.

It was recently stated that many patients have no response to triptans; complete pain relief is the exception rather than the rule.[17] How high then is the maximum effect of triptans? For oral triptans the maximum response for headache relief is approximately

Table 4.1 Qualitative and quantitative measures in acute and preventive migraine randomized clinical trials (RCTs; for details see text).

	Qualitative end-points	Quantitative end-points
Acute treatment RCTs	Pain free	Time to meaningful relief
	Sustained pain free	Time to pain free
	Headache relief	Speed of onset of action
	Consistency of pain free	Sum of Pain Intensity Differences
	Presence of nausea	VAS scales
	Presence of photophobia and phonophobia	50% reduction in VAS scale
	Global evaluation of treatment	HRQL related scales
	Incidence of adverse events	Usual activity loss
		Workplace loss of productivity
Preventive RCTs	Headache intensity	Headache frequency
	Incidence of adverse events	Migraine days
	Global evaluation of medicine	50% reduction in frequency
		Reduction to no or one attack per 4 weeks
		HRQL-related scales

HRQL, health-related quality of life; VAS, visual analogue score.

68% when headache is moderate or severe[4] and pain free is 70% when headache is mild with rizatriptan 10 mg.[16] The highest response rates were found after subcutaneous naratriptan.[18] Naratriptan 5 mg and 10 mg resulted in pain-free rates of 79% and 88%, respectively (Figure 4.1).[18] For subcutaneous sumatriptan 6 mg the pain-free rate was 55% (Figure 4.1).[18] Unfortunately naratriptan was for commercial reasons only developed further as an oral form in a low dose of 2.5 mg, which causes no more AEs than placebo,[3,4] the so-called 'user-friendly triptan'. So with parenteral naratriptan one gets near the maximum for pain free; and complete pain relief is the rule rather than the exception.

Also more strict success criteria than pain free have been suggested: *sustained pain free* (SPF) is pain free after 2 h, no relapse of headache within 24 h, and no use of escape medication.[3,8] The SPF varies from 14% for naratriptan 2.5 mg to 30% for rizatriptan 10 mg[3,19] when the headache is moderate or severe; and SPF increases to 60% after rizatriptan 10 mg when the headache is mild.[16] SPF is a suitable secondary efficacy measure in established migraine attacks in phase II and phase III. When treating patients in the mild phase of migraine SPF can be used as the primary efficacy measure.

Headache relief (formerly headache response) after 2 h has until recently been used as the primary end-point in most RCTs with triptans[3,4,19] and was used as the primary efficacy measure in a recent study on the effect of the CGRP antagonist BIB 4096 BS.[17] Headache relief is defined as a decrease in head pain from moderate (2) or severe (3) to none (0) or mild (1).[8,11] The therapeutic gain (percentage response after active treatment minus percentage response after placebo) for headache relief varies from 20% to 35% for oral triptans[3,19] and increases to 51% for subcutaneous sumatriptan.[4,5] Headache relief has been criticized because the different steps are not equal and the response rate depends on the initial severity of the treated attack.[20] Furthermore, patients want to be *pain free*.[2] With this efficacy measure it has been difficult to show that triptans are better than unspecific treatment[21] with one exception where sumatriptan was superior to tolfenamic acid.[22]

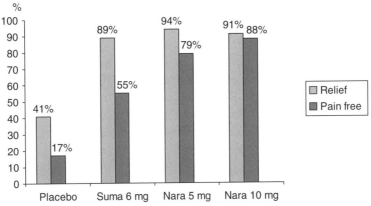

Fig. 4.1 The effect of placebo, subcutaneous sumatriptan (suma), and naratriptan (nara) on headache relief and pain free in one randomized controlled trial.[18]

Consistency of pain free has been suggested as a secondary efficacy parameter.[8] Consistency of pain free should be evaluated in modified-design crossover RCTs with placebo control. The optimal number of attacks for such consistency trials is five, and, in a double-blind design, four are treated with active medication and each of the first to the fifth, in five treatment groups, with placebo. A consistent response is then defined as pain free in three of four verum-treated attacks.[8] So far, there is no experience with this efficacy measure and it is most likely a very strict end-point with an estimated incidence of 20–24% with the triptans. Apart from this it is a very clinically relevant end-point.

Global evaluation of medicine (very poor, poor, no opinion, good, very good) has traditionally been used to let the patients judge the treatments.[8]

Functional disability has been rated as:[8] *none* (no disability: able to function normally), *mild* (performance of daily activities mildly impaired: can still do everything but with difficulties), *moderate* (performance of daily activities moderately impaired: unable to do some things), *severe* (performance of daily activities severely impaired: cannot do all or most things, bed rest may be necessary). Functional disability is a secondary efficacy measure in many RCTs. More patients were able to function normally after rizatriptan (39%) than after sumatriptan (32%).[23]

Presence of nausea/vomiting and no presence has normally been registered in RCT. Nausea can probably be graded in no, mild, moderate, and severe (and/or with vomiting) if the treatment is expected specifically to influence this. Nausea can also be evaluated on a 10-cm visual analogue (VAS) scale. Presence of *photophobia and phonophobia* is normally noted before and 2 h after treatment.

In addition to pain free after 2 h a measure of *no symptoms of migraine and normal function* after 2 h has been suggested as a more stringent efficacy measure.[24] For rizatriptan this symptom-free measure was found in more patients after rizatriptan 10 mg (31%) than after sumatriptan 100 mg (22%).[24]

AEs after triptans are a clinical problem and some patients cannot tolerate the AEs and have to stop the use of these drugs. After subcutaneous sumatriptan 6 mg there were 33% (95% confidence intervals (CI) 29 to 37%) more AEs than after placebo.[5] For oral sumatriptan 100 mg there were 16% (95% CI 13 to 19%) more AEs than for placebo,[5] whereas for naratriptan 2.5 mg and almotriptan 12.5 mg there were no more AEs than placebo.[3,5,19]

The Clinical Trial Subcommittee of the International Headache Society has suggested better ways for evaluating and reporting AEs (Tfelt-Hansen, personal communication). It is suggested to use health-related quality of life (HRQoL) scales to evaluate the benefit/tolerability ratio in RCTs in migraine.

Incidence of AEs should be recorded. Patients should report AEs at each time point at which efficacy is recorded (Tfelt-Hansen, personal communication). A standard open question should be used (e.g. 'Have you experienced any unusual or abnormal event or symptom? If so, what was it?'), and where relevant ask directly about specific AEs of interest (e.g. 'Have you experienced chest pain?'). Details about intensity should be asked for (using a scale of 0–10 or mild/moderate/severe) and, if possible, duration of each AE should be reported.

Workplace loss of productivity can be a suitable measure in acute RCTs. Subcutaneous sumatriptan resulted in 52% of patients returning to normal function within 2 h, whereas this was only the case in 9% of patients treated with placebo.[25]

Quantitative measures in acute migraine trials (see Table 4.1)

VAS scales have rarely been used in migraine RCTs.[26–28] In one RCT sumatriptan 100 mg (15 mm decrease after 2 h) was found comparable with diclofenac 50 mg (17 mm decrease).[26] Exact decreases on a VAS scale were greater after intravenous haloperidol 5 mg than after placebo in an emergency department in one RCT.[28] Based on a 50% decrease on a VAS scale subcutaneous sumatriptan (96%) was superior to intravenous acetylsalicylic acid lysinate (76%) and placebo (29%) (Figure 4.2).[27] The headache relief changed to the same degree: 91%, 74%, 24%, respectively.[27]

Time to *50% decrease* on a VAS scale for headache was used in a very large RCT ($n = 1743$)[29] comparing the combination of paracetamol (PAR), aspirin (ASA), and caffeine (CAF), with the single substances. The patients usually treated their migraine attacks (84%) or tension-type headache (13%) with over-the-counter drugs. The combination (PAR + ASA + CAF) was superior ($P < 0.01$) to the single substances and the combination of PAR and ASA.[29] What is the clinical relevance of these results? The global assessment of the treatment resulted in good or very good in 73.2% treated with PAR + ASA + CAF, and in 67.5% treated with ASA ($P < 0.01$).[29] There are thus some statistically highly significant results due to the many patients but the global evaluation indicates only a moderate difference.

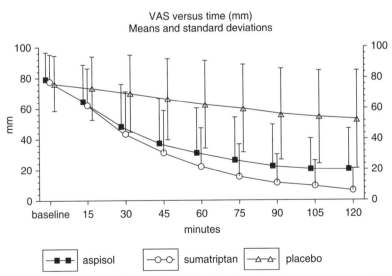

Fig. 4.2 Changes on a visual analogue scale (VAS) after placebo, subcutaneous sumatriptan, and intravenous acetylsalicylic acid lysinate (aspisol).[27]

Time to meaningful headache relief has been used in three studies.[30,31] Patients can be given a stopwatch starting at dosing and asked to register when they feel meaningful relief. In an open-label, randomized study the median time to meaningful relief was earlier for eletriptan 80 mg (84 min) than for rizatriptan 10 mg (93 min).[32] This efficacy measure is most likely to be suitable when the early onset of relief is the wanted effect, e.g. after intranasal administration.[30]

Rizatriptan has a somewhat quicker oral absorption than sumatriptan[5] and *speed of onset of effect* has been used as an efficacy parameter in rizatriptan versus sumatriptan and zolmitriptan (headache relief) and naratriptan (pain free) trials.[33–37] The RCTs have been analysed for headache relief with time-to-events analysis for headache relief up to 2 h. Such an analysis requires 200–400 patients in each treatment group because it is a very strict criterion when comparing two medium effective triptans such as rizatriptan and sumatriptan.[3,19,33,34] In three RCTs rizatriptan was superior to sumatriptan,[33,34] zolmitriptan,[36] and naratriptan,[37] whereas in one RCT no such earlier effect for rizatriptan 10 mg versus sumatriptan 50 mg could be observed.[35] It should be noted that this time-to-events analysis cannot distinguish between quicker onset and size of effect after 2 h.[38]

Sum of pain intensity differences (*SPIDs*) has been used in some RCTs in migraine but the results have rarely been published.[39] The results of SPID for four rizatriptan and sumatriptan RCTs has been compared with pain free.[39] It was concluded that SPIDs do not add anything more than pain free after 2 h.[39]

Time to onset of headache relief was measured in two large RCTs ($n = 2696$) with fast-disintegrating/rapid-release sumatriptan tablets.[40] Using a personal digital assistant patients indicated headache relief (mild or none) and pain free. Superiority for the 100 mg dose versus placebo was observed after 20 min and after 30 min for the 50 mg dose.[40] For pain free the results were 35 min (100 mg) and 48 min (50 mg), respectively.[40] This RCT thus demonstrated an early onset of effect of this novel sumatriptan formulation. The results for headache relief are, however, similar to the 30 min (the first time-point where patients grade their headache) for onset seen with other oral triptans in other RCTs.[4,5]

Usual activity loss can be used as an efficacy measure. Thus eletriptan (40 or 80 mg) treated patients were unable to perform their usual activity for a median period of 4 h. In contrast, the placebo-treated patients could not perform their usual activity for a median period of 9 h ($P < 0.001$).[41]

HRQoL scales are not in general use in acute migraine trials. They should be added because they reflect the impact of the migraine attack and the efficacy and tolerability of the drug. In one RCT the *Minor Symptoms Evaluation Profile* (MSEP)[42] was used to evaluate the effect of subcutaneous sumatriptan 8 mg.[43] It was shown that the general well-being of the patients was decreased by attacks and that this could be normalized with sumatriptan.[43] So the MSEP scale is sensitive enough to pick up the effect of a drug. MSEP is a generic scale and has the advantage that it can be used outside an attack to obtain a baseline. One can thus evaluate in the RCT whether the drug can revert the decreased well-being to the baseline. There are several headache-specific scales: MSQ (*Migraine specific QoL questionnaire*);[44,45] HDI (*Headache Disability Inventory*);[46] HImQ (*Headache Impact Questionnaire*);[47] and HIT (*Headache Impact Test*).[48] These scales should be suitable for use in acute migraine trials. Although statistically significant changes may frequently be seen with these HRQoL scales, a change of 10% or more is generally considered to have clinical relevance (Dahlöf, personal communication).

Conclusion for acute treatment

A quantitative end-point is not inherently a stricter end-point. Qualitative end-points such as pain free in established migraine attacks with moderate or severe headache should remain the primary efficacy end-point. It is what the patients want.[2] Sustained pain free is most likely too strict an end-point in most cases (response in only 20% after oral sumatriptan 100 mg[3,19]) and should for the moment be a secondary efficacy parameter. However, the response increases to 60% sustained pain free when used in mild headache after rizatriptan 10 mg.[16] Consistency of pain free should be used as a clinically relevant efficacy measure.[8]

Quantitative HRQoL scale should be used in acute RCTs in order to measure the total impact of the treatment and possible AEs.

Qualitative measures in preventive treatment randomized clinical trials (see Table 4.1)

It is from experience in a clinical setting that it can be seen in some patients that the intensity of attacks decreases with preventive treatment or the attacks can be treated more successfully after preventive treatment. This can be picked up by registration of *headache intensity* on a verbal scale: none, mild, moderate, and severe.[8]

The incidence of AEs and especially AE resulting in discontinuation is an important parameter in preventive RCTs. Clinical experience shows that many migraine patients discontinue treatment because of AEs (Task Force for better evaluation and reporting). This clinical experience is often not picked up in RCTs on migraine prevention. This is in most cases due to small sample size and in recent larger topiramate RCTs there were more AEs with active drugs than with placebo.[49–51] Recently, a task force of IHS has proposed how to evaluate and report AEs in migraine trials (Tfelt-Hansen, personal communication).

Global evaluation of medicine (very poor, poor, no opinion, good, very good) has traditionally been used to let the patients judge their treatments.[8]

Quantitative end-points in preventive treatment (see Table 4.1)

Current preventive treatment is unspecific and is not universally effective. Usually there is a 40–50% responder rate (50% decrease in attack frequency from baseline) to treatment in RCTs on migraine prophylaxis.[49–55]

The traditional primary efficacy parameter is *frequency of migraine attacks*. This parameter is intuitively a clinically relevant efficacy measure. It is what prevention is all about.

Responder rate is usually defined as a *50% reduction* in frequency of migraine attacks. This converts a quantitative parameter into a qualitative one and it is suitable for use in systematic reviews such as Cochrane Reviews. The responder rate is usually 40–50%. This parameter has been criticized because a decrease from six to three attacks is similar to two to one attacks with this parameter. In addition, if patients have decreases from six to three or four to two attacks they are respondes. Prophylaxis is, however, normally indicated if there are two to eight attacks per 4 weeks and in these patients there will still clinically be a need for prophylaxis. We therefore suggest that a response in RCTs should be defined as no or one attack per 4 weeks.

Because of the somewhat complicated definition of a migraine attack[8] the more simple *migraine days* per 4 weeks has been suggested as an efficacy measure. It is probably most useful in long-term phase III or phase IV RCTs.

HRQoL scales (both generic and migraine specific scales, see above) should be used in preventive RCTs in migraine. In addition, the MIDAS *(Migraine Disability Assessment)* scale[56] can be used. The use of these scales will take into account both efficacy and the impact of AEs.

Conclusions for preventive migraine treatment

In preventive RCTs migraine frequency should remain the primary end-point. Migraine days is an alternative that can be used in long-term RCTs and extension studies.

In clinical practice preventive treatment of migraine is indicated if the patient has two to eight attacks per month that cannot be treated satisfactorily with acute treatment. In my view a reasonable and acceptable goal, from a clinical point of view, would be no or one migraine attack per month. Responders should therefore be re-defined as patients with no or only one attack per month. This will be a very strict criterion for the prevention of migraine and can for the moment only be used as a secondary efficacy measure. If we get more specific and more effective drugs in the future it could probably be a primary efficacy measure.

Quantitative HRQoL scales should be used in preventive RCTs because they are most likely to reflect the patients' need. Their sensitivity remains to be tested. They should be secondary efficacy measures in preventive migraine RCTs.

References

1. Lipton RB, Bigal ME, Stewart WF (2005) Clinical trials of acute treatment for migraine including multiple attacks studies of pain, disability, and health-related quality of life. *Neurology* 65(Suppl. 4), S50–8.
2. Lipton RB, Hamelsky SW, Dayno JM (2002) What do patients with migraine want from acute migraine therapy? *Headache* 42 (Suppl. 1), 3–9.
3. Ferrari MD, Roon KI, Lipton RB, Goadsby PJ (2001) Oral triptans (serotonin 5-HT$_{1B/1D}$ agonists) in acute migraine: a meta-analysis of 53 trials. *Lancet* 358, 1668–75.

4. Tfelt-Hansen P, De Vries P, Saxena PR (2000) Triptans in migraine. A comparative review of pharmacology, pharmacokinetics and efficacy. *Drugs* 60, 1259–87.

5. Saxena PR, Tfelt-Hansen P (2006) Triptans, 5HT1B/1D agonists in the acute treatment of migraine. In: Olesen J, Goadsby PJ, Ramadan NM, Tfelt-Hansen P, Welch KMA (eds) *The Headaches*, 3rd edn, pp. 469–503. Lippincott Williams & Wilkins, Philadelphia, PA.

6. Dahlöf CGH, Solomon GD (2006) Impact of the headache on the individual and family. In: Olesen J, Goadsby PJ, Ramadan NM, Tfelt-Hansen P, Welch KMA (eds) *The Headaches*, 3rd edn, pp. 27–34. Lippincott Williams & Wilkins, Philadelphia, PA.

7. Tfelt-Hansen P, Bach F, Daugaard D, Tsiropoulos I, Riddersholm B (2006) Treatment with sumatriptan 50 mg in the mild phase of migraine attacks in patients with infrequent attacks. A randomised, double-blind, placebo-controlled study. *J Headache Pain* 7, 389–94.

8. International Headache Society Clinical Trial Subcommittee (2000) Guidelines for controlled trials of drugs in migraine. Second edition. *Cephalalgia* 20, 765–86.

9. Tfelt-Hansen P (2004) The methodology of prophylactic trials. Discussion summary. In: Olesen J, Silberstein SD, Tfelt-Hansen P (eds) *Preventive Pharmacotherapy of Headache Disorders*, pp. 29–30. Oxford University Press, New York.

10. International Headache Society Committee on Clinical Trials in Migraine (1991) Guidelines for controlled trials of drugs in migraine. First edition. *Cephalalgia* 11, 1–12.

11. Pilgrim AJ (1991) Methodology of clinical trials of sumatriptan in migraine and cluster headache. *Eur J Neurol* 31, 295.

12. Tfelt-Hansen P (1998) Efficacy and adverse events of subcutaneous, oral and intranasal sumatriptan used for migraine treatment, a systematic review based on number needed to treat. *Cephalalgia* 18, 532–8.

13. Klapper J, Lucas C, Rosjo O, Charlesworth B; ZODIAC Study Group (2004) Benefits of treating highly disabled migraine patients with zolmitriptan while pain is mild. *Cephalalgia* 24, 918–24.

14. Winner P, Landy S, Richardson M, Ames M (2005) Early intervention in migraine with sumatriptan tablets 50 mg versus 100 mg: a pooled analysis of data from six trials. *Clin Ther* 27, 1785–94.

15. Nett R, Landy S, Schackelford S, Richardson MS, Ames M, Lener M (2003) Pain-free efficacy after treatment with sumatriptan in the mild phase of menstrually associated migraine. *Obstet Gynecol* 102, 835–42.

16. Mathew NT, Kailasam J, Meadors I (2004) Early treatment of migraine with rizatriptan, a placebo-controlled study. *Headache* 44, 669–73.

17. Olesen J, Diener H-C, Husstedt IW, Goadsby PJ, Hall D, Meier U, Pollentier S, Lesko LM, for the BIBN 4096 BS Clinical Proof of Concept Study Group (2004) Calcitonin gene-related peptide receptor antagonist BIBN 4096 BS for the acute treatment of migraine. *N Engl J Med* 350, 1104–10.

18. Dahlöf C, Hogenhuis L, Olesen J, *et al.* (1998) Early clinical experience with subcutaneous naratriptan in the acute treatment of migraine: a dose-ranging study. *Eur J Neurol* 5, 469–77.

19. Ferrari MD, Goadsby PJ, Roon KI, Lipton RB (2002) Triptans (serotonin, 5-HT1B/1D agonists) in migraine: detailed results and methods of meta-analysis of 53 trials. *Cephalalgia* 22, 633–58.

20. Tfelt-Hansen P, Schoenen J, Lauret D (1997) Success rates of combined oral lysine acetylsalicylate and metoclopramide, oral sumatriptan, and placebo depend on initial headache severity. A preliminary retrospective analysis. In: Olesen J, Tfelt-Hansen P (eds) *6th International Headache Research Seminar. Headache Treatment. Trial Methodology and New Drugs*, pp. 103–6. Lippincott-Raven, New York.

21. Lipton RB, Bigal ME, Goadsby PJ (2004) Double-blind clinical trials of oral triptans vs other classes of acute migraine medication—a review. *Cephalalgia* 24, 321–32.

22. Tfelt-Hansen P (2006) Triptans vs. other classes of migraine medication. *Cephalalgia* 26, 628.

23. Bussone G, D'Amico, McCarroll KA, Gerth W, Lines CR (2002) Restoring migraine sufferers ability to function normally, a comparison of rizatriptan and other triptans in randomized trials. *Eur J Neurol* 48, 172–7.
24. Adelman JV, Lipton RB, Ferrari MD, Diener H-C, McCarroll KA, Vandormael K, Lines CR (2001) Comparison of rizatriptan and other triptans on stringent measures of efficacy. *Neurology* 57, 1377–83.
25. Cady RC, Ryan R, Jhingran P, O'Quinn S, Pait DG (1998) Sumatriptan injection reduces productivity loss during migraine attacks. Results of a double-blind, placebo-controlled trial. *Arch Intern Med* 158, 1013–18.
26. (1999) Acute treatment of migraine attacks: efficacy and safety of a nonsteriodal anti-inflammatory drug, diclofenac-potassium, in comparison to oral sumatriptan and placebo. The Diclofenac-K/Sumatriptan Migraine Study Group. *Cephalalgia* 19, 232–40.
27. Diener HC for the ASASUMAMIG Study Group (1999) Efficacy and safety of intravenous acetylsalicylic acid lysinate compared to subcutaneous sumatriptan and parenteral placebo in the acute treatment of migraine. A double-blind, double-dummy, randomized, multicenter, parallel group study. *Cephalalgia* 19, 581–8.
28. Honkaniemi J, Liimatainen S, Rainesalo S, Sulavuori S (2006) Haloperidol in the acute treatment of migraine, a randomized, double-blind, placebo-controlled study. *Headache* 46, 781–7.
29. Diener HC, Pfaffenrath V, Pageler L, Peil H, Aicher B (2005) The fixed combination of acetylsalicylic acid, paracetamol and caffeine is more effective than single substances and dual combination for the treatment of headache, a multicentre, randomized, double-blind, single-dose, placebo-controlled parallel group study. *Cephalalgia* 25, 776–87.
30. Ryan R, Elkind A, Baker CC, Mullican W, Debussey BS, Asgharnejad M (1997) Sumatriptan nasal spray for the acute treatment of migraine, results of two clinical studies. *Neurology* 49, 1225–30.
31. Goldstein J, Silberstein SD, Saper JR, Ryan Jr RE, Lipton RB (2006) Acetaminophen, aspirin, and caffeine in combination versus ibuprofen for acute migraine, results from a multicenter, double-blind, randomized, parallel-group, single-dose, placebo-controlled study. *Headache* 46, 444–53.
32. Sunshine A, Muthern SA, Olson N, Elkind A, Almas S, Sikes C (2006) Comparative sensitivity of stopwatch methodology and conventional pain assessment measures for detecting early response to triptans in migraine, results of a randomized, open-labeled pilot study. *Clin Ther* 28, 1107–15.
33. Goldstein J, Ryan R, Jiang K, Geston A, Block GA, Lines C (1998) Crossover comparison of rizatriptan 5 mg and 10 mg versus sumatriptan 25 mg and 50 mg in migraine. Rizatriptan Protocol 046 Study Group. *Headache* 38, 737–47.
34. Tfelt-Hansen P, Teall J, Rodriguez F, Giacovazzo M, Paz J, Malbecq W, Block GA, Reines SA, Visser WH on behalf of the Rizatriptan 030 Study Group (1998) Oral rizatriptan versus oral sumatriptan: A direct comparative study in the acute treatment of migraine. *Headache* 38, 748–55.
35. Kolodny A, Polis A, Battisti WP, Hohnson-Prattn L, Skobieranda F, Rizatriptan 052 Study Group (2004) Comparison of rizatriptan 5 mg and 19 mg tablets and sumatriptan 25 mg and 50 mg tablets. *Cephalalgia* 24, 540–6.
36. Pascual J, Vega P, Diener HC, Allen C, Vrijens F, Patel K (2000) Comparison of rizatriptan 10 mg vs. zolmitriptan 2.5 mg in the acute treatment of migraine: Rizatriptan-Zolmitriptan Study Group. *Cephalalgia* 20, 455–61.
37. Bomhof MAM, Paz J, Legg N, Allen C, Vandormael K, Patel K (1999) Comparison of rizatriptan 10 mg vs. naratriptan 2.5 mg in migraine. *Eur J Neurol* 42, 171–9.
38. Tfelt-Hansen P (2000) A comment on time-to-event analysis for headache relief. *Cephalalgia* 20; 255–6.
39. Tfelt-Hansen P, McCarroll K, Lines C (2002) Sum of Pain Intensity Differences (SPID) in migraine trials. A comment based on four rizatriptan trials. *Cephalalgia* 22, 664–6.

40. Sheftell FD, Dahlöf CG, Brandes JL, Agosti R, Jones MW, Barets PS (2005) Two replicate random-ized, double-blind, placebo-controlled trials of the time to onset of headache relief in the acute treatment of migraine with a fast-disintegrating/rapid-release formulation of sumatriptan tablets. *Clin Ther* 27, 407–17.

41. Wells NE, Steiner TJ (2000) Effectiveness of eletriptan in reducing time loss caused by migraine attacks. *Pharmacoeconomics* 18, 557–66.

42. Dahlöf C (1990) Minor Symptoms Evaluation (MSE) Profile-a questionnaire for assessment of subjective CNS-related symptoms. *Scand J Prim Health Care Suppl* 1(6), 19–25.

43. Dahlöf C, Edwards C, Toth A (1992) Sumatriptan injection is superior to placebo in the acute treatment of migraine with regard to both efficacy and general well-being. *Cephalalgia* 12, 214–20.

44. Wagner TH, Patrick DL, Galer BS, Berzon RA (1996) A new instrument to assess the long-term quality of life effects from migraine, development and psychometric testing of the MSQOL. *Headache* 36(8), 484–92.

45. Jhingran P, Osterhaus JT, Miller DW, Lee JT, Kirchdoerfer L (1998) Development and validation of the Migraine-Specific Quality of Life Questionnaire. *Headache* 38(4), 295–302.

46. Jacobson GP, Ramadan NM, Aggarwal SK, Newman CW (1994) The Henry Ford Hospital Headache Disability Inventory (HDI). *Neurology* 44(5), 837–42.

47. Stewart WF, Lipton RB, Simon D, Von Korff M, Liberman J (1998) Reliability of an illness severity measure for headache in a population sample of migraine sufferers. *Cephalalgia* 18, 44–51.

48. Kosinski M, Bayliss MS, Bjorner JB, *et al.* (2003) A six-item short-form survey for measuring headache impact: the HIT-6. *Qual Life Res* 12(8), 963–74.

49. Diener HC, Tfelt-Hansen P, Dahlöf C, *et al.* (2004) Topiramate in migraine prophylaxis. Results from a placebo-controlled trial with propranolol as an active control. *Eur Neurol* 251, 943–50.

50. Brandes JL, Saper JR, Diamond M, *et al.* (2004) Topiramate for migraine prevention, a randomized controlled trial. *JAMA* 291, 965–73.

51. Silberstein SD, Neto W, Schmitt JJ, Jacobs D; MIGR-001 Study Group (2004) Topiramate in migraine prevention: results of a large controlled study. *Arch Neurol* 61, 480–95.

52. Tfelt-Hansen P, Rolan P (2006) β-Adrenoceptor blocking drugs in migraine prophylaxis. In: Olesen J, Goadsby PJ, Ramadan NM, Tfelt-Hansen P, Welch KMA (eds). *The Headaches*, 3rd edn, pp. 519–28. Lippincott Williams & Wilkins, Philadelphia, PA.

53. Toda N, Tfelt-Hansen P (2006) Calcium antagonists in migraine prophylaxis. In: Olesen J, Goadsby PJ, Ramadan NM, Tfelt-Hansen P, Welch KMA (eds). *The Headaches*, 3rd edn, pp. 539–44. Lippincott Williams & Wilkins, Philadelphia, PA.

54. Tfelt-Hansen P, Saxena PR (2006) Antiserotonin drugs in migraine prophylaxis. In: Olesen J, Goadsby PJ, Ramadan NM, Tfelt-Hansen P, Welch KMA (eds). *The Headaches*, 3rd edn, pp. 529–37. Lippincott Williams & Wilkins, Philadelphia, PA.

55. Silberstein SD, Tfelt-Hansen P (2006) Antiepileptic drugs in migraine prophylaxis. In: Olesen J, Goadsby PJ, Ramadan NM, Tfelt-Hansen P, Welch KMA (eds). *The Headaches*, 3rd edn, pp. 545–51. Lippincott Williams & Wilkins, Philadelphia, PA.

56. Stewart WF, Lipton RB, Dowson AJ, Sawyer J (2001) Development and testing of the Migraine Disability Assessment (MIDAS) Questionnaire to assess headache-related disability. *Neurology* 56 (6 Suppl. 1), S20–8.

5

Health-related quality of life and similar end-points

Carl G.H. Dahlöf

Introduction

Migraine is an inherited, episodic, chronic neurological disease characterized by recurrent episodes of severe throbbing headaches associated with nausea and increased sensitivity to sound and light, which typically affects the sufferers during their most productive years.[1–14] During an attack, people with severe migraine are almost completely incapacitated by a throbbing headache, nausea and/or vomiting and increased sensitivity to l ight and sound. Severe migraine attacks are very disabling and the World Health Organization (WHO) ranks migraine among the most disabling medical illnesses in the world, with acute attacks causing as much disability as quadriplegia, psychosis, and dementia.[15,16]

More than 600 million (11%) of the world population (6.7 billion) suffer from migraine, which places a heavy economic burden on both the individual and society.[17] Migraine attacks obstruct family obligations and social plans, result in absenteeism from work, impair the ability to perform normal tasks at home, school, or in the workplace, produce suffering and emotional stress, and impair health-related quality of life.[2–4,6–12,18–20] Every day about 2 million individuals in Europe have to go through a migraine attack, which per annum burden the European economy by 27 billion Euros.[21] In fact, migraine and other headaches account for 32% of the total costs (health-care, direct non-medical and indirect) for all neurological diseases in Europe.[21]

The mean attack frequency of the general population of migraineurs is about one attack per month but the distribution is markedly skewed, where some migraineurs have a few attacks per year, whereas others experience several attacks per month. In a Swedish epidemiological study 27% of the migraineurs accounted for 68% of the total number of migraine attacks.[22] This would indicate that about one-third of the migrainous population are more afflicted than the others. Similar findings have been demonstrated in the USA where 38% of male migraineurs and 51% of female migraineurs accounted for 90% and 93% of all work loss (Lost Work Day Equivalents = LWDEs) due to migraine, respectively.[23]

Migraine attacks can have a profound effect on the day-to-day life and well-being of the sufferer. In the long term, migraine may cause profound emotional changes and result in coping strategies that interfere with working, social, and family life, and many normal daily activities. Almost all, if not all, migraineurs take medications, whether non-prescription or prescription, in an attempt to rapidly relieve the most debilitating symptoms of the migraine attack—pain, nausea, phonophobia, and photophobia.[19,24–26] Many migraineurs would also benefit from preventive medication, in particular the most badly affected (one-third), but generally less than 10% are presently using prophylactic medication. Increased use of improved and well-executed treatment strategies should lead to increased benefits for patients with reduction in the personal and societal burden of migraine.

Stricter success criteria in acute and prevention trials in migraine have been suggested to be used in the development of new drugs (see Chapter 4). Although much of the burden of migraine stems from the symptoms of the attack, migraineurs may also suffer from migraine between attacks.[19,27] Consequently, we should aim to establish the full impact of migraine on the patient's lifestyle and well-being.[28] Assessment of health-related quality of life (HRQoL) has over the years become an important addition to the methods used to evaluate the personal impact of diseases.[4,25,29,30] HRQoL is assessed using questionnaires that combine a subjective perception of the sufferer's life situation and an objective assessment of health factors. The impact of migraine is usually measured through self-administered questionnaires. The questionnaires may be generic or specific to a particular disease. Generic questionnaires are suitable for comparisons between study populations and different diseases, whereas disease-specific questionnaires best assess problems associated with a single disease. An ideal questionnaire has to be reliable, valid, and you should be able to complete it within 5 minutes. The questionnaire has to measure individual patients at all levels of severity (from mild to severe impact), has to enable comparisons of scores across questionnaires, and finally has to have the sensitivity to track changes over time.

Health-related quality of life and disability outcome measures in migraine

The full impact of migraine is not easy to measure. Depending on the definition of HRQoL used or the aspects of disability we are interested in, the instruments can be focused to the patient's emotional well-being, headache severity, and ability to cope with headaches or work productivity. Some instruments have been developed to quantify migraine disability and also to improve communication between patients and health-care professionals.[4,25]

Some of the assessment tools have the restriction of disability meaning minutes, hours, or days during which work, school, or home activities were missed/affected by 50% or more. Although restriction of activities from a time perspective has high face validity, research in other therapeutic areas has suggested that it may be a challenge for patients to accurately recall time missed beyond 2–4 weeks. In addition, some of the currently available assessment tools are not likely to demonstrate changes over time due to different migraine interventions.

There are a number of validated instruments that have been developed to quantify disability: the Migraine-Specific Quality of Life Questionnaire (MSQ);[31,32] the Subjective Symptom Assessment Profile (SSAP);[33] the Minor Symptoms Evaluation Profile (MSEP);[34] the Short-form 36 (SF-36);[20,35–37] the Headache Disability Inventory (HDI);[38,39] the Headache Impact Questionnaire (HImQ);[40,41] Migraine Disability Assessment Questionnaire (MIDAS);[42–44] the Headache Impact Test (HIT);[45,46] and the Migraine Attack Severity Scale (MIGSEV);[47,48] all of which use different distinctive approaches to measurement. Principal differences among questionnaires are reflected in their methods of administration, which can be anything from Internet/computerized to paper-based self-administered evaluations. With respect to recall periods, they can differ from the first 24 h of the migraine attack to considering the last 1–3 month period with migraine attacks. A simple comparison of some of these validated instruments is demonstrated in Table 5.1.

The success of medications and other treatments dictates the extent of the sufferer's immediate disability, which may range from beginning to resume activities within hours to being immobilized in bed for days—arising only with the urge to vomit. Despite the treatment used, total recovery still seems to follow the natural duration of the attack. We developed a questionnaire for measuring disability and patients' quality of life during the migraine attack, i.e. the Minor Symptoms Evaluation Profile-acute (MSEP-acute) (Figure 5.1).[49] Figure 5.1 clearly shows the difference between patients' answers in the MSEP-acute questionnaire done between and during migraine attacks, when the answers were left-shifted at baseline and right-shifted toward 'deterioration' during the attack. While placebo did not change these results (middle), a subcutaneous injection of sumatriptan caused an improvement and shifted the answers toward baseline values obtained outside the migraine attacks (see Figure 5.1).

Another illustrative example of using the self-administered standardized questionnaires is the Subjective Symptom Assessment Profile (SSAP) test, developed for general well-being evaluation of migraine patients and other patient categories (Figure 5.2).[33] In Figure 5.2, through the SSAP diagram, it can be demonstrated that the area of symptoms between migraineurs without migraine attack is larger than that of age- and sex-matched controls.

Table 5.1 Content of widely used headache impact questionnaires.

	HDI	HImQ	MIDAS	MSQ	HIT-6™
Pain (frequency/severity)		X	X		X
Role functioning	X	X	X	X	X
Social functioning	X	X	X	X	X
Energy/fatigue				X	X
Cognition	X			X	X
Emotional distress	X			X	X

HDI, Headache Disability Inventory; HImQ, Headache Impact Questionnaire; MIDAS, Migraine Disability Assessment Questionnaire; MSQ, Migraine-Specific Quality of Life Questionnaire; HIT-6™ Headache Impact Test.

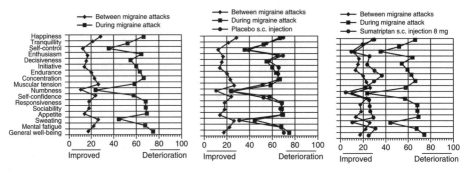

Fig. 5.1 The Minor Symptoms Evaluation Profile-acute (MSEP-acute) assessments before and after acute migraine treatment with sumatriptan 8 mg subcutaneous injection and placebo.[49]

From this evaluation it appears that migraine affects the symptom profile of the migraineurs also during days when they are not suffering attacks. Thus, in addition to the disability perceived during the migraine attack, it seems that some impairment is also experienced between the attacks.[27,50,51] The unpredictability of migraine and anxiety about future attacks often thus has an interictal influence. When a population-based sample of migraineurs were asked about recovery, 43%, 43%, and 9% respectively (4% no response) stated that they recovered 'completely', 'more or less', and 'not at all' between the attacks.[19] In other words, less than half recovered fully between the attacks.

Moreover, there are other questionnaires, such as the SF-36, which by evaluating eight different dimensions enables us to compare quality of life in migraineurs with that of

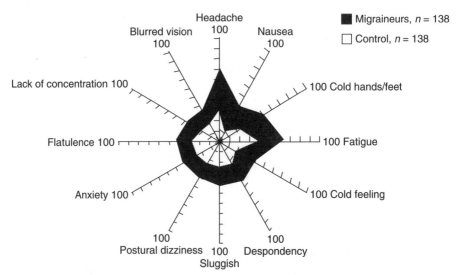

Fig. 5.2 Results of Subjective Symptom Assessment Profile (SSAP) questionnaires test, widely used to compare well-being of migraine patients between attacks with that of an age- and sex-matched control group.[27]

patients with other diseases. Subjects ($n = 845$) were surveyed 2–6 months after participation in a placebo-controlled clinical trial and asked to complete a questionnaire, including the SF-36 Health Survey, a migraine severity measurement scale, and demographics. Results were adjusted for severity of illness and comorbidities. Scores were compared with responses to the same survey by the US sample and by patients with other chronic conditions, such as depression and osteoarthritis (Figure 5.3).[20]

In a recent similar study a subsample of migraine sufferers were evaluated with a new, even shorter generic health survey, the SF-8 Health Survey (SF-8), an alternate form that uses one question to measure each of the eight SF-36 domains.[52] Data from 7557 participants surveyed via the Internet and mail were used to document the burden of migraine on HRQoL and to compare the relative burden of migraine with other chronic conditions using the SF-8. The HRQoL of migraineurs was similar to those with congestive heart failure, hypertension, and diabetes, and is better than those with depression.[52] In addition, migraine sufferers experienced better physical health but worse mental health than those with osteoarthritis. These results support previous research indicating that the burden of migraine on functional health and well-being is considerable and comparable with other chronic conditions known to have substantial impact on HRQoL.

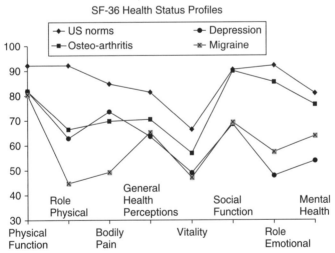

Fig. 5.3 Results of the Short-form 36® (SF-36) questionnaire test, widely used for comparing and evaluating eight different dimensions in migraineurs with those in patients with other diseases.[20] SF-36 measures quality of life in eight different aspects: physical functioning, role-physical function, bodily pain, general health, vitality, social function, role-emotional, and mental health. ◆ Reflects the norm for the general US population. ✳ Reflects the scores in patients with migraine, whereas ● and ■ lines reflect the scores in patients with depression and osteoarthritis, respectively. Migraine patients have the lowest physical functioning and bodily pain scores but the general health perception is also low. However, patients with depression have the lowest score in social functioning, role-emotional well-being, and mental health.

Socio-economic factors

An evaluation of the full impact of migraine on patients and society is necessary to account for socio-economic aspects of direct health-care cost that may include hospitalization, office and emergency room visits, and drug administration. Apart from the direct costs, hidden indirect costs such as loss of productivity at work also exist. If we compare direct versus indirect cost, normally we can observe that the indirect cost is about 70–80% of the total costs. From a patient's perspective, the loss of time due to headache disability in social, leisure, and family activities also contributes to impair their quality of life. It is, however, difficult to translate migraineurs' health-related quality of life and disability due to their migraine *per se* into money. Accordingly, it is not always easy to demonstrate substantial benefits of migraine therapy on headache disability.[50] This could possibly be due to the fact that most disability is suffered at home, whereas the majority of tests are addressing the impact of disability on work performance, school performance, etc. In addition, absenteeism from work or school is very limited (about 6 days per year out of 98.4 days with migraine per year).[53] These data suggest that while migraineurs do attend work, school etc. during many of their attacks they do so with reduced functional status—a scenario often described as 'presenteeism'. A recent telephone survey that was conducted of a random sample ($n = 4007$) of the population aged 16–65 years of mainland England demonstrated that an estimated 5.7 working days were lost per year for every working or student migraineur, although the most disabled 10% accounted for 85% of the total.[53] All together, these factors make it difficult to evaluate the real burden of migraine and to extrapolate the total costs of their migraine attacks.

A retrospective study using linked medical and pharmacy claims data that allowed identification of families and individuals with migraine indicates that the total health-care costs of a family with a migraineur were 70% higher than those of non-migraine family, with most of the difference concentrated in outpatient costs.[12] Migraine families incur far higher direct and indirect health-care costs than non-migraine families, with variation depending on which family member is the clinically detected migraineur and possible co-morbid conditions.[12,54]

Impact of headache therapy on disability

The impact of short-term treatment for migraine attacks on HRQoL was evaluated in an open prospective 6-month study at the Gothenburg Migraine Clinic.[27] Socio-economic factors, subjective symptoms, and general well-being/quality of life were evaluated by self-administered questionnaires in 99 patients with migraine with or without aura in accordance with the classification of the International Headache Society. Short-term treatment comprising conventional therapy or subcutaneous sumatriptan reduced number of days per month with migraine, absenteeism from work, and migraine-associated symptoms, but did not significantly improve general well-being between attacks.[27]

A prospective, observational study without control group assessed the outcomes of migraineurs in a mixed model staff/independent practice association managed care organization for patients previously diagnosed as having migraine who received their first prescription for sumatriptan.[55] Data collected included medical as well as pharmacy claims and patient surveys to measure changes in satisfaction, health-related quality of life, workplace productivity, and non-workplace activity after sumatriptan therapy was initiated. A total of 178 patients completed the study. Results obtained from 178 patients showed significant decreases in the mean number of migraine-related physician office visits, emergency department visits, and medical procedures in the 6 months after sumatriptan therapy compared with the 6 months before sumatriptan was used ($P < 0.05$).[55] There were also improvements in patient satisfaction and significant reductions in time lost from workplace productivity and non-workplace activity.

Unfortunately, there is very limited double-blind and controlled prospective data on the effects of headache therapy on disability in this respect. A prospective sequential multinational (five countries) study was to concurrently evaluate the effects of subcutaneous sumatriptan on clinical parameters, HRQoL measures, workplace productivity, and patient satisfaction.[50] Patients ($n = 58$, aged 18–65 years) diagnosed with moderate to severe migraine treated their symptoms for 24 weeks with subcutaneous sumatriptan after a 12-week period of treating symptoms with their customary (non-sumatriptan) therapy. Patients used diary cards to record information concerning the effects of migraine on workplace productivity and non-workplace activity time. The average workplace productivity time lost was 23.4 h per patient during 12 weeks of customary therapy, compared with 7.2 and 5.8 h per patient during the first and second 12-week periods of sumatriptan therapy, respectively. An average of 9.3 h of non-workplace activity time was lost per patient during the customary therapy phase, compared with 3.2 and 2.8 h during the first and second 12-week periods of sumatriptan therapy, respectively. Treatment of migraine with subcutaneous sumatriptan compared with customary therapy was associated with an average gain per patient of approximately 16 h of workplace productivity time and 6 h of non-workplace activity time, over a 3-month period.[50]

In a phase III, multinational, randomized clinical trial, 692 patients treated a migraine attack with eletriptan 40 mg or 80 mg, or placebo.[56] Patients responded to a questionnaire seeking information concerning the amount of time lost from usual activities during the attack. Time loss assessments were made 24 h after the last dose taken and recorded in a diary. Patients receiving either dose of the active compound were unable to perform their usual activities for a median period of 4 h compared with 9 h experienced by those taking placebo. This difference was highly statistically significant ($P < 0.001$).[56] The time saving associated with eletriptan usage reflected the differences in efficacy findings in the clinical component of the study.

Studies detailing the specific impact of migraine preventive therapy on daily activities are limited. Topiramate is approved in approximately 30 countries for the prophylaxis (prevention) of migraine headache in adults. In three pivotal trials, changes in mean Migraine-Specific Questionnaire (MSQ) and Medical Outcome Study Short Form 36 (SF-36) scores from baseline to each assessment point during the double-blind phase were calculated for pooled intent-to-treat patients. Topiramate 100 mg/day significantly improved all three MSQ domains throughout the double-blind phase compared with placebo ($P = 0.024$ at week 8, $P < 0.001$ at weeks 16 and 26 for Role Prevention; $P < 0.001$ for Role Restriction and Emotional Function, all time-points).[57] Topiramate 100 mg/day also significantly improved the SF-36 physical component scores (PCS) throughout the double-blind phase compared with placebo ($P < 0.001$, all time-points), and significantly improved the mental component scores (MCS) at week 26 ($P = 0.043$). The greatest topiramate-associated improvements on SF-36 subscales were seen for bodily pain and general health perceptions ($P < 0.05$; weeks 8, 16, and 26), and physical functioning, vitality, role-physical, and social functioning ($P < 0.05$; weeks 16 and 26). Topiramate-associated improvements on the disease-specific MSQ were stronger than on the generic SF-36 scale, which is not surprising given that generic scales tend to measure constructs that are not necessarily affected by a specific disease.

The Genetic Epidemiology of Migraine (GEM) study revealed that patient function was inversely related to migraine attack frequency ($P < 0.0002$) with those suffering from a high frequency of attacks reporting diminished physical, mental, and social functioning.[58] In the analysis of the topiramate study, patients who experienced $\geq 50\%$ decreases in monthly migraine frequency on either topiramate or placebo ($\geq 50\%$ responders) experienced significantly more improvement in their functioning levels than those patients who experienced $< 50\%$ decreases in monthly migraine frequency. This result indicates that reducing monthly migraine frequency is associated with improved patient ability to carry out daily activities.

Assessing disability in clinical practice

Presently, the magnitude of impact of headache and migraine is generally measured by two of the most useful and reliable patient disability and life quality questionnaires, the Migraine Disability Assessment Questionnaire (MIDAS) and the Internet-based Headache Impact Test (HIT) (Table 5.1).

Migraine Disability Assessment

The MIDAS questionnaire is a brief, self-administered questionnaire designed to quantify headache-related disability.[42–44] Headache sufferers answer five questions, noting the number of days, in the past 3 months, of activity limitations due to migraine. The MIDAS score is the sum of missed work or school days, missed household chores days, and missed non-work activity days, and days at work or school plus days of house-hold chores where productivity was reduced by half or more in the last 3 months. The MIDAS scores are then categorized by disability level: little or no disability (0–5), mild disability (6–10), moderate disability (11–20), and severe disability (20+).[42]

The reliability and internal consistency of the MIDAS score is high, as tested in a population-based sample of headache sufferers where MIDAS scores are substantially higher in migraine cases than in non-migraine cases, supporting the validity of the measurement.[44] In addition, Stewart et al.[44] conducted another trial in order to examine the test–retest reliability and internal consistency of the overall MIDAS score using population-based samples of migraine sufferers across the USA and UK. A total of 97 migraine-headache sufferers from the USA and 100 from the UK completed the MIDAS questionnaire twice in an average of 3 weeks apart from one another. The result of this first international population-based study to assess the reliability of disability-related scores for migraine shows that the reliability and internal consistency of the MIDAS is similar to those of other migraine questionnaires. However, the MIDAS requires fewer questions, is easier to score, and provides intuitively meaningful information on lost days of activity.[44]

Headache Impact Test

The HIT is a tool to measure the impact that headaches have on a person's ability. It is a new Internet-based test that has been implemented to assess the wide effects of migraine by quantifying the impact of headache frequency and severity on migraineurs' lives (available at: www.headachetest.com). HIT is a dynamic, computer-adaptive questionnaire, which has been shown to be reliable, sensitive, and valid for clinical settings. The HIT scores show the effect that headaches have on patients' normal life and the ability to function with respect to their treatment.[46] HIT was developed by a team of international headache experts from neurology and primary care medicine in collaboration with the psychometricians who developed the SF-36 health assessment tool. In fact, HIT was adapted from widely used headache impact measures that were validated independently for the purpose of HIT creating. Thus, this test was developed from a number of established measurement tools that have been used successfully for years. The HIT includes 54 questions that assess pain, disability, and affective distress presented through a standardized scoring range of 36–78.[46] From the final score on a 1–2-min questionnaire, HIT yields a very accurate description of the impact that headaches have on patients' life and ability to function. HIT is a widely used headache impact questionnaire able to consider at the same time frequency and severity of pain, role and social functioning, energy, fatigue, cognition, and emotional distress, producing a more accurate estimate of individual patient scores. HIT assessments also meet standards based on clinical criteria by estimating the severity of headache impacts sensitive to changes in severity over time.

A paper-based, shorter version of the HIT questionnaire has been developed for people without access to the Internet or without computer knowledge.[46] This standardized short paper version of HIT, called HIT-6TM, is based on six questions and functions as well as the standard HIT version. Data on headache characteristics and treatment regimen are available from 4287 subjects who completed HIT-6TM in the Landmark study.[4,59] The results of the Landmark study also clearly show that the burden of headache may be translated into frequency or severity.[4]

Both MIDAS and HIT are scientifically valid measures of migraine severity and have the potential to improve communication between patients and physicians, assess migraine severity, and act as outcome measures to monitor treatment efficacy. However, HIT is considered to be the most reliable method for evaluating an individual patient's progress over time with greater accessibility and coverage of the spectrum of headache than MIDAS.

Conclusions

Although most people suffer from different types of headaches, the severity of their pain is often not communicated properly to their doctors. Research shows that when doctors understand exactly how headaches are affecting their patients, they are able to provide a better and fully successful treatment programme. In particular, migraine can be difficult to manage in primary care, where it is under-recognized, underdiagnosed, and under-treated. Migraine care could only be improved by incorporating assessments of migraine impact into management strategies. Research has shown that measurements of headache-related disability, together with assessments of pain intensity, headache frequency, tiredness, mood alterations, and cognition, can be used to assess the impact of migraine on sufferers' lives and society.

Increased use of tools for assessment of HRQoL and disability in combination with well-executed treatment strategies would most likely lead to increased benefits for patients with a reduction in the personal and societal burden of migraine.

References

1. Headache Classification Committee of the International Headache Society (2004) The International Classification of Headache Disorders: 2nd edition. *Cephalalgia* 24 (Suppl. 1), 9–160.
2. Lipton RB, Bigal ME, Diamond M, Freitag F, Reed ML, Stewart WF (2007) Migraine prevalence, disease burden, and the need for preventive therapy. *Neurology* 68(5), 343–9.
3. Stovner LJ, Hagen K (2006) Prevalence, burden, and cost of headache disorders. *Curr Opin Neurol* 19(3), 281–5.
4. Dahlöf CGH, Solomon GD (2006) Impact of headache on the individual and family. In: Olesen J, Goadsby PJ, Ramadan NM, Tfelt-Hansen P, Welch KMA (eds) *The Headaches*, 3rd edn, pp. 27–34. Lippincott Williams & Wilkins, Philadelphia, PA.
5. Lipton RB, Bigal ME (2005) Migraine: epidemiology, impact, and risk factors for progression. *Headache* 45 Suppl 1, S3–13.
6. Edvinsson L, Uddman R (2005) Neurobiology in primary headaches. *Brain Res Brain Res Rev* 48(3), 438–56.
7. Dueland AN, Leira R, Cabelli ST (2005) The impact of migraine on psychological well-being of young women and their communication with physicians about migraine: a multinational study. *Curr Med Res Opin* 21(8), 1297–305.
8. Pradalier A, Auray JP, El Hasnaoui A, *et al.* (2004) Economic impact of migraine and other episodic headaches in France: data from the GRIM2000 study. *Pharmacoeconomics* 22(15), 985–99.
9. MacGregor EA, Brandes J, Eikermann A, Giammarco R (2004) Impact of migraine on patients and their families, the Migraine And Zolmitriptan Evaluation (MAZE) survey–Phase III. *Curr Med Res Opin* 20(7), 1143–50.
10. Bussone G, Usai S, Grazzi L, Rigamonti A, Solari A, D'Amico D (2004) Disability and quality of life in different primary headaches, results from Italian studies. *Neurol Sci* 25(3), S105–7.
11. Bigal ME, Lipton RB, Stewart WF (2004) The epidemiology and impact of migraine. *Curr Neurol Neurosci Rep* 4(2), 98–104.
12. Stang PE, Crown WH, Bizier R, Chatterton ML, White R (2004) The family impact and costs of migraine. *Am J Manag Care* 10(5), 313–20.
13. Silberstein SD (2004) Migraine. *Lancet* 363(9406), 381–91.

14. Goadsby PJ, Lipton RB, Ferrari MD (2002) Migraine–current understanding and treatment. *N Engl J Med* 346(4), 257–70.

15. Lopez AD, Murray CC (1998) The global burden of disease, 1990–2020. *Nat Med* 4(11), 1241–3.

16. Menken M, Munsat TL, Toole JF (2000) The global burden of disease study, implications for neurology. The ambulatory workload of office-based neurologists, implications of the National Ambulatory Medical Care Survey. *Arch Neurol* 57(3), 418–20.

17. Stovner LJ, Hagen K, Jensen R, *et al.* (2007) The global burden of headache: a documentation of headache prevalence and disability worldwide. *Cephalalgia* 27, 193–210.

18. Lipton RB, Stewart WF, Diamond S, Diamond ML, Reed M (2001) Prevalence and burden of migraine in the United States: data from the American Migraine Study II. *Headache* 41(7), 646–57.

19. Linde M, Dahlöf C (2004) Attitudes and burden of disease among self-considered migraineurs–a nation-wide population-based survey in Sweden. *Cephalalgia* 24(6), 455–65.

20. Osterhaus JT, Townsend RJ, Gandek B, Ware JE Jr (1994) Measuring the functional status and well-being of patients with migraine headache. *Headache* 34(6), 337–43.

21. Berg J, Stovner LJ (2005) Cost of migraine and other headaches in Europe. *Eur J Neurol* 12 (Suppl 1), 59–62.

22. Dahlöf C, Linde M (2001) One-year prevalence of migraine in Sweden: a population-based study in adults. *Cephalalgia* 21(6), 664–71.

23. Stewart WF, Lipton RB, Simon D (1996) Work-related disability: results from the American migraine study. *Cephalalgia* 16(4), 231–8.

24. Lipton RB, Silberstein SD (2001) The role of headache-related disability in migraine management: implications for headache treatment guidelines. *Neurology* 56(6 Suppl 1), S35–42.

25. Dahlöf CG (2003) Measuring disability and quality of life in migraine. *Drugs Today* 39, 17–23.

26. MacGregor EA, Brandes J, Eikermann A (2003) Migraine prevalence and treatment patterns: the global Migraine and Zolmitriptan Evaluation survey. *Headache* 43, 19–26.

27. Dahlöf CG (1995) Health-related quality of life under six months' treatment of migraine–an open clinic-based longitudinal study. *Cephalalgia* 15(5), 414–22.

28. Dimenäs ES, Dahlöf CG, Jern SC, Wiklund IK (1990) Defining quality of life in medicine. *Scand J Prim Health-care* Suppl 1, 7–10.

29. Dahlöf C (1993) Assessment of health-related quality of life in migraine. *Cephalalgia* 13(4), 233–7.

30. Lipton RB, Stewart WF (1995) Health-related quality of life in headache research. *Headache* 35(8), 447–8.

31. Jhingran P, Davis SM, LaVange LM, Miller DW, Helms RW (1998) MSQ: Migraine-Specific Quality-of-Life Questionnaire. Further investigation of the factor structure. *Pharmacoeconomics* 13(6), 707–17.

32. Jhingran P, Osterhaus JT, Miller DW, Lee JT, Kirchdoerfer L (1998) Development and validation of the Migraine-Specific Quality of Life Questionnaire. *Headache* 38(4), 295–302.

33. Dimenäs ES, Wiklund IK, Dahlöf CG, Lindvall KG, Olofsson BK, De Faire UH (1989) Differences in the subjective well-being and symptoms of normotensives, borderline hypertensives and hypertensives. *J Hypertens* 7(11), 885–90.

34. Dahlöf C (1990) Minor Symptoms Evaluation (MSE) Profile–a questionnaire for assessment of subjective CNS-related symptoms. *Scand J Prim Health-care* Suppl 1, 19–25.

35. Ware JE Jr, Sherbourne CD (1992) The MOS 36-item short-form health survey (SF-36). I. Conceptual framework and item selection. *Med Care* 30(6), 473–83.

36. McHorney CA, Ware JE Jr, Lu JF, Sherbourne CD (1994) The MOS 36-item Short-Form Health Survey (SF-36): III. Tests of data quality, scaling assumptions, and reliability across diverse patient groups. *Med Care* 32, 40–66.

37. McHorney CA, Ware JE Jr, Raczek AE (1993) The MOS 36-Item Short-Form Health Survey (SF-36): II. Psychometric and clinical tests of validity in measuring physical and mental health constructs. *Med Care* 31(3), 247–63.

38. Jacobson GP, Ramadan NM, Aggarwal SK, Newman CW (1994) The Henry Ford Hospital Headache Disability Inventory (HDI). *Neurology* 44(5), 837–42.

39. Jacobson GP, Ramadan NM, Norris L, Newman CW (1995) Headache disability inventory (HDI), short-term test–retest reliability and spouse perceptions. *Headache* 35(9), 534–9.

40. Stewart WF, Lipton RB, Simon D, Liberman J, Von Korff M (1999) Validity of an illness severity measure for headache in a population sample of migraine sufferers. *Pain* 79(2–3), 291–301.

41. Stewart WF, Lipton RB, Simon D, Von Korff M, Liberman J (1998) Reliability of an illness severity measure for headache in a population sample of migraine sufferers. *Cephalalgia* 18, 44–51.

42. Stewart WF, Lipton RB, Dowson AJ, Sawyer J (2001) Development and testing of the Migraine Disability Assessment (MIDAS) Questionnaire to assess headache-related disability. *Neurology* 56(6 Suppl 1), S20–8.

43. Stewart WF, Lipton RB, Kolodner KB, Sawyer J, Lee C, Liberman JN (2000) Validity of the Migraine Disability Assessment (MIDAS) score in comparison to a diary-based measure in a population sample of migraine sufferers. *Pain* 88, 41–52.

44. Stewart WF, Lipton RB, Whyte J, *et al.* (1999) An international study to assess reliability of the Migraine Disability Assessment (MIDAS) score. *Neurology* 53(5), 988–94.

45. Bjorner JB, Kosinski M, Ware JE Jr (2003) Using item response theory to calibrate the Headache Impact Test (HIT) to the metric of traditional headache scales. *Qual Life Res* 12(8), 981–1002.

46. Ware JE Jr, Kosinski M, Bjorner JB, *et al.* (2003) Applications of computerized adaptive testing (CAT) to the assessment of headache impact. *Qual Life Res* 12(8), 935–52.

47. El Hasnaoui A, Vray M, Blin P, Nachit-Ouinekh F, Boureau F (2004) Assessment of migraine severity using the MIGSEV scale, relationship to migraine features and quality of life. *Cephalalgia* 24(4), 262–70.

48. El Hasnaoui A, Vray M, Richard A, Nachit-Ouinekh F, Boureau F (2003) Assessing the severity of migraine, development of the MIGSEV scale. *Headache* 43(6), 628–35.

49. Dahlöf C, Edwards C, Toth A (1992) Sumatriptan injection is superior to placebo in the acute treatment of migraine—with regard to both efficacy and general well-being. *Cephalalgia* 12(4), 214–20.

50. Cortelli P, Dahlöf C, Bouchard J, *et al.* (1997) A multinational investigation of the impact of subcutaneous sumatriptan. III: Workplace productivity and non-workplace activity. *Pharmacoeconomics* 1, 35–42.

51. Lipton RB, Hamelsky SW, Kolodner KB, Steiner TJ, Stewart WF (2000) Migraine, quality of life, and depression: a population-based case-control study. *Neurology* 55(5), 629–35.

52. Turner-Bowker DM, Bayliss MS, Ware JE Jr, Kosinski M (2003) Usefulness of the SF-8 Health Survey for comparing the impact of migraine and other conditions. *Qual Life Res* 12(8), 1003–12.

53. Steiner TJ, Scher AI, Stewart WF, Kolodner K, Liberman J, Lipton RB (2003) The prevalence and disability burden of adult migraine in England and their relationships to age, gender and ethnicity. *Cephalalgia* 23(7), 519–27.

54. Pesa J, Lage MJ (2004) The medical costs of migraine and comorbid anxiety and depression. *Headache* 44(6), 562–70.

55. Lofland JH, Johnson NE, Batenhorst AS, Nash DB (1999) Changes in resource use and outcomes for patients with migraine treated with sumatriptan: a managed care perspective. *Arch Intern Med* 159(8), 857–63.

56. Wells NE, Steiner TJ (2000) Effectiveness of eletriptan in reducing time loss caused by migraine attacks. *Pharmacoeconomics* 18(6), 557–66.

57. Dahlöf C, Loder E, Diamond M, Rupnow M, Papadopoulos G, Mao L (2007) The impact of migraine prevention on daily activities: a longitudinal and responder analysis from three topiramate placebo-controlled clinical trials. *Health and Quality of Life Outcomes*, in press.

58. Terwindt GM, Ferrari MD, Tijhuis M, Groenen SM, Picavet HS, Launer LJ (2000) The impact of migraine on quality of life in the general population: the GEM study. *Neurology* 55(5), 624–9.

59. Tepper SJ, Dahlöf CG, Dowson A, *et al.* (2004) Prevalence and diagnosis of migraine in patients consulting their physician with a complaint of headache: data from the landmark study. *Headache* 44(9), 856–64.

6

Clinically relevant designs and outcome measures for acute migraine trials

Michel D. Ferrari and Hille Koppen

When comparing the results for the use of triptans in acute migraine trials and the clinical perception gained from clinical experience, there seems to be a mismatch. Very few if any randomized controlled clinical trials have convincingly demonstrated superiority for efficacy of triptans compared with that of analgesics or non-steroidal anti-inflammatory drugs.[1] This clearly contrasts with clinical experience. A possible explanation is that the design and outcome measures currently used in acute migraine trials (i.e. pain free at 2 h) do not fully reflect what is needed in clinical practice.

When asked, patients want their migraine headaches to be relieved completely, with a rapid onset of the improvement and without recurrence of the headache and without major side-effects.[2] Thus reduction of pain severity at 2 h as a primary trial end-point does not fully reflect patient needs. As an example, in an open-label preference study comparing an oral triptan with subcutaneous sumatriptan in a cross-over design, 51% preferred the oral triptan as compared with only 43% for subcutaneous sumatriptan despite the much higher pain-free rates at 2 h for the latter. Main drivers for the preference for the oral triptan were lack of adverse events and a longer duration of action.

It should be noted that just reporting percentages for recurrence rates, without the associated initial pain relief rates, is meaningless.[3] Recurrence is a conditional response and low recurrence rates may for instance be found in agents with low initial relief rates indicating that very few patients were actually helped by taking the drug.

The best way of capturing patients' needs of fast and complete improvement without recurrence and side-effects is sustained pain free. This is defined as: no pain at 2 h post-dose, no recurrence of any pain, and no use of escape medication 2–24 h post-dose. This measure is simple, clinically relevant, and suitable to use both in early treatment trials and in traditional trial designs where patients are asked to treat only when the headache is of moderate or severe intensity.[4] On the other hand, major drawbacks of using sustained pain free as the primary efficacy end-point in acute migraine trials are the difficulty of explaining the concept of recurrence and the reality of low absolute efficacy numbers (20–30% at most), which is being perceived as low efficacy.

Traditionally triptan trials require patients to treat migraine attacks only when the headache is moderate to severe. Although there are good methodological reasons for this rather artificial design, in clinical practice patients may treat their migraine attacks differently. Recently, several studies have been published that study the efficacy of early treatment. When early treatment with triptans is studied, several methodological and clinical pitfalls need to be considered. Studies comparing patients who treat mild headaches and patients who treat severe headaches run the risk of actually comparing two different study populations. When asked to treat early, migraine patients may accidentally treat short migraine or tension-type headache. It is obvious that as success rates are highly dependent on the chosen end-point and design, treating early is an attractive approach for achieving higher efficacy rates. For an optimal and clinically relevant comparison of early versus late treatment, sustained pain free should be used as the outcome measure and only one type of patients (either slowly progressing or those with rapidly progressing attacks) should be included. The design would ideally be a four-arm parallel-group design with random allocation of the patients to one of four treatments: (1) early with placebo; (2) early with verum; (3) late with placebo; (4) late with verum.[4] The therapeutic gain of verum minus placebo for early treatment should then be compared with the therapeutic gain of verum minus placebo for late treatment.

In conclusion, current trial designs and primary outcome measures do not seem to reflect clinical reality and needs. The use of sustained pain free would be a much better outcome measure that can be used in both traditional and so-called early treatment trials.

References

1. Lipton RB, Bigal ME, Goadsby PJ (2004) Double-blind clinical trials of oral triptans vs other classes of acute migraine medication—a review. *Cephalalgia* 24, 321–32.
2. Lipton RB, Stewart WF (1999) Acute migraine therapy: do doctors understand what patients want from therapy. *Headache* 39, s20–6.
3. Ferrari M (1999) How to assess and compare drugs in the management of migraine: success rates in terms of response and recurrence. *Cephalalgia* 19 (Suppl. 23), 2–4.
4. Ferrari MD (2004) Should we advise patients to treat migraine attacks early? *Cephalalgia* 24, 915–17.

7

Effectiveness of different steroid dosage in Tolosa–Hunt syndrome with different phenotypes: some critical points about the new International Headache Society classification

E. Marchioni, S. Colnaghi, M. Versino,
A. Pichiecchio, E. Tavazzi, and G. Nappi

Introduction

The Tolosa–Hunt syndrome (THS) consists of one or more episodes of unilateral orbital pain associated with the paresis of at least one oculomotor nerve and magnetic resonance imaging (MRI) or biopsy demonstration of inflammatory granulomas in the cavernous sinus and/or orbital apex. International Headache Society (IHS) classification codes THS in paragraph 13.16 and highlights the importance of steroid efficacy within 72 h from onset.[1,2] However, no further details have been provided about the dosage, route of administration, and duration of steroid course. We describe two cases of THS that the diagnostic criteria of the present IHS fail to define fully.

Design

This is in the form of a report of two cases.

Description of cases

Case 1

A 40-year-old man presented with a subacute retro-orbital pain that was followed 1 day later by the appearance of vertical diplopia due to a right superior rectus paresis, right lid ptosis, and hypoaesthesia of the first and second trigeminal branch territory (Figure 7.1). The fat-suppressed (SPIR) gadolinium-enhanced MRI showed the inflammatory pathological tissue inside the right cavernous sinus and the orbital apex (Figure 7.2). The pain disappeared 1 day after starting oral prednisone (75 mg/day), while the ptosis fully recovered in 2 months, and diplopia persisted only on up-gaze together with a light hypoaesthesia. Four months later the patient was symptom-free, MRI was normalized, and steroid medication was tapered.

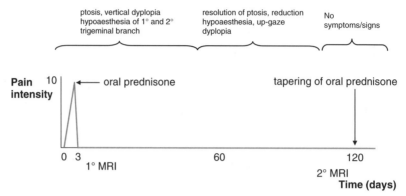

Fig. 7.1 Time-related clinical events in case 1.

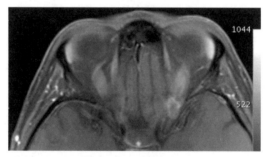

Fig. 7.2 Magnetic resonance imaging findings in case 1.

Case 2

A 33-year-old woman complained of acute left orbital pain and vertical diplopia (Figure 7.3). SPIR MRI showed inflammatory pathological tissue inside the orbital apex with partial involvement of the rectus superior muscle (Figure 7.4). An intravenous 6-methyl-prednisolone (6-MP) cycle was started for a total of 8 g distributed in 10 days. Pain was fully resolved within 84 h from the onset of treatment, and diplopia showed a marked attenuation. A few days after the shift from intravenous 6-MP to oral prednisone (75 mg/day) the pain relapsed showing a fluctuating course for at least 1 month, when a cycle of high-dose 6-MP was restarted with resolution of pain. MRI was performed 3 and 5 months after the disease onset, showing a reduction of the lesion volume of the orbital apex paralleling the improvement of pain.

Comments

We report here two cases of painful ophthalmoplegia sharing a good response to different doses of steroid, and a long-lasting ophthalmoplegia together with MRI persistence of inflammatory granulomas. In the second patient only high-dose 6-MP produced a satisfactory effect. The partial III cranial nerve impairment (cavernous sinus) and the direct

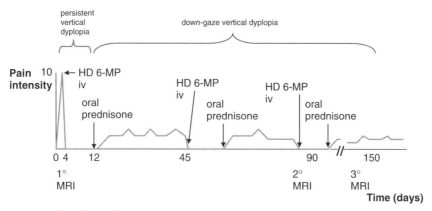

Fig. 7.3 Time-related clinical events in case 2.

muscular involvement of the superior rectus (orbital apex) were, respectively, the causes of ophthalmoplegia in the first and in the second patient. Both conditions, despite their clear relationship to the paragraph of THS (13.16), could not be fully classified on the basis of the IHS criteria for this topic. In our opinion the main critical points of IHS (see Table 7.1) are the following: (1) the criterion D, stating the resolution of pain and paresis within 72 h, seems too rigid and not supported by the literature data (the 'adequate dosage' of steroid, cited in the same point, is rather vague), and in our opinion high-dose 6-MP could be considered as a valid alternative to the generally used oral prednisone[3]; (2) oculomotor nerves and muscles could separately cause diplopia, but this point is not adequately explained.

The IHS classification in the comments states that the inflammatory lesion could be both in the cavernous sinus or in the orbit. Consequently, one could argue that it includes under the same code both the THS and the so-called orbital pseudotumour. In our opinion, this choice should be better indicated because of its relevant prognostic implication.

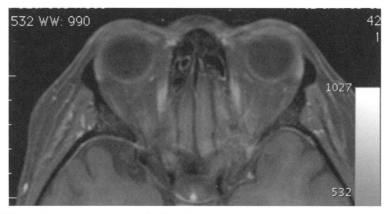

Fig. 7.4 Magnetic resonance imaging findings in case 2.

Table 7.1 International Headache Society classification of Tolosa–Hunt syndrome (13.16).

Description
Episodic orbital pain associated with paralysis of one or more of the third, fourth, and/or sixth cranial nerves, which usually resolves spontaneously but tends to relapse and remit.

Criteria
A One or more episodes of unilateral orbital pain persisting for weeks if untreated
B Paresis of one or more of the third, fourth and/or sixth cranial nerves and/or demonstration of granuloma by magnetic resonance imaging or biopsy
C Paresis coincides with the onset of pain or follows it within 2 weeks
D Pain and paresis resolve within 72 h when treated adequately with corticosteroids
E Other causes have been excluded by appropriate investigations

Note: other causes of painful ophthalmoplegia include tumours, vasculitis, basal meningitis, sarcoid, diabetes mellitus, and ophthalmoplegic 'migraine'.
Comments: Some reported cases of Tolosa–Hunt syndrome had additional involvement of the trigeminal nerve (commonly the first division) or optic, facial, or acoustic nerves. Sympathetic innervation of the pupil is occasionally affected. The syndrome has been caused by granulomatous material in the cavernous sinus, superior orbital fissure or orbit in some biopsied cases. Careful follow-up is required to exclude other possible causes of painful ophthalmoplegia.

Future targets

Creation of a THS database to address the following issues:

(a) definition of appropriate MRI techniques to localize the site of the lesion (orbit; apex; sinus);

(b) the effect of different steroid dosage and route of administration;

(c) relapse rate;

(d) subgroups prognosis based on (a) and (b).

References

1. Headache Classification Committee of the International Headache Society (2004) The International Classification of Headache Disorders: 2nd edition. *Cephalaigia* 24 (Suppl. 1), 1–160.
2. La Mantia L, *et al.* (2006) Tolosa-Hunt syndrome: critical literature review based on IHS 2004 criteria. *Cephalalgia* 26(7), 772–81.
3. Colnaghi S, *et al.* (2006) SPIR MRI usefulness for management of steroid treatment in Tolosa-Hunt syndrome. *Neurol Sci* 27, 137–9.

8

Discussion summary: Trials methodology

Jes Olesen

The major issue in this discussion was to determine the best possible end-point in trials of acute migraine. Tfelt-Hansen has presented evidence supporting the so-called complete response, i.e. one dose of the drug results in a pain-free state within 2 h and this pain-free state is maintained for at least 24 h without further intake of drugs. There was general agreement that this is a very tough end-point resulting in a low success rate with triptans. From a methodological point of view, the end-point is quite good because it has an extremely low placebo effect and thus results in a fairly large therapeutic gain. Because of the relatively low success rate it may also leave more room for improvement over the triptans when new drugs are introduced. However, there is considerable disadvantage of this end-point in the testing of new drugs for registration purposes. It was suggested that if this had been the primary end-point in the triptan trials, then triptans may never have entered the market and certainly they would have had an extremely difficult time getting reimbursement. From the commercial side of companies it was stated that practising physicians go for simple end-points and a high success rate. Companies did not believe that it would be easy to sell a new drug with a 20–30% success rate due to an extremely tough end-point. A possible compromise might be that the usual success criteria are preserved for studies leading to registration of new drugs where the question is mainly to show superiority over placebo and perhaps comparability with existing treatment. In the further development of such a new compound, attempts to demonstrate superiority over existing treatments could with advantage use the complete response. Opinions about this compromise remained divided. Michel Ferrari stressed in particular in his presentation that the issue of recurrence becomes meaningless with the usual success criteria because recurrence depends entirely on the size of the therapeutic response. As an example, if success with placebo is only 10%, then the recurrence rate with placebo could easily be 3 or 4%, which sounds good but of course has no meaning. Numbers needed to treat was another concept discussed. This concept is excellent for the comparison of active drugs but it gives no intuitive meaning to practising physicians. In general, doctors are not used to the concept and cannot understand that a drug can be worthwhile if it is necessary to treat four or five patients to have one success.

Quality of life becomes increasingly important in the development of new drugs. Carl Dahlöf presented data showing that, even outside an attack, the quality of life is considerably decreased by migraine. He also stressed that only a small fraction of migraine attacks lead to absence from work, although this is the major cost parameter in the calculation of the cost of migraine. Because of this low number of attacks leading to absence, there have never been any trials documenting that triptans have actually led to less absenteeism from work. On the other hand, there is plenty of evidence demonstrating that they have a significant positive effect on the quality of life of the sufferers. In longitudinal population-based studies it seems that absenteeism from work has not decreased after the introduction of triptans. This may partly be due to an increasing prevalence of migraine but it may also reflect that although attacks are better treated, patients still don't feel quite fit for work. It was suggested that to have real impact on the societal cost of migraine, better prophylactic drugs are needed. If attack frequency is reduced then it follows that absenteeism from work will be reduced to the same extent. It is expected that there will be an increasing pressure on companies to document the cost-effectiveness of their compounds in the future, and this was expected to be easier for prophylactic drugs than for acute drugs.

Lastly, novel designs for migraine drug trials were discussed. Using migraine patients already in phase 1 studies or combining phase 1 studies with studies of surrogate measures would be one way of saving cost and time. The need for better animal and human models is obvious. In previous studies using the nitroglycerine model in migraine patients, pretreatment with either propranolol or valproate had been given versus placebo and patients then exposed to nitroglycerine. The propranolol study was negative while the valproate study was positive. The conclusion was that models may be of use but that much more work is required to develop sufficiently sensitive and specific models for the testing of prophylactic drugs. Models may not be positive for all prophylactic drugs, depending on their mechanism of action. In phase 2, adaptive designs versus more classical designs were discussed. There was evidence from the pharma industry that adaptive designs may save approximately 15% in terms of time, but they are more difficult and costly. Designs that are less fancy than the one employed in the study of BIBN 4096 BS are perhaps more cost-effective. Another approach is to use multiple doses, each given to a relatively small group of sufferers, for example between 10 and 20 patients in a parallel fashion. This will not give enough power to distinguish statistically between the different doses, but it would be enough to show a dose–response relationship and to identify the two or three doses to take forward in phase 3 trials.

Jes Olesen mentioned that there is now an initiative under the European Brain Council to analyse the whole drug development process and to introduce completely new aspects resulting in a faster drug development. This is all driven by a desire from patient organizations to have access to novel drugs faster.

Nitric oxide and spreading depression modulators

9

Inducible nitric oxide synthase and development of new migraine treatments

Boris A. Chizh

Nitric oxide and inducible nitric oxide synthase

Nitric oxide (NO) is a diffusible, short-acting, and highly reactive molecule that can mediate intercellular communication and trigger a range of intracellular cascades throughout the body. NO is produced from L-arginine by NO synthases (NOS). Of the three NOS isoforms, the neuronal (nNOS or type I) and endothelial (eNOS or type III) ones are widely expressed constitutively and play important parts in neurotransmission and vascular tone, respectively.[1,2] In contrast, constitutive expression levels of the inducible isoform (iNOS) are low and can be dramatically upregulated by tissue injury and inflammation. This makes selective iNOS inhibition an attractive therapeutic approach, as the low constitutive expression implies a low risk of effects on normal physiological processes. Furthermore, in contrast to the other isoforms, iNOS is capable of producing large (nanomolar versus picomolar) quantities of NO in a calmodulin-independent fashion.[1,2] This suggests a greater relative functional role of iNOS under inflammatory conditions. As neurogenic inflammation appears to be important in migraine pathophysiology,[3] selective iNOS inhibition seems to be an attractive target for developing new antimigraine treatments.

Nitric oxide, inducible nitric oxide synthase, and migraine pathophysiology

Interest in NOS inhibitors for migraine originates primarily from the evidence that exogenous NO donors, such as glyceryl trinitrate (GTN), can cause headache in humans. GTN infusion evokes an immediate headache in healthy subjects; this is most likely associated with a direct vasodilatation and secondary nociceptor activation by exogenous NO.[4–6] In addition, NO can directly activate nociceptors.[7] This suggests that endogenous NO may have a similar action on blood vessels and perivascular nerve endings in spontaneous headache pain.[5,8] In migraineurs, GTN infusion can cause a biphasic headache, with a second phase resembling a migraine attack in quality and duration.[9,10] The delayed migraine-like headache following GTN infusion may involve upregulation of iNOS in the meninges and release of endogenous NO. Thus, *in vivo* experiments have shown that a brief infusion of GTN can cause vasodilatation and increased meningeal blood flow *in vivo*, and can lead to a sustained meningeal release of NO.[11] Furthermore, a similar brief infusion of GTN resulted in upregulation of iNOS mRNA and protein, and an inflammatory response in the dura with the time course consistent with that of the delayed GTN-induced headache in migraineurs.[12] Importantly, the inflammation was suppressed by a selective iNOS inhibitor.[12] *In vitro* data demonstrate that iNOS upregulation may be involved in the cellular response of trigeminal neurones to stress.[13] In the clinic, both iNOS mRNA and protein have been found to be upregulated in serial samples of jugular blood monocytes of migraine patients; the time course of this upregulation closely matched the development and resolution of the headache.[14] These data suggest a more universal role for iNOS in the pathophysiology of different stages of migraine headache.

Initiation and cortical spreading depression

NO may also be responsible for the coupling between abnormal brain neuronal activity and changes in cranial vascular tone during the initial phases preceding the migraine headache attack. Cortical spreading depression (CSD), a mechanism thought to be responsible for the initiation of headache in migraineurs,[15,16] appears to involve NO release. Thus, experimentally evoked CSD in animals has been shown to cause NO release and vasodilatation.[11,17,18] This effect could be blocked by non-selective NOS inhibition.[19]

Nitric oxide and the vicious circle

NO production can trigger an upregulation and increased release from trigeminal afferents of other potent algogens and vasodilators; this mechanism may involve iNOS. *In vitro* experiments, treatment of trigeminal neurones with NO donors led to overexpression of iNOS and greatly enhanced synthesis and release of calcitonin gene-related peptide (CGRP).[20] This peptide appears to play a key role in the neurovascular events underlying migraine headache.[21,22] The NO-triggered CGRP release may involve the formation of prostaglandins.[23] There is a well-established cross-talk between iNOS and another inducible enzyme known to play a key role in inflammation, cyclooxygenase-2 (COX2).[24,25] The importance of this mechanism is further supported by the finding that inflammatory hyperalgesia and prostaglandin E_2 formation are substantially reduced, and that the antihyperalgesic effect of the COX inhibitor indomethacin is absent, in iNOS knock-out animals.[26]

Taken together, these data suggest that NO release following iNOS activation in the initial stages of migraine headache may trigger a cascade of release of vasoactive and inflammatory mediators, such as CGRP and prostaglandins, leading to further vasodilatation, activation of perivascular nerve fibres, and formation of a 'vicious circle' of trigeminal activation during the attack.

Evidence with nitric oxide antagonists

Preclinically, non-selective NOS inhibitors have been shown to attenuate neurogenic vasodilatation and/or plasma extravasation in migraine models.[27] There is also some evidence with iNOS-selective inhibitors suggesting that neurogenic inflammation in the meninges may involve this isoform (e.g. references 12 and 28, but cf. 29). It should be borne in mind that the *in vivo* selectivity of some of these tool inhibitors may be limited.

In the clinic, the non-selective NOS inhibitor L-NMMA has been shown to attenuate acute migraine and tension-type headache.[30,31] Furthermore, the NO scavenger hydroxocobalamin has shown prophylactic efficacy in a pilot clinical study.[32] Although these clinical data do not pinpoint the involvement of specific NOS isoforms, they are generally consistent with the preclinical evidence on the importance of NO and the role of iNOS at different stages of migraine pathophysiology. On the other hand, eNOS-mediated vascular mechanisms cannot be ruled out, as suggested by reports of elevated blood pressure following the administration of L-NMMA in those studies.

Selective inducible nitric oxide synthase inhibitors

Several companies have been developing selective iNOS inhibitors for a range of indications. Several potent and selective iNOS inhibitors have been identified.[33] GW274150 and GW273629 are potent and highly selective iNOS inhibitors in human recombinant and in rat native tissue NOS assays.[34] This selectivity appears to be preserved *in vivo*. Thus, no change in blood pressure was observed in control animals with these compounds, whereas the endotoxin-evoked hypotension (presumed to involve iNOS induction and iNOS-mediated NO release) was dose-dependently reversed by GW273629.

Preclinical effects: inflammatory pain

Consistent with the role of iNOS in inflammation, iNOS upregulation has been demonstrated in preclinical models of inflammatory pain, and its selective inhibitors have shown efficacy. Thus, immunohistochemically detected iNOS was upregulated in the paw after Freund's Complete Adjuvant injection, correlated with the behavioural hyperalgesia.[35] The selective iNOS inhibitor GW274150 reduced nitrite levels in the inflamed paw, inflammation, and hyperalgesia in a dose-dependent manner. The compound also alleviated the allodynia associated with perineural inflammation in a model of neuropathic pain, presumably via a peripheral mechanism.[35]

Inducible nitric oxide synthase selective inhibitors in humans

Some iNOS selective inhibitors have reached clinical phases of development. GW273629 has been found to be safe and well tolerated in migraine patients, and comparable peripheral exposure levels were achieved both during and outsite of the attack.[36] At these doses that are predicted to be pharmacologically active, no effects on vital signs, including blood pressure, were observed, suggesting selectivity of iNOS inhibition.

Conclusions and perspectives

NO production plays a key role at different levels of migraine pathogenesis, from coupling abnormal brain activity with vascular events to the formation of vicious circle of trigeminal nociceptor activation. Thus, there appears to be a strong rationale for NO inhibition for both prophylactic and acute treatment of migraine. Although there are not enough data to unequivocally indicate the most important NOS isoform, iNOS appears to be a likely candidate enzyme responsible for migraine headache. Furthermore, the wide constitutive expression of eNOS and nNOS poses risks of cardiovascular and central nervous system side-effects with non-selective inhibitors. The appeal of selective iNOS inhibition is in its low constitutive expression, which implies a low risk of effects on physiological processes, and its profound upregulation under conditions of inflammation. Selective iNOS inhibitors have been developed and shown efficacy in preclinical inflammatory states; results of clinical trials in migraine patients are awaited.

Acknowledgements

The contribution of Drs Joanne Palmer, Jo Hunter, and Martin Lunnon of GSK and Professor Jan De Hoon of Leuven University is greatly appreciated.

References

1. Alderton WK, Cooper CE, Knowles RG (2001) Nitric oxide synthases: structure, function and inhibition. *Biochem J* 357, 593–615.
2. Knowles RG, Moncada S (1994) Nitric oxide synthases in mammals. *Biochem J* 298, 249–58.
3. Waeber C, Moskowitz MA (2005) Migraine as an inflammatory disorder. *Neurology* 64, S9–15.
4. Ashina M, Bendtsen L, Jensen R, Sakai F, Olesen J (2000) Possible mechanisms of glyceryl-trinitrate-induced immediate headache in patients with chronic tension-type headache. *Cephalalgia* 20, 919–24.
5. Olesen J, Jansen-Olesen I (2000) Nitric oxide mechanisms in migraine. *Pathol Biol (Paris)* 48, 648–57.
6. Thomsen LL, Olesen J (1998) Nitric oxide theory of migraine. *Clin Neurosci* 5, 28–33.
7. Anbar M, Gratt BM (1997) Role of nitric oxide in the physiopathology of pain. *J Pain Symptom Manage* 14, 225–54.
8. Thomsen LL, Olesen J (2001) Nitric oxide in primary headaches. *Curr Opin Neurol* 14, 315–21.
9. Christiansen I, Daugaard D, Lykke TL, Olesen J (2000) Glyceryl trinitrate induced headache in migraineurs—relation to attack frequency. *Eur J Neurol* 7, 405–11.
10. Christiansen I, Thomsen LL, Daugaard D, Ulrich V, Olesen J (1999) Glyceryl trinitrate induces attacks of migraine without aura in sufferers of migraine with aura. *Cephalalgia* 19, 660–7.
11. Read SJ, Smith MI, Hunter AJ, Parsons AA (1997) Enhanced nitric oxide release during cortical spreading depression following infusion of glyceryl trinitrate in the anaesthetized cat. *Cephalalgia* 17, 159–65.
12. Reuter U, Bolay H, Jansen-Olesen I, Chiarugi A, Sanchez dR, Letourneau R *et al.* (2001) Delayed inflammation in rat meninges: implications for migraine pathophysiology. *Brain* 124, 2490–502.
13. Jansen-Olesen I, Zhou M, Zinck T, Xu CB, Edvinsson L (2005) Expression of inducible nitric oxide synthase in trigeminal ganglion cells during culture. *Basic Clin Pharmacol Toxicol* 97, 355–63.
14. Sarchielli P, Floridi A, Mancini ML, *et al.* (2006) NF-kappaB activity and iNOS expression in monocytes from internal jugular blood of migraine without aura patients during attacks. *Cephalalgia* 26, 1071–9.
15. Dalkara T, Zervas NT, Moskowitz MA (2006) From spreading depression to the trigeminovascular system. *Neurol Sci* 27 (Suppl. 2), S86–90.

16. Bolay H, Moskowitz MA (2005) The emerging importance of cortical spreading depression in migraine headache. *Rev Neurol (Paris)* 161, 655–7.

17. Read SJ, Smith MI, Hunter AJ, Upton N, Parsons AA (2000) SB-220453, a potential novel antimigraine agent, inhibits nitric oxide release following induction of cortical spreading depression in the anaesthetized cat. *Cephalalgia* 20, 92–9.

18. Read SJ, Parsons AA (2000) Sumatriptan modifies cortical free radical release during cortical spreading depression. A novel antimigraine action for sumatriptan? *Brain Res* 870, 44–53.

19. Read SJ, Smith MI, Hunter AJ, Parsons AA (1997) The dynamics of nitric oxide release measured directly and in real time following repeated waves of cortical spreading depression in the anaesthetised cat. *Neurosci Lett* 232, 127–30.

20. Bellamy J, Bowen EJ, Russo AF, Durham PL (2006) Nitric oxide regulation of calcitonin gene-related peptide gene expression in rat trigeminal ganglia neurons. *Eur J Neurosci* 23, 2057–66.

21. Moskowitz MA, Cutrer FM (1996) CGRP: blood flow and more? *Cephalalgia* 16, 287.

22. Ramadan NM, Buchanan TM (2006) New and future migraine therapy. *Pharmacol Ther* 112, 199–212.

23. Holzer P, Jocic M, Peskar BA (1995) Mediation by prostaglandins of the nitric oxide-induced neurogenic vasodilatation in rat skin. *Br J Pharmacol* 116, 2365–70.

24. Perez-Sala D, Lamas S (2001) Regulation of cyclooxygenase-2 expression by nitric oxide in cells. *Antioxid Redox Signal* 3, 231–48.

25. Tsatsanis C, Androulidaki A, Venihaki M, Margioris AN (2006) Signalling networks regulating cyclooxygenase-2. *Int J Biochem Cell Biol* 38, 1654–61.

26. Guhring H, Gorig M, Ates M, *et al.* (2000) Suppressed injury-induced rise in spinal prostaglandin E2 production and reduced early thermal hyperalgesia in iNOS-deficient mice. *J Neurosci* 20, 6714–20.

27. Peitl B, Nemeth J, Szolcsanyi J, Szilvassy Z, Porszasz R (2004) Sensory nitrergic meningeal vasodilatation and non-nitrergic plasma extravasation in anaesthesized rats. *Eur J Pharmacol* 497, 293–9.

28. Reuter U, Chiarugi A, Bolay H, Moskowitz MA (2002) Nuclear factor-kappaB as a molecular target for migraine therapy. *Ann Neurol* 51, 507–16.

29. Akerman S, Williamson DJ, Kaube H, Goadsby PJ (2002) Nitric oxide synthase inhibitors can antagonize neurogenic and calcitonin gene-related peptide induced dilation of dural meningeal vessels. *Br J Pharmacol* 137, 62–8.

30. Lassen LH, Ashina M, Christiansen I, *et al.* (1998) Nitric oxide synthase inhibition: a new principle in the treatment of migraine attacks. *Cephalalgia* 18, 27–32.

31. Ashina M (2002) Nitric oxide synthase inhibitors for the treatment of chronic tension-type headache. *Expert Opin Pharmacother* 3, 395–9.

32. van der Kuy PH, Merkus FW, Lohman JJ, ter Berg JW, Hooymans PM (2002) Hydroxocobalamin, a nitric oxide scavenger, in the prophylaxis of migraine: an open, pilot study. *Cephalalgia* 22, 513–19.

33. Salerno L, Sorrenti V, Di Giacomo C, Romeo G, Siracusa MA (2002) Progress in the development of selective nitric oxide synthase (NOS) inhibitors. *Curr Pharm Design* 8, 177–200.

34. Alderton WK, Angell AD, Craig C, *et al.* (2005) GW274150 and GW273629 are potent and highly selective inhibitors of inducible nitric oxide synthase *in vitro* and *in vivo*. *Br J Pharmacol* 145, 301–12.

35. De Alba J, Clayton NM, Collins SD, Colthup P, Chessell I, Knowles RG (2006) GW274150, a novel and highly selective inhibitor of the inducible isoform of nitric oxide synthase (iNOS), shows analgesic effects in rat models of inflammatory and neuropathic pain. *Pain* 120, 170–81.

36. de Hoon JN, Depre M, Guillard F, *et al.* (2007) iNOS inhibition in acute migraine: pharmacokinetic characteristics, safety and tolerability of GW273629. *Cephalalgia* 27, 721.

10

Mechanisms of cortical spreading depression as targets for migraine therapy

Kevin C. Brennan and Andrew C. Charles

Since its original description more than 60 years ago, cortical spreading depression (CSD) has been a central focus of migraine research. But despite decades of investigation, the specific cellular mechanisms of CSD, the extent to which it occurs in humans, and the role that it plays in migraine remain controversial. Research on CSD has yet to directly identify any new therapies for migraine. This may soon change, however, as recent advances in the understanding of the molecular, cellular, and pharmacological mechanisms of CSD and related cortical phenomena lead to new therapeutic approaches that target these mechanisms.

Cortical spreading depression and migraine

CSD was originally reported by Leão in 1944 as a propagated electrophysiological event that spread across large areas of cortex at rates of approximately 3 mm/min. Because its temporal and spatial characteristics are consistent with the clinical features of migraine aura, it was immediately hypothesized that CSD is a fundamental pathophysiological mechanism of migraine. Multiple recording modalities have subsequently shown similar propagated waves of altered brain activity and blood flow in animal models and humans with migraine.[1–4] The similarities between these waves and the electrophysiological events of CSD have led to the assumption that they are all the same phenomena—but this may not be the case. There may in fact be multiple inter-related but distinct cellular mechanisms underlying slowly propagated cortical waves. While CSD clearly involves changes in neuronal excitability, there may also be distinct glial and vascular waves that play a part in migraine. Distinct mechanisms for slowly propagated neuronal, glial, and vascular signalling may therefore represent individual targets for migraine therapy.

Despite the remarkably similar features of CSD and the clinical and imaging features of migraine aura, there are significant questions regarding the occurrence of classical CSD in human migraine. First, the typical EEG changes of CSD have not been observed in patients with migraine. While it has been suggested that this is because surface EEG does not have the sensitivity to detect CSD,[5,6] it seems likely that surface EEG should be able to detect at least some of the profound changes in neuronal activity that are associated with classical CSD in animal models. CSD is a propagated wave of massive neuronal excitation followed by sustained inhibition, accompanied by marked ionic fluxes and adenosine triphosphate (ATP) and glucose utilization.[7,8] A negative DC (direct current) potential shift consistent with CSD has been observed in migraine patients with magnetoencephalography.[9] However, it is not clear why the EEG amplitude attenuation associated with classical CSD would not be detected with surface EEG in migraine patients. It is also difficult to reconcile this extreme electrophysiological event with the relatively minor neurological dysfunction that occurs in many patients with migraine aura. While certain forms of migraine, such as familial hemiplegic migraine, are accompanied by significant neurological deficits, the majority of patients with migraine aura have mild symptoms relative to what would be expected with the dramatic changes in neuronal activity that occur with classical CSD. And at least one positron emission tomography study has demonstrated CSD-like propagation of oligaemia in a patient who did not have any clear aura symptoms.[2] These observations raise the possibility that there are waves of vascular and possibly glial activity that could occur in migraine that do not necessarily involve the extensive changes in neuronal activity that are seen with classical CSD in animal models.

Intercellular calcium signalling in astrocytes

A non-neuronal phenomenon that has been observed to propagate with very similar temporal and spatial characteristics *in vitro* is intercellular calcium waves in astrocytes.[10] Astrocytes have been traditionally viewed as playing a primarily supportive role in the central nervous system. However, *in vitro* imaging studies demonstrate that astrocytes are capable of extensive, active intercellular signalling. Astrocytes show waves of increased intracellular calcium concentration that can be evoked by stimulation of one or a few cells and communicated to hundreds of neighbouring cells over long distances (Figure 10.1).[11] This intercellular Ca^{2+} signalling in astrocytes may be involved in active modulation of neuronal signalling and vascular tone.[12] Astrocytes have functional receptors for most neurotransmitters and neuromodulators. In addition, they are capable of active release of transmitters via multiple mechanisms.[12] Through these mechanisms, they are able to both respond to synaptic neuronal signalling and actively modulate it.[13] Astrocytes also have a close structural relationship with the vasculature, by virtue of endfeet that wrap around vessels. Astrocyte calcium signalling has been reported to directly cause changes in vascular tone, through release of vasoactive messengers and regulation of extracellular K^+.[14–17]

Astrocytes are therefore ideally positioned to mediate phenomena associated with migraine. They can modulate both neuronal activity and vascular activity in a spatially propagated fashion that is consistent with the changes in brain activity and clinical symptomatology of migraine. Astrocyte waves could therefore provide an explanation for the occurrence of spreading changes in cortical activity that may occur in the absence of significant neurological symptoms. Because astrocyte Ca^{2+} waves may not necessarily be associated with large alterations in neuronal activity, they could represent a mechanism for clinical and imaging phenomena of migraine that occur in the absence of the severity of neurological deficits that one would expect with classical CSD.

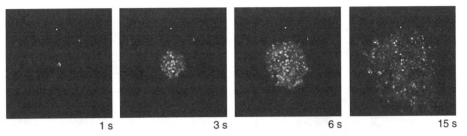

1 s   3 s   6 s   15 s

Fig. 10.1 Intercellular calcium wave in astrocyte culture. Image sequence shows response to mechanical stimulation of a single cell in a microscopic field of cultured astrocytes (500 × 500 μM) loaded with the fluorescent calcium indicator fluo-4. A wave of increased fluorescence (corresponding to an increase in intracellular calcium concentration) spreads concentrically from the stimulated cell to hundreds of surrounding cells, with a propagation rate that is very similar to that of cortical spreading depression.

In brain slice preparations, Ca^{2+} waves in astrocytes consistently occur in association with CSD.[18–20] A recent study has also reported that astrocyte Ca^{2+} waves also occur with CSD *in vivo*, where they appear to mediate vasoconstriction associated with the CSD wavefront.[21] However, the occurrence of CSD can be pharmacologically dissociated from astrocyte calcium signalling. CSD can occur in the absence of astrocyte calcium waves, and vice versa.[18–21] One possibility is that they share a common mechanism for initiation and/or propagation, but that additional factors specific to each individual process are required for their independent occurrence. And although they may not have a requisite interdependence, there are multiple potential mechanisms by which the two phenomena could interact with clinically important consequences.

Our initial studies suggested that intercellular calcium signalling in astrocytes occurred via gap junctions between cells, because the propagation of calcium waves was correlated with the expression of connexin43, the primary gap junction protein in astrocytes.[22] However, studies by our group and a variety of others have established that a primary mechanism for the propagation of intercellular calcium waves is the release of ATP and the subsequent activation of purinergic receptors on neighbouring cells.[23–25] This extracellular mechanism for the intercellular propagation of calcium waves can be reconciled with the involvement of connexins by the observation that connexin channels not only create gap junctions between cells, they also serve as a pathway of release of signalling molecules from astrocytes. We and others have provided evidence that undocked connexin channels, or connexin 'hemichannels', represent a pathway for release of ATP from astrocytes.[23,25] They may also be a pathway for release of glutamate from astrocytes.[26] Alternative pathways for release of ATP and glutamate include other membrane channels, a regulated vesicular mechanism of release, or reversal of transporters.[27–31] Regardless of the specific release pathway, it is clear that astrocytes release substantial quantities of ATP and glutamate associated with intercellular Ca^{2+} signalling. Astrocytes also express high levels of Ca^{2+}-activated K^+ channels,[32,33] suggesting that Ca^{2+} waves could be associated with propagated efflux of K^+. Finally, astrocyte Ca^{2+}

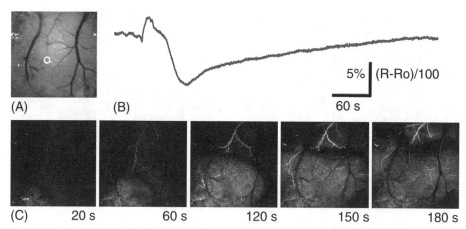

(A)   (B)   5% | (R-Ro)/100   60 s

(C)   20 s   60 s   120 s   150 s   180 s

Fig. 10.2 Optical intrinsic signal imaging of cortical spreading depression (CSD). (A) Mouse cortex visualized through thinned skull (image scale 2.4 × 2.4 mm). White circle shows region of interest used for reflectance measurement shown in (B). (B) Line trace shows change in reflectance versus time following CSD evoked by ejection of KCl from a micropipette. CSD is associated with a multiphasic change in reflectance that corresponds with the electrophysiological changes of CSD (not shown). (C) Image sequence showing propagation of reflectance changes associated with CSD. CSD was evoked at time 0 s. Each image in the sequence represents the absolute difference in reflectance at the specified time compared with 0 s. A multiphasic wave of reflectance change propagates concentrically from the site of the stimulus. Arteriolar dilation propagates ahead of the parenchymal CSD wavefront.

waves have been observed to be associated with propagated increases in intracellular Na^+ concentration.[34] It has been proposed that this represents a mechanism for spatial co-ordination of energy metabolism.[34,35]

Optical imaging of cortical spreading depression

Multiple approaches have been used to investigate CSD in animal models. Optical intrinsic signal(OIS) imaging is particularly well suited to the investigation of CSD, as it allows high spatiotemporal resolution with the wide field of view necessary to analyse a phenomenon that can spread across a whole cerebral hemisphere. OIS exploits the fact that changes in cerebral metabolic activity and blood flow result in changes in reflected light.[36] Different wavelengths emphasize different components of the signal. For example, OIS at 570 nm, an isosbestic point where oxy- and deoxyhaemoglobin absorption is equal, yields an image dominated by changes in blood volume, with signal changes very similar to what is seen with laser Doppler or speckle flowmetry. At 610 nm, deoxyhaemoglobin absorption is greater than oxyhaemoglobin absorption; the resulting image is blood oxygenation level dependent in a manner comparable with BOLD (blood oxygen level dependent) functional magnetic resonance imaging. At wavelengths above 700 nm, haemoglobin absorption drops off dramatically, and light scatter changes, likely caused by neuronal depolarization and swelling, dominate.[36–38]

OIS imaging has been used for several years to investigate the physiology of CSD in experimental models.[36,39,40] CSD is associated with a wave of change in OIS that propagates across the cortex at approximately 3 mm/min, and whose wavefront is correlated with negative DC shift of CSD.[36,40] The OIS signal change associated with CSD is multiphasic; imaging with white light excitation reveals an initial decrease in reflectance (darkening) followed by an increase, and a subsequent larger decrease in signal. The signal then recovers to baseline, or in some cases overshoots above baseline before eventually recovering. This response is highly replicable within species, although there is some species-to-species variation. For example, in mice the second phase of the signal change is much larger than that observed in rats, possibly corresponding to a greater decrease in perfusion near the CSD wavefront.[41,42]

Intrinsic conduction of arteriolar dilation associated with cortical spreading depression

In addition to imaging changes in parenchymal signal, the high spatial resolution of OIS allows accurate measurement of changes in arteriolar calibre that accompany CSD.

It has long been known that changes in arteriolar diameter occur at the cortical surface during CSD.[43] Again, there is some variation in this response from species to species, but dilation of arterioles is consistently observed in rodents during CSD. While it has been assumed that such CSD-associated vascular changes represent a purely passive response to activity in the underlying parenchyma, we have found that arteriolar dilation propagates with an intrinsic velocity that is greater than that of the OIS changes in surrounding tissue.[42] This means that arteriolar dilation may occur up to hundreds of microns and tens of seconds before arrival of the CSD OIS wavefront and accompanying DC potential shift. This arteriolar dilation preceding the CSD wavefront can follow a circuitous path along individual vessels, indicating that it is not simply the result of a circumferentially propagating signal ahead of the CSD wave that is not detected by OIS imaging or electrophysiological recording. We have also found that arteriolar changes can propagate into brain regions that remained unaffected by CSD throughout the experiment.[42] These findings indicate that there is an intrinsic mechanism for vascular conduction associated with CSD. This mechanism could be important in migraine, as trigeminally innervated cortical surface vessels have long been thought to be a pathway by which CSD could evoke migraine pain.

Gender differences in thresholds for cortical spreading depression

Our models of CSD enable accurate and reproducible quantification of thresholds for induction of CSD. We have used two different approaches to examine CSD thresholds. The first is microejection of controlled quantities of KCl with a picopump, and the second is tetanic electrical stimulation. Each of these techniques can be reliably used to determine the threshold for induction of CSD, allowing comparison of CSD thresholds between groups of animals under different conditions. Examination of the threshold for induction of CSD in female versus male mice revealed a rather surprising finding: the threshold for induction of CSD is consistently lower in female mice than in males.[44] Although we did not monitor the oestrous cycle in the animals that were used for these observations, it is likely that they were sampled at different times in the oestrous cycle or were non-cycling (as commonly occurs in mice housed four to a cage, as was done with our subjects). This means that the lower threshold for induction of CSD in females versus males may be at least in part independent of the cyclical fluctuations in hormones associated with the oestrous cycle, indicating an increased excitability of the female brain that may underlie the increased prevalence of migraine in women.

Targeting mechanisms of cortical spreading depression and other cortical waves for migraine preventive therapy

Multiple lines of evidence indicate that CSD in rodents is a legitimate model for identification of new migraine therapies. First, expression of known human migraine genes in mice results in alterations in CSD consistent with an increased brain excitability that is hypothesized to underlie migraine.[45] A transgenic mouse expressing one of the calcium channel mutations associated with a form of familial hemiplegic migraine in humans shows a reduced threshold for CSD, as well as an increased rate of CSD propagation.[45] We have found that a mouse expressing a gene responsible for familial advanced sleep phase syndrome in a family whose affected members also have migraine with aura also shows a reduced threshold for CSD as well as altered vascular responses to CSD (unpublished data). These findings indicate that known and potential migraine genes alter the properties of CSD in mice. Another important piece of evidence supporting CSD in rodents as a model for migraine is the finding that diverse pharmacological agents known to be effective in the prevention of migraine all inhibit spreading depression in rats.[46,47] While the involvement of intercellular astrocyte signalling in migraine is highly speculative, the possibility that this process occurs either in parallel with CSD, or possibly independently of CSD, suggests that this may also be an appealing target to pursue for migraine therapy.

Calcium channel antagonists

The recent demonstration that a mutation in a P/Q-type calcium channel is responsible for a form of familial hemiplegic migraine indicates that this type of channel, which is believed to play a primary role in the regulation of neuronal synaptic transmitter release, can play a role in migraine.[48] The subsequent finding that mice expressing this mutation have a reduced threshold for the induction of CSD provides critical evidence that genetic mechanisms in migraine patients can result in an increased propensity for propagated waves of altered cortical excitability.[45] A role for P/Q calcium channels in migraine is supported by observations that inhibitors of these channels modulate CSD *in vitro*.[49] Calcium channel blockers have been used for many years as migraine preventive agents.

While it has been widely assumed that these drugs were working primarily by modulating vascular tone, the evidence described above has shifted attention to their potential modulation of neuronal excitability and transmitter release. In order for calcium channel blockers to target these mechanisms, they must cross the blood–brain barrier in sufficient concentrations to alter neuronal activity. Thus, the blood–brain barrier permeability of calcium channel blockers could be a key determinant of their therapeutic efficacy for migraine. The selectivity of calcium channel blockers for P/Q channels could also be an important feature required for their efficacy as migraine preventive treatments. There are currently no calcium channel blockers in clinical use that selectively target P/Q channels.

Glutamate receptor antagonists

Glutamate receptors are an important potential target for migraine therapy based on multiple sites of action, both in the cortex and in the trigeminal nociceptive pathway. Glutamate receptor agonists can evoke CSD, and conversely NMDA receptor antagonists can inhibit CSD evoked by other stimuli.[50–52] Most glutamate receptor antagonists have had limited clinical application because of significant side-effects. These adverse effects, including hallucinations and sedation, likely result from interference with the critical functions of normal excitatory neurotransmission. However, there are some glutamate receptor antagonists that are generally well tolerated. One example is memantine. Memantine, a derivative of amantadine, is currently approved by the FDA in the USA for the treatment of Alzheimer's disease. Like other NMDA antagonists, it has been reported to inhibit CSD in rats.[53] Attention regarding its therapeutic mechanism has been focused primarily on its modulation of NMDA receptor channels, but it also inhibits nicotinic acetylcholine receptors and 5HT3 receptors *in vitro*. Memantine has been reported to be a low affinity, open channel blocker of NMDA receptors with a fast off-rate. It has been proposed that these characteristics of NMDA receptor modulation result in inhibition of 'excessive' activity of the receptor, with relative sparing of the normal function of the receptor, which plays a crucial part in physiological brain function. This could explain why, in contrast to other NMDA receptor antagonists that have substantial side-effects, memantine is generally very well tolerated.

Our initial clinical experience with memantine as a preventive agent in migraine has been promising. We have now treated over 100 patients with this compound, and an unblinded, uncontrolled case review of some of these patients suggests that it has had efficacy in preventing migraine in a significant number of patients who had previously failed with many other treatment approaches. Significant side-effects were uncommon. While these observations are highly preliminary, and potentially confounded by substantial recall bias and placebo effect, they are none the less encouraging because of the refractory patient population that was studied, the generally good tolerability of the treatment, and the appealing rationale for a mechanism of action via the inhibition of CSD. Our observations suggest that memantine and potentially other low affinity glutamate receptor antagonists should be studied in well designed trials as migraine preventive agents.

Potential glial targets for migraine therapy

As discussed above, there is circumstantial evidence implicating intercellular signalling in astrocytes as a mechanism in migraine. Astrocyte calcium waves occur with CSD, and may mediate vascular changes accompanying the CSD wave.[21] The identification of a familial hemiplegic migraine mutation in a Na/K ATPase that in adults is expressed primarily in astrocytes provides strong support for the idea that astrocytes may play a key role in migraine.[54,55] Inhibitors of connexin channels, which are a pathway for intercellular signalling in astrocytes, may represent a novel migraine preventive treatment approach. Fenamates, some of which are in clinical use as anti-inflammatories, are connexin channel blockers that also block intercellular calcium waves and ATP release in astrocytes.[25,56] These compounds have been shown to be effective in the acute treatment of migraine,[57,58] but there are no published studies of their efficacy as migraine preventive agents. Another connexin channel blocker that is a compound of interest as a migraine preventive agent is tonabersat. Tonabersat has been found to block gap junctions, in addition to inhibiting CSD.[59,60] Studies of this drug as a migraine preventive agent are underway, as is further investigation of its potential mechanisms of action. The substantial quantities of ATP that are released in association with intercellular calcium waves in astrocytes (and by extension, also probably with CSD) raise the possibility that purinergic receptor modulators could also be treatments for migraine. ATP has been implicated as a mediator of pain in a variety of models. ATP at low concentrations activates trigeminal neurons *in vitro* (unpublished data). A speculative hypothesis is that ATP released by astrocytes could activate trigeminal afferents involved in the generation of migraine pain. ATP released by astrocytes is metabolized by extracellular nucleotideases to adenosine, such that this could be another important astrocyte-released extracellular messenger. Caffeine, which is well known to be a modulator of migraine, and is an adenosine receptor antagonist, is a component of several migraine abortive preparations. Purinergic receptor antagonists are therefore another potential migraine treatment approach that targets astrocyte signalling.

Astrocyte signalling has been reported to modulate vascular function via release of eicosanoids and modulation of extracellular K^+.[14–17,61] Inhibitors of astrocyte cyclooxygenases or other enzymes in the pathways for generation of astrocyte released vasoactive messengers could therefore be targets for migraine therapy based on this mechanism. In addition to the Na/K ATPase, calcium activated K^+ channels may be important in the contribution of astrocytes to increases in extracellular K^+ that may influence brain activity and vascular tone. Inhibitors of these channels could therefore be considered as therapeutic agents.

Vascular mechanisms of cortical spreading depression as therapeutic targets

Dilation of brain and meningeal vessels has for some time been considered to be a primary mediator of migraine pain, and multiple therapies have been believed to exert their therapeutic effects primarily as vasoconstrictors. But optical imaging indicates that the changes in vascular tone associated with CSD are complex and multiphasic. In addition, functional imaging in patients with migraine has primarily shown propagated decreases in blood flow, consistent with vasoconstriction rather than vasodilation, in some cases even during the pain phase of the attack.[1–4] Our studies also suggest that there is an intrinsic vascular mechanism for propagation of vasomotor changes associated with CSD, raising the possibility that the blood vessels may actively contribute to CSD as opposed to simply responding passively to the activity of the brain parenchyma.[42] Taken together, these observations suggest that the focus on vasoconstriction as a primary mechanism for migraine therapy may be too simplistic, and that other types of vasomodulators might also have significant therapeutic effects.

Gender-based susceptibility to cortical spreading depression as a therapeutic target

Although it is well known that the frequency of migraine is linked to hormonal changes in women, the roles of individual hormones and the potential contribution of non-hormonal factors based on sex chromosomal differences remain poorly understood. Our observation of a reduced threshold for CSD in female versus male mice[44] opens the possibility that this may be a model for studying therapeutic approaches that may specifically target migraine in women. Investigations to determine the effects of chronic versus cyclical hormone levels as well as sex chromosome effects on CSD in female and male mice may identify new treatments based on specific mechanisms of gender differences.

Conclusions

High-resolution microscopic imaging techniques are powerful tools for investigation of potential migraine mechanisms in animal models. These techniques have been used to demonstrate how specific astrocytic and vascular signalling pathways could play key roles in migraine. The use of these imaging and electrophysiological techniques to reliably and reproducibly quantify thresholds for induction of CSD under different conditions has the potential to greatly expand our understanding of the factors that influence the susceptibility to migraine, and to develop new treatments that modulate this susceptibility. Ongoing studies to characterize CSD and intercellular calcium signalling in transgenic models for migraine, under different gender-related conditions, and in the presence of novel therapeutic compounds, may result in significant advances in our ability to understand and treat this exceptionally common and disabling disorder.

References

1. Olesen J, Larsen B, Lauritzen M (1981) Focal hyperemia followed by spreading oligemia and impaired activation of rCBF in classic migraine. *Ann Neurol* 9, 344–52.
2. Woods RP, Iacoboni M, Mazziotta JC (1994) Bilateral spreading cerebral hypoperfusion during spontaneous migraine headache. *N Engl J Med* 331, 1689–92.

3. Cao Y, Welch KM, Aurora S, Vikingstad EM (1999) Functional MRI-BOLD of visually triggered headache in patients with migraine. *Arch Neurol* 56, 548–54.

4. Hadjikhani N, Sanchez del Rio M, Wu O, Schwartz D, Bakker D, Fischl B, Kwong KK, Cutrer FM, Rosen BR, Tootell RBH, Sorensen AG, Moskowitz MA (2001) Mechanisms of migraine aura revealed by functional MRI in human visual cortex. *Proc Natl Acad Sci USA* 98, 4687–92.

5. Strong AJ, Dardis R (2005) Depolarisation phenomena in traumatic and ischaemic brain injury. *Adv Tech Stand Neurosurg* 30, 3–49.

6. Fabricius M, Fuhr S, Bhatia R, Boutelle M, Hashemi P, Strong AJ, Lauritzen M (2006) Cortical spreading depression and peri-infarct depolarization in acutely injured human cerebral cortex. *Brain* 129, 778–90.

7. Gorji A (2001) Spreading depression: a review of the clinical relevance. *Brain Res Rev* 38, 33–60.

8. Somjen GG (2001) Mechanisms of spreading depression and hypoxic spreading depression-like depolarization. *Physiol Rev* 81, 1065–96.

9. Bowyer SM, Aurora SK, Moran JE, Tepley N, Welch KMA (2001) Magnetoencephalographic fields from patients with spontaneous and induced migraine aura. *Ann Neurol* 50, 582–7.

10. Charles AC, Merrill JE, Dirksen ER, Sanderson MJ (1991) Intercellular signaling in glial cells: calcium waves and oscillations in response to mechanical stimulation and glutamate. *Neuron* 6, 983–92.

11. Charles A (1998) Intercellular calcium waves in glia. *Glia* 24, 39–49.

12. Haydon PG, Carmignoto G (2006) Astrocyte control of synaptic transmission and neurovascular coupling. *Physiol Rev* 86, 1009–31.

13. Wang X, Lou N, Xu Q, Tian GF, Peng WG, Han X, Kang J, Takano T, Nedergaard M (2006) Astrocytic Ca^{2+} signaling evoked by sensory stimulation *in vivo*. *Nat Neurosci* 9, 816–23.

14. Zonta M, Angulo MC, Gobbo S, Rosengarten B, Hossmann KA, Pozzan T, Carmignoto G (2003) Neuron-to-astrocyte signaling is central to the dynamic control of brain microcirculation. *Nat Neurosci* 6, 43–50.

15. Mulligan SJ, MacVicar BA (2004) Calcium transients in astrocyte endfeet cause cerebrovascular constrictions. *Nature* 431, 195–9.

16. Filosa JA, Bonev AD, Straub SV, Meredith AL, Wilkerson MK, Aldrich RW, Nelson MT (2006) Local potassium signaling couples neuronal activity to vasodilation in the brain. *Nat Neurosci* 9, 1397–403.

17. Takano T, Tian GF, Peng W, Lou N, Libionka W, Han X, Nedergaard M (2006) Astrocyte-mediated control of cerebral blood flow. *Nat Neurosci* 9, 260–7.

18. Basarsky TA, Duffy SN, Andrew RD, MacVicar BA (1998) Imaging spreading depression and associated intracellular calcium waves in brain slices. *J Neurosci* 18, 7189–99.

19. Kunkler PE, Kraig RP (1998) Calcium waves precede electrophysiological changes of spreading depression in hippocampal organ cultures. *J Neurosci* 18, 3416–25.

20. Peters O, Schipke CG, Hashimoto Y, Kettenmann H (2003) Different mechanisms promote astrocyte Ca^{2+} waves and spreading depression in the mouse neocortex. *J Neurosci* 23, 9888–96.

21. Chuquet J, Hollender L, Nimchinsky EA (2007) High-resolution *in vivo* imaging of the neurovascular unit during spreading depression. *J Neurosci* 27, 4036–44.

22. Charles A, Naus C, Zhu D, Kidder G, Dirksen E, Sanderson M (1992) Intercellular calcium signaling via gap junctions in glioma cells. *J Cell Biol* 118, 195–201.

23. Cotrina ML, Lin JH, Alves-Rodrigues A, Liu S, Li J, Azmi-Ghadimi H, Kang J, Naus CC, Nedergaard M (1998) Connexins regulate calcium signaling by controlling ATP release. *Proc Natl Acad Sci USA* 95, 15735–40.

24. Guthrie PB, Knappenberger J, Segal M, Bennett MV, Charles AC, Kater SB (1999) ATP released from astrocytes mediates glial calcium waves. *J Neurosci* 19, 520–8.

25. Stout CE, Costantin JL, Naus CC, Charles AC (2002) Intercellular calcium signaling in astrocytes via ATP release through connexin hemichannels. *J Biol Chem* 277, 10482–8.

26. Ye Z-C, Wyeth MS, Baltan-Tekkok S, Ransom BR (2003) Functional hemichannels in astrocytes: a novel mechanism of glutamate release. *J Neurosci* 23, 3588–96.

27. Araque A, Li N, Doyle RT, Haydon PG (2000) SNARE protein-dependent glutamate release from astrocytes. *J Neurosci* 20, 666–73.

28. Coco S, Calegari F, Pravettoni E, Pozzi D, Taverna E, Rosa P, Matteoli M, Verderio C (2003) Storage and release of ATP from astrocytes in culture. *J Biol Chem* 278, 1354–62.

29. Bezzi P, Gundersen V, Galbete JL, Seifert G, Steinhauser C, Pilati E, Volterra A (2004) Astrocytes contain a vesicular compartment that is competent for regulated exocytosis of glutamate. *Nature Neuroscience* 7, 613–20.

30. Montana V, Malarkey EB, Verderio C, Matteoli M, Parpura V (2006) Vesicular transmitter release from astrocytes. *Glia* 54, 700–15.

31. Jourdain P, Bergersen LH, Bhaukaurally K, Bezzi P, Santello M, Domercq M, Matute C, Tonello F, Gundersen V, Volterra A (2007) Glutamate exocytosis from astrocytes controls synaptic strength. *Nature Neuroscience* 10, 331–9.

32. Price DL, Ludwig JW, Mi H, Schwarz TL, Ellisman MH (2002) Distribution of rSlo Ca^{2+}-activated K^+ channels in rat astrocyte perivascular endfeet. *Brain Res* 956, 183–93.

33. Gebremedhin D, Yamaura K, Zhang C, Bylund J, Koehler RC, Harder DR (2003) Metabotropic glutamate receptor activation enhances the activities of two types of Ca^{2+}-activated K^+ channels in rat hippocampal astrocytes. *J Neurosci* 23, 1678–87.

34. Bernardinelli Y, Magistretti PJ, Chatton J-Y (2004) Astrocytes generate Na^+-mediated metabolic waves. *Proc Natl Acad Sci USA* 101, 14937–42.

35. Charles A (2005) Reaching out beyond the synapse: glial intercellular waves coordinate metabolism. *Sci STKE* 2005, pe6.

36. Ba AM, Guiou M, Pouratian N, Muthialu A, Rex DE, Cannestra AF, Chen JW, Toga AW (2002) Multiwavelength optical intrinsic signal imaging of cortical spreading depression. *J Neurophysiol* 88, 2726–35.

37. Frostig RD, Lieke EE, Ts'o DY, Grinvald A (1990) Cortical functional architecture and local coupling between neuronal activity and the microcirculation revealed by *in vivo* high-resolution optical imaging of intrinsic signals. *Proc Natl Acad Sci USA* 87, 6082–6.

38. Fayuk D, Aitken PG, Somjen GG, Turner DA (2002) Two different mechanisms underlie reversible, intrinsic optical signals in rat hippocampal slices. *J Neurophysiol* 87, 1924–37.

39. O'Farrell AM, Rex DE, Muthialu A, Pouratian N, Wong GK, Cannestra AF, Chen JW, Toga AW (2000) Characterization of optical intrinsic signals and blood volume during cortical spreading depression. *Neuroreport* 11, 2121–5.

40. Guiou M, Sheth S, Nemoto M, Walker M, Pouratian N, Ba A, Toga AW (2005) Cortical spreading depression produces long-term disruption of activity-related changes in cerebral blood volume and neurovascular coupling. *J Biomed Opt* 10, 11004.

41. Ayata C, Shin HK, Salomone S, Ozdemir-Gursoy Y, Boas DA, Dunn AK, Moskowitz MA (2004) Pronounced hypoperfusion during spreading depression in mouse cortex. *J Cereb Blood Flow Metab* 24, 1172–82.

42. Brennan KC, Beltran-Parrazal L, Lopez-Valdes HE, Theriot J, Toga AW, Charles AC (2007) Distinct vascular conduction with cortical spreading depression. *J Neurophysiol* 96, 443–51.

43. Leão AAP (1944) Spreading depression of activity in the cerebral cortex. *J Neurophysiol* 7, 359–90.

44. Brennan KC, Romero-Reyes MR, Lopez-Valdes HE, Arnold AP, Charles AC (2007) Reduced threshold for cortical spreading depression in female mice. *Ann Neurol* 61, 603–6.

45. van den Maagdenberg AMJM, Pietrobon D, Pizzorusso T, Kaja S, Broos LAM, Cesetti T, van de Ven RCG, Tottene A, van der Kaa J, Plomp JJ (2004) A cacna1a knockin migraine mouse model with increased susceptibility to cortical spreading depression. *Neuron* 41, 701–10.

46. Akerman S, Goadsby PJ (2005) Topiramate inhibits cortical spreading depression in rat and cat: impact in migraine aura. *Neuroreport* 16, 1383–7.

47. Ayata C, Jin H, Kudo C, Dalkara T, Moskowitz MA (2006) Suppression of cortical spreading depression in migraine prophylaxis. *Ann Neurol* 59, 652–61.

48. Ophoff RA, Terwindt GM, Vergouwe MN, van Eijk R, Oefner PJ, Hoffman SM, Lamerdin JE, Mohrenweiser HW, Bulman DE, Ferrari M, Haan J, Lindhout D, van Ommen GJ, Hofker MH, Ferrari MD, Frants RR (1996) Familial hemiplegic migraine and episodic ataxia type-2 are caused by mutations in the Ca^{2+} channel gene CACNL1A4. *Cell* 87, 543–52.

49. Kunkler PE, Kraig RP (2004) P/Q Ca^{2+} channel blockade stops spreading depression and related pyramidal neuronal Ca^{2+} rise in hippocampal organ culture. *Hippocampus* 14, 356–67.

50. Hernandez-Caceres J, Macias-Gonzalez R, Brozek G, Bures J (1987) Systemic ketamine blocks cortical spreading depression but does not delay the onset of terminal anoxic depolarization in rats. *Brain Res* 437, 360–4.

51. Lauritzen M, Hansen A (1992) The effect of glutamate receptor blockade on anoxic depolarization and cortical spreading depression. *J Cereb Blood Flow Metab* 12, 223–9.

52. Gressens P, Spedding M, Gigler G, Kertesz S, Villa P, Medja F, Williamson T, Kapus G, Levay G, Szenasi G (2005) The effects of AMPA receptor antagonists in models of stroke and neurodegeneration. *Eur J Pharmacol* 519, 58–67.

53. Peeters M, Gunthorpe MJ, Strijbos PJ, Goldsmith P, Upton N, James MF (2007) Effects of pan- and subtype-selective NMDA receptor antagonists on cortical spreading depression in the rat: therapeutic potential for migraine. *J Pharmacol Exp Ther* 321, 564–72.

54. De Fusco M, Marconi R, Silvestri L, Atorino L, Rampoldi L, Morgante L, Ballabio A, Aridon P, Casari G (2003) Haploinsufficiency of ATP1A2 encoding the Na^+/K^+ pump alpha2 subunit associated with familial hemiplegic migraine type 2. *Nat Genet* 33, 192–6.

55. Vanmolkot KRJ, Kors EE, Turk U, Turkdogan D, Keyser A, Broos LAM, Kia SK, van den Heuvel JJMW, Black DF, Haan J, Frants RR, Barone V, Ferrari MD, Casari G, Koenderink JB, van den Maagdenberg AMJM (2006) Two de novo mutations in the Na,K-ATPase gene ATP1A2 associated with pure familial hemiplegic migraine. *Eur J Hum Genet* 14, 555–60.

56. Eskandari S, Zampighi GA, Leung DW, Wright EM, Loo DD (2002) Inhibition of gap junction hemichannels by chloride channel blockers. *J Membr Biol* 185, 93–102.

57. Diener HC, Montagna P, Gacs G, Lyczak P, Schumann G, Zoller B, Mulder LJ, Siegel J, Edson K (2006) Efficacy and tolerability of diclofenac potassium sachets in migraine: a randomized, double-blind, cross-over study in comparison with diclofenac potassium tablets and placebo. *Cephalalgia* 26, 537–47.

58. Vecsei L, Gallacchi G, Sagi I, Semjen J, Tajti J, Szok D, Muller M, Vadass P, Kerekgyarto M (2007) Diclofenac epolamine is effective in the treatment of acute migraine attacks. A randomized, crossover, double blind, placebo-controlled, clinical study. *Cephalalgia* 27, 29–34.

59. Bradley DP, Smith MI, Netsiri C, Smith JM, Bockhorst KHJ, Hall LD, Huang CLH, Leslie RA, Parsons AA, James MF (2001) Diffusion-weighted MRI used to detect *in vivo* modulation of cortical spreading depression: comparison of sumatriptan and tonabersat. *Exp Neurol* 172, 342–53.

60. Read SJ, Hirst WD, Upton N, Parsons AA (2001) Cortical spreading depression produces increased cGMP levels in cortex and brain stem that is inhibited by tonabersat (SB-220453) but not sumatriptan. *Brain Res* 891, 69–77.

61. Metea MR, Newman EA (2006) Glial cells dilate and constrict blood vessels: a mechanism of neurovascular coupling. *J Neurosci* 26, 2862–70.

11

Tonabersat

Peter R. Blower and Paul C. Sharpe

Introduction

Migraine is now considered to be a complex disorder of the brain, manifesting as the well-known attacks of headache and associated symptoms of nausea/vomiting, photophobia, and phonophobia.[1] The ultimate aim of migraine treatments is to prevent symptoms completely but they generally fall far short of this goal. Therapeutic strategies for migraine include acute treatment for all patients and prophylaxis for patients who experience frequent and/or severe attacks.[2] One therapeutic class of acute treatments is the triptans, which are effective and generally well tolerated in most patients[3] and have been used successfully in the clinic for more than 15 years. However, it may take up to 2 h to derive optimal benefit from triptan tablets and only about 50–70% of patients respond following treatment,[2] leaving many patients with a suboptimal response. Historically, prophylaxis has not been regarded as a favourable option because of the lack of effective prophylactic agents that are free from frequent unwanted side-effects.

Anticonvulsants (topiramate and valproate) and beta-blockers are the most commonly used migraine prophylactics but, as with acute triptan therapy, only about half of patients respond well to these treatments.[2,4] In patients who usually experience around a dozen migraine days per month, this level of prophylactic efficacy represents 1 week free from migraine per month and brings them significantly closer to the therapeutic ideal of freedom from symptoms. It also suggests that an increased prescription of prophylactic drugs is desirable. Results from a large recent survey[5] conducted in the USA indicated that prophylaxis should be offered in 26% of migraine sufferers and should be considered in a further 13%, yet it is currently prescribed in a mere 12–13% of migraineurs.[5,6] Taken together, published data would justify a greater use of prophylactic medications in clinical practice and emphasize that new prophylactic drugs with good efficacy and tolerability profiles are urgently needed.

This chapter reviews pharmacological and initial clinical data on tonabersat (formerly SB-220453, Minster Pharmaceuticals plc, Saffron Walden, UK), a novel, migraine prophylactic agent that targets receptors in the brain.

Rationale for development

Recent evidence indicates that migraine is a form of sensory dysmodulation, i.e. a system failure of normal sensory processing. Brain imaging studies during migraine attacks have firmly established that reproducible changes occur in brainstem regions, including those involved in sensory modulation.[1] Cortical spreading depression (CSD) is a slowly propagating, transient disturbance in electroencephalographic activity that is implicated in the neurophysiological disturbances associated with migraine, especially aura.[7] Migraine headache follows CSD, possibly after nitric oxide release (the putative 'migraine mediator') and activation of the trigeminal vascular system. Recent research has focused on new potential prophylactic treatments that target either CSD inhibition or the trigeminovascular system.[1] Tonabersat affects both.

Preclinical pharmacology of tonabersat

Receptor pharmacology

Tonabersat is a novel benzoylamino-benzopyran compound with potent anticonvulsant activity.[8–11] It selectively and specifically binds to a unique stereo-selective site in the central nervous system (pKi 7.9) and has negligible effect on several other known anticonvulsant mechanisms. Furthermore, many other drugs (including sumatriptan, anticonvulsants, amino acid analogues, and modulators of Na$^+$/K$^+$ channels) are inactive at the tonabersat binding site. Additionally, tonabersat has shown no activity when tested in more than 80 different binding assays, including those for amino acid analogues, Na$^+$/K$^+$ channels, and a variety of adrenoceptors and other neurotransmitter receptors. Tonabersat does not act via any previously established mechanism of anticonvulsant (e.g. sodium channels, glutamatergic and GABAergic neurotransmission) or antimigraine activity. The tonabersat binding site is present in the brain of several species (including primate and human) but there is no evidence for binding in rat peripheral tissues. The greatest degree of binding occurs in superficial layers of the cerebral cortex and the granule cell layer of the cerebellar cortex; there is moderate binding in the dentate gyrus of the hippocampus. Studies using a close structural analogue, carabersat, indicate that tonabersat and related compounds act at neuronal gap junctions, connections between the cytoplasmic spaces of adjacent neurons, or adjacent neurons and glia, that allow molecules and ions to pass between them.

Mechanism of action

Research in animals has demonstrated the potent inhibitory effects of tonabersat on both CSD and trigeminal nerve stimulation, and its absence of effects on cardiovascular function. A study in the anaesthetized cat investigated the effects of tonabersat on the generation and propagation of repetitive CSD.[12] Vehicle or tonabersat (1, 3, or 10 mg/kg) was administered intraperitoneally (i.p.) 90 min prior to induction of CSD by KCl in the suprasylvian gyrus. Tonabersat produced dose-related inhibition of the number of events in the suprasylvian gyrus and adjacent marginal gyrus (Figure 11.1) and the period of repetitive CSD activity (Figure 11.2). Tonabersat also reduced CSD-related repetitive pial vasodilatation but had no effect on resting haemodynamics. A second study evaluated changes in nitric oxide metabolism (using the marker cGMP) post-CSD in the rat

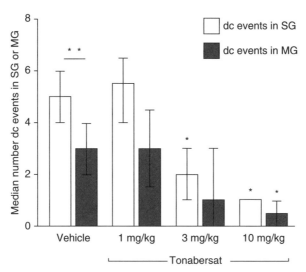

Fig. 11.1 Effects of tonabersat on the number of episodes of cortical spreading depression in the suprasylvian gyrus (SG) and marginal gyrus (MG) of the cat. Data shown represent median and range (25–75%), n = 5–7. Vehicle and tonabersat given intraperitoneally 90 min before KCl. *P < 0.01 versus corresponding gyri in vehicle group (Mann–Whitney test). **P < 0.05 between gyri within group (Mann–Whitney test). Reproduced from *Cephalalgia*, 20, Smith MI *et al*. Repetitive cortical spreading depression in a gyrencephalic feline brain: inhibition by the novel benzoy-lamino-benzopyran SB-220453 (2000), pp. 549 & 550, with permission from Blackwell Publishing.

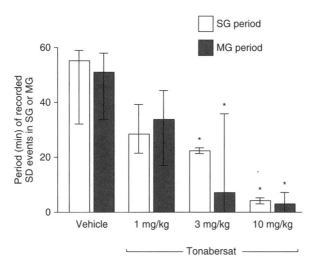

Fig. 11.2 Duration of spreading depression (SD) activity in the suprasylvian gyrus (SG) and marginal gyrus (MG) of the cat. Data shown represent median and range (25–75%), n = 5–7. Vehicle and tonabersat given intraperitoneally 90 min before KCl. *P < 0.05 versus correspon-ding gyri in vehicle group (Mann–Whitney test). Reproduced from *Cephalalgia*, 20, Smith MI *et al*. Repetitive cortical spreading depression in a gyrencephalic feline brain: inhibition by the novel benzoylamino-benzopyran SB-220453 (2000), pp. 549 & 550, with permission from Blackwell Publishing.

following pretreatment with vehicle, tonabersat 10 mg/kg, or sumatriptan 300 µg/kg.[13] Tonabersat inhibited the generation of CSD events and associated nitric oxide release following a cortical KCl stimulus. In the vehicle-treated group a median of eight depolarizations were observed. Tonabersat significantly reduced the number of these events while sumatriptan had no effect. Three days following KCl application, CSD in vehicle-treated animals produced a highly significant elevation in the concentration of brain stem cGMP. This elevation was abolished by pretreatment with tonabersat but not sumatriptan. In a similar study,[14] this group investigated the protective effects of tonabersat in the anaesthetized cat. Nitric oxide was released for a median time of 59 min in vehicle-treated animals, but tonabersat (1, 3, and 10 mg/kg i.p.) reduced this in a dose-dependent manner (Figure 11.3). At the highest dose (10 mg/kg) nitric oxide release was reduced to 5 min.

Data from a study in rats demonstrated that tonabersat abolished trigeminal nerve ganglion-induced plasma protein extravasation in a dose-dependent fashion.[8] Administration of tonabersat 3 and 10 mg/kg i.p. significantly ($P < 0.05$) reduced the extravasation ratio, which compares the degree of plasma protein extravasation from stimulated versus non-stimulated tissue (Figure 11.4). A further study investigated the activity of tonabersat in a model of trigeminal parasympathetic neurovascular reflexes in the anaesthetized cat.[15] Stimulation of the trigeminal nerve ganglion increased carotid blood flow by 65% and reduced vascular resistance by 41% with minimal effect on blood pressure and no effect on heart rate. Intravenous infusion of tonabersat 3.4 µmol/h and

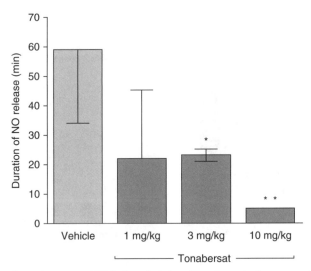

Fig. 11.3 Effects of tonabersat on CSD-induced nitric oxide release in the suprasylvian gyrus (SG) of the cat. Data shown represent median total durations of nitric oxide (NO) release; vehicle and tonabersat given intraperitoneally 90 min before KCl, $n = 4$–7. *$P < 0.05$, **$P < 0.01$ vs. corresponding gyri in vehicle group (Mann–Whitney test). Reproduced from *Cephalalgia*, 20, Read SJ, Smith MI, Hunter AJ, *et al*. SB-220453, a potential novel antimigraine agent, inhibits nitric oxide release following induction of cortical spreading depression in the anaesthetized cat (2000), pp. 92–99, with permission from Blackwell Publishing.

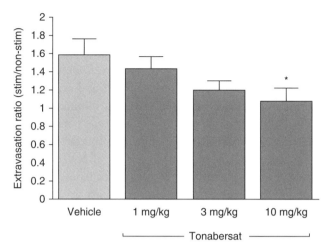

Fig. 11.4 Effects of tonabersat on trigeminal nerve-induced protein extravasation in rat dura mater. Data represent mean ± standard error of mean; n = 6–8. *P < 0.05 versus vehicle group (Mann–Whitney test). Reproduced from *Bioorganic and Medicinal Chemistry Letters*, 9(2), Chan WN, Evans JM, Hadley MS, *et al*. Identification of (-)-cis-6-acetyl-4S-(3-choro-4-fluoro-benzoy-lamino)-3,4-dihydro-2,2-dimethyl-2H-benzo-[b]pyran-3S-ol as a potential antimigraine agent, (1999), pp.6, with permission from Elsevier.
stim = stimulated; non-stim = non-stimulated.

11.5 µmol/h produced time-related reductions in the stimulation-induced responses with a maximal inhibition (relative to control) of about 30% at 2 and 4 h, respectively. Following intraduodenal administration of tonabersat, the maximal inhibition of the responses was 55% at 2 h (Figure 11.5). There were no effects on resting blood pressure, heart rate, carotid blood flow, or carotid vascular resistance following tonabersat administration. These data demonstrate blockade of trigeminal parasympathetic

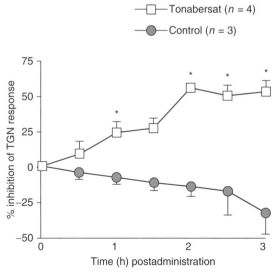

Fig. 11.5 Effects of intraduodenal administration of tonabersat (10 mg/kg) on trigeminal nerve stimulation (TGN)-induced carotid vasodilatation in the cat;[15] Reproduced from *The British Journal of Pharmacology*, 132, Parsons AA, Bingham S, Raval P, *et al*. Tonabersat (SB-220453) a novel benzopyran with anticonvulsant properties attenuates trigeminal nerve-induced neurovascular reflexes, pp.1549–57, with permission from Macmillan Publishers Ltd.

reflexes with tonabersat. It has also been shown that, in contrast to sumatriptan, tonabersat has no contractile effects on isolated human coronary or cranial blood vessels.[16]

In summary, tonabersat has a novel mechanism of action, acting to inhibit markedly the chemically evoked repetitive CSD and associated nitric oxide release, and to block trigeminal (sensory) nerve stimulation-evoked inflammation and neurovascular reflexes. In addition, it is devoid of cardiovascular effects and has minimal liability for inducing neurological deficits. This pharmacological profile suggests a potential therapeutic role in the treatment of migraine, blocking the neurological processes that lead to trigeminal activation and pain generation, but without contractile effects on blood vessels and the potential for cardiovascular side-effects. Tonabersat therefore intervenes at a much earlier stage in the migraine pathophysiological cascade than other drugs such as triptans, non-steroidal anti-inflammatory drugs, and calcitonin gene-related peptide antagonists.

Clinical pharmacology of tonabersat

The pharmacokinetics of tonabersat in man has been evaluated in six studies of healthy subjects and one of migraine patients.[17] Two drug interaction studies[17] have also been conducted. Following a single dose (2–80 mg), tonabersat absorption was fairly rapid: median T_{max} values occurred 2–3 h post-dose; and values for C_{max} and AUC were generally dose proportional. Following repeat dosing, the steady-state plasma concentration of tonabersat was approximately twofold higher than following a single dose. Absorption was delayed by a high-fat meal, although food had no effect on overall systemic exposure. However, absorption during a migraine attack was variable and tended to be delayed.

After dosing approximately 5% of tonabersat is converted by cytosolic carbonyl reductase enzymes to the principle metabolite, SB-277726, but most remains unchanged. Tonabersat is highly bound (98.2%) to human plasma proteins in a concentration-independent manner. During elimination, the plasma concentration of tonabersat declines in an approximately bi-exponential manner with an average $t_{1/2}$ of 24–40 h. Clearance of tonabersat is predominantly by hepatic metabolism and urinary concentrations are negligible. Although CYP 450 3A induction was reported in rats and mice and *in vitro* following tonabersat, there was no evidence of CYP 450 3A induction in humans.[17] Interaction studies showed that tonabersat did not induce metabolism of the oral contraceptive pill and that there was no interaction with sumatriptan.[17]

In summary, the tonabersat clinical pharmacological data are favourable for an antimigraine drug. Absorption was relatively rapid and linear over a wide dose range giving the drug some potential as an acute treatment but with the limitation of delayed absorption during the migraine attack, presumably due to gastric stasis. The relatively long $t_{1/2}$ gives tonabersat a favourable profile for daily dosing and use as a prophylactic agent. A large proportion of the migraine population comprises young women, so the lack of interaction with oral contraceptives is reassuring.

Clinical studies with tonabersat

Following characterization of its pharmacokinetics, tonabersat was first investigated as an acute treatment for migraine.[17] Three placebo-controlled studies investigated single, oral doses of tonabersat (15 mg and 40 mg) for treating moderate-to-severe headache. In one study, tonabersat 15 mg and 40 mg were significantly superior to placebo in terms of the proportion of patients reporting headache relief after 2 h, but these results were not replicated in the other two studies. All studies were confounded by the prior use of sumatriptan, with prior use of the drug resulting in an apparent reduced response to tonabersat. Tonabersat had similar efficacy to sumatriptan in patients who had not previously used a triptan. A fourth study investigated tonabersat 80 mg taken during the migraine aura to prevent or ameliorate subsequent headache, but the drug was not shown to be effective for this indication. These data indicate that tonabersat is only moderately effective as an acute treatment for migraine. The reasons for this may include the plasma C_{max} values for tonabersat occurring later than the 2-h efficacy time point, which is exacerbated because tonabersat is absorbed slowly during the migraine attack. These pharmacokinetic features of tonabersat are not likely to be relevant to prophylaxis, while the long plasma half-life makes once-a-day, preventative dosing logical. The efficacy and tolerability of tonabersat in the prophylaxis of migraine has been evaluated in one placebo-controlled, phase II proof-of-concept study, and full data from this study are due to be reported shortly. Further phase IIb clinical studies are planned to investigate fully the dose–response, efficacy, and tolerability of the drug.

Safety and tolerability of tonabersat

Pharmacological safety assessments[17] in animals revealed no problems likely to be relevant to treatment in humans. In addition to the cardiovascular safety data described above,[15,16] supratherapeutic doses of tonabersat given to rats (up to 300 mg/kg) and dogs (up to 60 mg/kg) had no toxicologically significant effects on cardiovascular, renal, or respiratory function. Overall, toxicological and long-term exposure studies demonstrated no effects likely to limit administration to migraine sufferers. In addition, there was no evidence of carcinogenicity (2-year dosing studies in rat and mouse) or genotoxicity and no effect on fertility or foetal development.

In humans, tonabersat has been administered to 55 healthy subjects and 809 migraine patients in single oral doses of up to 80 mg, and to 46 healthy subjects in repeat doses (for up to 7 days) of up to 80 mg.[17] Tonabersat was generally well tolerated in healthy subjects and migraine patients; most adverse events occurred more frequently in active than placebo groups, were mild or moderate in intensity, and resolved rapidly. Adverse events were reported by 18%, 19%, and 29% of healthy subjects taking placebo, tonabersat 20 mg, and tonabersat 40 mg, respectively. The most common side-effects reported were headache (8.4%, 4.7%, and 8.3%, respectively) and dizziness (2.4%, 2.4%, and 5.6%, respectively). Among the migraine patients in this study, 26.3% of those taking placebo, 36.3% of those taking tonabersat 40 mg, and 39.9% of those taking tonabersat 80 mg reported adverse event(s). Most common were: dizziness (4.0%, 8.7%, and 16.2%, respectively), nausea (5.6%, 8.9%, and 9%, respectively), somnolence (1.9%, 6.1%, and 5.2%, respectively) and vertigo (0.5%, 4.2%, and 3.9%, respectively). No significant changes in vital signs, ECGs, or laboratory assessments were reported following tonabersat administration.

Conclusions

Migraine treatment is currently suboptimal: acute treatments are not completely effective and prophylactic treatments are insufficiently prescribed, perhaps because of the side-effect profiles of currently available prophylactic drugs. New, effective, and well-tolerated prophylactic treatments are urgently needed. Tonabersat is the first in a novel class of benzopyran anticonvulsant compounds with a pharmacological profile supporting its potential to treat migraine. It has a unique central nervous system binding site, thought to be at the neuronal gap junction. Tonabersat has potent inhibitory effects on CSD and trigeminal nerve stimulation, both implicated in the postulated mechanisms for migraine pathogenesis. However, tonabersat has no deleterious cardiovascular effects and is inactive at binding sites associated with standard antimigraine drugs. Tonabersat is relatively slowly absorbed in humans during migraine attacks, is mostly tightly bound to plasma proteins, and is cleared primarily by hepatic metabolism. It has a long plasma half-life making it suitable for once-daily dosing. The slow absorption of tonabersat probably explains its moderate effectiveness as an acute treatment for migraine, but its pharmacokinetic profile is likely to provide much greater potential in prophylaxis. Tonabersat is well tolerated in healthy subjects and migraine patients. The most frequently reported adverse events are dizziness, nausea, somnolence, and vertigo, which are typically mild and transient. The first placebo-controlled clinical study on tonabersat in migraine prophylaxis is now complete and data will be published in the near future.

References

1. Goadsby PJ (2007) Recent advances in understanding migraine mechanisms, molecules and therapeutics. *Trends Mol Med* 13, 39–44.
2. Silberstein SD, for the US Headache Consortium (2000) Practice parameter: evidence-based guidelines for migraine headache (an evidence-based review). Report of the Quality Standards Subcommittee of the American Academy of Neurology. *Neurology* 55, 754–62.
3. Ferrari MD, Roon KI, Lipton RB, Goadsby PJ (2001) Oral triptans (serotonin 5-HT$_{1B/1D}$ agonists) in acute migraine treatment: a meta-analysis of 53 trials. *Lancet* 358, 1668–75.
4. Silberstein SD (2005) Topiramate in migraine prevention. *Headache* 45 (Suppl. 1), S57–65.
5. Lipton RB, Bigal ME, Diamond M, *et al.* (2007) Migraine prevalence, disease burden, and the need for preventive therapy. *Neurology* 68, 343–9.
6. Diamond S, Bigal ME, Silberstein SD, *et al.* (2007) Patterns of diagnosis and acute and preventive treatment for migraine in the United States: results from the American Migraine Prevalence and Prevention Study. *Headache* 47, 355–63.
7. Moskowitz MA, MacFarlane R (1993) Neurovascular and molecular mechanisms in migraine headaches. *Cerebrovasc Brain Metab Rev* 5, 159–177.
8. Chan WN, Evans JM, Hadley MS, *et al.* (1999) Identification of (–)-cis-6-acetyl-4S-(3-choro-4-fluoro-benzoylamino)-3,4-dihydro-2,2-dimethyl-2H-benzo-[b]pyran-3S-ol as a potential antimigraine agent. *Bioorg Med Chem Lett* 9, 285–90.
9. Herdon HJ, Jerman JC, Stean TO, *et al.* (1997) Characterisation of the binding of [3H]-SB-204269, a radiolabelled form of the new anticonvulsant B-204269, to a novel binding site in rat brain membranes. *Br J Pharmacol* 121, 1687–91.

10. Upton N, Blackburn TP, Campbell CA, *et al.* (1997) Profile of SB-204269, a mechanistically novel anticonvulsant drug, in rat models of focal and generalized epileptic seizures. *Br J Pharmacol* 121, 1679–86.

11. Upton N, Thompson M (2000) SB-204269 and related novel antiepileptic agents. *Prog Med Chem* 37, 177–200.

12. Smith MI, Read SJ, Chan WN, *et al.* (2000) Repetitive cortical spreading depression in a gyrencephalic feline brain: inhibition by the novel benzoylamino-benzopyran SB-220453. *Cephalalgia* 20, 546–53.

13. Read SJ, Hirst WD, Upton N, Parsons AA (2001) Cortical spreading depression produces increased cGMP levels in cortex and brain stem that is inhibited by tonabersat (SB-220453) but not sumatriptan. *Brain Res* 891, 69–77.

14. Read SJ, Smith MI, Hunter AJ, Upton N, Parsons AA (2000) SB-220453, a potential novel antimigraine agent, inhibits nitric oxide release following induction of cortical spreading depression in the anaesthetized cat. *Cephalalgia* 20, 92–9.

15. Parsons AA, Bingham S, Raval P, *et al.* (2001) Tonabersat (SB-220453) a novel benzopyran with anticonvulsant properties attenuates trigeminal nerve-induced neurovascular reflexes. *Br J Pharmacol* 132, 1549–57.

16. Maassen VanDenBrink A, van den Broek RW, de Vries R, *et al.* (2000) The potential anti-migraine compound SB-220453 does not contract human isolated blood vessels or myocardium; a comparison with sumatriptan. *Cephalalgia* 20, 538–45.

17. Minster Pharmaceuticals plc., data on file.

12

Discussion summary: Nitric oxide and spreading depression modulators

Nabih Ramadan

In relation to the presentation of Boris Chizh it was asked whether there is indeed evidence that inducible nitric oxide synthase is activated during migraine aura. The fact that nitric oxide production is turned on by cortical spreading depression strongly suggests that, and there is also other indirect evidence. Whether inducible nitric oxide synthase is turned on during attacks without an aura is much less certain. In the pharmacokinetic studies there was a nice demonstration of the influence of an acute migraine attack on the absorption of orally administrated drugs. Almost 40% reduction was seen and this of course confirmed previous observations. The question of efficacy of the GlaxoSmithKline (GSK) substance had not been presented but after questions from the audience it was mentioned that a full analysis is not yet available and it is not yet in the public domain. It was then asked whether the whole programme has been disbanded but there is still ongoing activity trying to develop inducible nitric oxide synthase inhibitors for migraine and perhaps other headaches. There are several development candidates and there is no guarantee that the candidate tested in previous studies will be the candidate in possible future studies.

The discussion then turned to neuronal nitric oxide synthase (nNOS) inhibiting drugs. It was first asked why a small Canadian biotech company had been successful in developing highly selective nNOS inhibitors when a number of other companies, including big pharma companies, had been unsuccessful. The answer was partly that this small company has excellent medicinal chemists, partly that it had been possible to learn from past experience in other companies and, finally, that the crystal structure of the enzymes had become known and could be used for modelling. The acute allodynia caused by triptans was mentioned, and it was asked whether nNOS inhibitors possibly had the same activity. This is not the case and it is actually the hope that these compounds would alleviate both early and late allodynia caused by a migraine attack. If nNOS inhibition has this effect, it supports the development of nNOS selective compounds with a 5-hydroxytryptamine 1B/1D activity. The prevention of sensitization might in theory lead to less recurrence too. Andrew Charles had demonstrated the existence of several different kinds of waves in the cerebral cortex and their interrelation. It was asked whether any of the known prophylactic migraine drugs had any effect on these waves. Systematic studies of these compounds had not yet been conducted but preliminary data would indicate that topiramate may have such an effect. It was also asked why calcium waves apparently did not influence the cerebral vasculature in the reported experiments while the Moskowitz group had found that cortical spreading depression wire activation of metalloproteinases could open the blood–brain barrier and thus influence dural nociceptors. The difference is partly explained by the time-scale, which is very short in the experiments of Andrew Charles and much longer in the experiments of the Moskowitz group. The latter has used repetitive cortical spreading depressions while Charles used a single wave. The next issue was whether calcium waves can perhaps be visualized *in vivo*. Maiken Nedergaard has recently published a study where she was able to show calcium waves. It is still too early to decide whether these waves have a vascular correlate that can perhaps be picked up using near infrared spectroscopy. Charles had reported positive effects of memantine in migraine patients in an open label study. The doses used were titrated slowly. A few patients responded to 5 mg × 2, the majority to 10 mg × 2, and a few had to have 15 mg × 2. In 20 cluster headache patients there were also promising results. This goes along with a clear activity of memantine on calcium waves.

Turning to tonabersat it was asked what the mechanism of action could be in the early phases of cortical spreading depression and particularly what the mechanism could be in blocking neurogenic inflammation – the answer was that all of this work was 10 years old. A lot of work had been done at that time but no mechanism had been discovered. It is clear that the binding site is very specific and totally different from any other known binding site. Saxena had tried the compound several years ago in many different tissues and largely found that it had no effect outside the brain. Doods had studied the effect of the calcitonin gene-related peptide blocker BIBN4096BS, which totally inhibited neurogenic inflammation but the relevance to tonabersat was uncertain.

Lastly, the clinical results of the tonabersat trial were discussed. There was a very low dropout rate in the active group, and literally no side-effects. This suggested that the dose had been too low. The dose was set as half of the single dose used for treating acute migraine attacks with escalation to 40 mg, i.e. the most commonly used dose for acute migraine attacks and still only half of the maximum dose used in previous studies. This was because of a fear of accumulation with chronic use. Now the result had shown that there was room for increasing the dose in future studies. The main result of the prophylactic trial was that all outcome parameters were better on tonabersat than on placebo but only a single end-point was significant. It was pointed out that the data analysis was not yet complete and that full results will be presented properly later this year.

Session IV

Calcitonin gene-related peptide and 5-hydroxytryptamine modulators

13

Calcitonin gene-related peptide: relevance for migraine

Jes Olesen and Inger Jansen-Olesen

Migraine is a disorder without any patho-anatomical correlate. This has made the scientific study of migraine difficult but, on the other hand, holds the promise that the condition may be fully reversible by adequate pharmacological intervention. The origin of nociceptive activity in migraine is in all likelihood the sensory nerve terminals around blood vessels in the brain and/or in the extracranial tissues of the head. Considerable interest has therefore been directed towards identifying signalling molecules in the perivascular nerves and in the blood vessels of the head as well as identifying their receptors and related mechanisms such as ion channels and second messengers. For this purpose animal models are important but, because of species differences, human studies are indispensable. It is from a combination of animal experimental studies and human studies that evidence has been accumulating to suggest that calcitonin gene-related peptide (CGRP) may be crucial in migraine. The following chapter will give an outline of the different studies that have led to the current high level of interest in CGRP antagonism as a possible new treatment principle in migraine.

From a historical point of view, Lars Edvinsson was the driving force behind the elucidation of CGRP's distribution in the cranial circulation (Figure 13.1) and in the evaluation of its basic effects and receptor mechanisms[1–6] (Figure 13.2). His basic studies led him to suggest that CGRP may play a part in migraine pathophysiology. This was later confirmed in human studies.[7–9]

Calcitonin gene-related peptide and its receptors

CGRP was cloned by Amara and co-workers in 1982 and is a 37 amino acid peptide with amino and carboxyl terminals.[10] Based on rat CGRP, the human homologue was isolated in 1984.[11] It is present in an α and a β form that derive from separate genes.[12] The two CGRP subtypes are in general equally distributed within the central and peripheral nervous system.[12,13] However, the amount of mRNA for α-CGRP is ten times higher and the actual concentration of α-CGRP is three to six times higher in the trigeminal ganglion and the primary sensory neurons and nerve terminals.[12,14] CGRP is most abundant in the posterior horn and in primary sensory neurons of the spinal cord and in the trigeminal system where it is co-localized with substance P.[15] CGRP-containing nerve fibres have been identified throughout the cardiovascular system[16,17] but they are primarily located

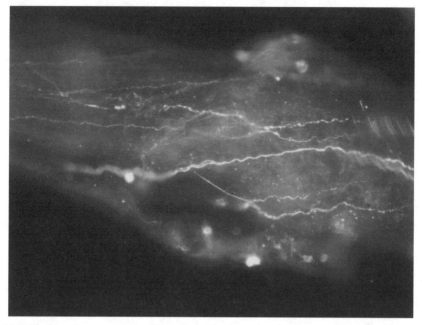

Fig. 13.1 Whole-mount preparation from rat cerebral arteries showing a moderately dense network of nerve fibres containing calcitonin gene-related peptide. Reproduced with courtesy of Helle Wulf.

in sensory nerve terminals around blood vessels and more so in the cranial circulation.[6] Circulating CGRP is found in human plasma.[18–20] It can be released by electrical stimulation of sensory nerves.[19] Bradykinins have been shown to increase CGRP release[21–23] and so may prostaglandins.[24]

CGRP receptors that are blocked by CGRP$_{8-37}$ were previously called CGRP$_1$ receptors and those not blocked were called CGRP$_2$ receptors.[25,26] The molecular biology of the CGRP$_2$ receptors has not been worked out; thus there is still an uncertain nature of this receptor. Furthermore, the use of peptide antagonists to classify CGRP receptors has subsequently been criticized and as experimental conditions may change the actions of these peptides their ability to reliably discriminate between CGRP receptor subtypes will be limited.[27] CGRP receptors comprise the calcitonin-receptor-like receptor (CALCRL) co-expressed with a receptor activity-modifying protein (RAMP).[28] The latter are small proteins containing a single membrane spanning domain, a large extracellular domain, and a short cytoplasm domain. Co-expression of CALCRL with RAMP1 forms CGRP receptors, whereas co-expression with RAMP2 or RAMP3 forms receptors for adrenomedullin.[29,30] It has been suggested that functional CGRP receptors may require another protein called receptor component protein (RCP).[31]

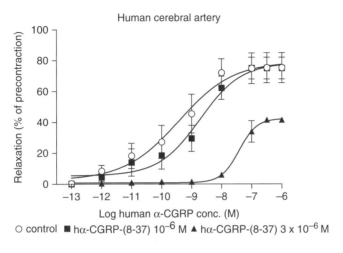

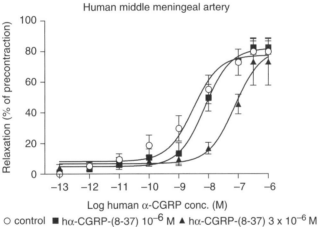

Fig. 13.2 Relaxant responses in human cerebral and middle meningeal arteries pre-contracted by 3×10^{-6} M prostaglandin F_{2a} to the cumulative application of human α-CGRP with and without the antagonist human α-CGRP$_{8-37}$ (10^{-6} M – 3×10^{-6} M). Values given represent mean ± SEM, $n = 4–11$. CGRP, calcitonin gene-related peptide. Reproduced from the *European Journal of Pharmacology*, 481(2–3), Jansen-Olesen, *et al.* In-depth characterization of CGRP receptors in human intracranial arteries (2003), pp. 207–216 with permission from Elsevier.

Function of calcitonin gene-related peptide

Infused intravenously, CGRP causes marked increase in heart rate, a decrease in blood pressure, and flushing of the face as well as headache.[32–34] These responses are dose-dependent and limited by the systemic vascular effects. Infusion of CGRP also causes a slight increase in cerebral blood flow and slight dilatation of the middle cerebral artery in humans while the superficial temporal artery is markedly dilated.[34] Infusion of the CGRP antagonist olcegepant has no effect on systemic haemodynamic parameters in humans,[35] illustrating that CGRP is not normally leaking out of perivascular nerve terminals and that CGRP does not participate in the multiple dilator and constrictor actions that tightly control normal vascular diameter. Pretreatment with olcegepant totally and completely abolished all effects of infused CGRP in humans.[34] Animal experimental studies have demonstrated strong vasodilator action of CGRP on isolated blood vessels and in a close cranial window model in the rat. In the latter model, CGRP dilated the middle meningeal artery while an effect on brain arteries was probably secondary to systemic blood pressure decrease.[36] In studies with perfused cerebral arteries, CGRP was only active from the adventitial side and not when given intraluminally.[37,38] Like in humans the blocker olcegepant completely blocked any effect of CGRP infusion in rats.[36]

Calcitonin gene-related peptide in blood

CGRP levels in blood have generally been very stable and only a few diseases are known to alter circulating CGRP levels. It therefore created enormous interest, when it was first published that CGRP was increased in the external jugular venous blood but not in cubital fossa blood during a migraine attack.[8] When measured in another group of patients after sumatriptan treatment, CGRP was normal in both studies. Values in patients were compared with values in a control group and no intrapatient comparison was made.[8,39] Subsequently, an Italian study also found increased CGRP in external jugular blood but, in contrast to the study of Goadsby *et al.*, also in blood from the cubital fossa.[40] Based on animal studies plus the presumed increase of CGRP during migraine, Boehringer Ingelheim developed the first selective non-peptide CGRP antagonist, olcegepant, also known as BIBN4096BS.

Glyceryl trinitrate induces attacks in migraine sufferers.[41] We therefore measured CGRP in the jugular venous blood before and after glyceryl trinitrate in rat but found no difference.[42] These studies led us to consider that the published literature on CGRP release needed to be further studied. While the initial studies were all comparing patient data with historic controls, we used patients as their own controls by studying CGRP in the external jugular and cubital fossa blood during attack as well as outside of attack. In this study we found no indication of increased CGRP during attack. To guard against any difference in assay, we used the exact same assay as in the previous studies plus another better validated assay. We did extensive analyses of these materials showing that duration of attack, age or sex of patients, severity of pain, and other factors were not associated with increased CGRP. It therefore remains an open question whether CGRP is ever increased during migraine attack and, if so, under which circumstances and in which patients it may be increased.[20] One major difference between our study and the previous studies was that we took blood in the patient's own home under considerably more comfortable conditions than in the previous study where patients had been desperate enough to go to an emergency room with their migraine attack.[8] The latter situation could be considerably more stressful and stress is known to increase CGRP.[43] If that was the explanation one would, however, expect CGRP to increase both in external jugular venous blood and in cubital fossa blood.

Is calcitonin gene-related peptide able to activate nociceptors?

CGRP is present within nociceptive pathways both peripherally and in the central nervous system. However, the role of CGRP in nociception is not fully understood. We were unable to show any nociceptive effect of CGRP when injected intradermally in human subjects, and CGRP did not even have an additive effect when combined with nociceptive substances.[44] Similarly, CGRP applied to dura mater was unable to sensitize peripheral sensory nerve endings and also unable to sensitize nociceptive neurons in the brain.[45] It remains unclear, therefore, how CGRP could be involved in the nociceptive mechanisms of migraine. One possible mechanism that does not seem to be involved is neurogenic inflammation. Although stimulation of the trigeminal ganglion results in leaking of plasma proteins from the vascular space into the dura mater (neurogenic inflammation) this is not caused by CGRP but by liberation of substance P. Consistent with this, the plasma extravasation was abolished in tachykinin neurokinin 1 receptor knockout mice after mustard oil application while vasodilatation was enhanced. In α-CGRP knockout mice, mustard oil caused plasma extravasation and vasodilatation that was inhibited by treatment with a neurokinin 1 receptor.[46]

Calcitonin gene-related peptide can induce migraine headache

CGRP infusion into normal experimental subjects reliably causes mild headache concomitant with vascular responses as described above.[34] When CGRP was infused into subjects with migraine without aura, it induced a more pronounced headache followed by a delayed increase in headache. Three of ten subjects fulfilled all the criteria for migraine without aura attack according to the International Headache Society. In patients where the headache did not quite fulfil criteria for migraine, it was still migraine-like.[47] The study demonstrated beyond doubt that, with regard to headache and migraine, CGRP is a nociceptive molecule. However, the site of this action remains uncertain. There were slight but significant changes in cerebral blood flow and in the diameter of the middle cerebral artery. In addition another study showed that the superficial temporal artery dilated markedly after CGRP infusion.[34] Unfortunately the middle meningeal artery could not be measured in these human studies, but it is likely that it was markedly dilated because it bears more resemblance to the superficial temporal artery than to the cerebral arteries. Another important fact is that the non-peptide CGRP receptor antagonist olcegepant completely prevented CGRP induced headache.[34] Olcegepant is a large water-soluble molecule that does not readily pass the blood–brain barrier. However, it is an extremely potent molecule and the dose used clinically is high compared with doses used to block arterial dilatation in experimental studies.[9,34–36] Therefore, an intracerebral site of action of olcegepant cannot be ruled out. However, if this is true a lower dose of olcegepant should be sufficient to block peripheral CGRP effects. In a recent study, the effect of compound 3, an equipotent analogue of olcegepant, blocked the increase in dermal blood flow after topical application of capsaicin. In rhesus monkey a maximum inhibition was observed at 30 μg/kg or 2.1 mg/70 kg, which corresponds well to the dose (2.5 mg) used in humans.[48]

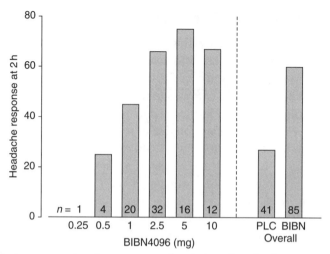

Fig. 13.3 Headache response (moderate or severe headache at baseline becoming nil or mild at 2 hours post-dose) rates for each dose of BIBN4096 tested, the placebo response rate, and the pooled active drug rate.

Calcitonin gene-related peptide receptor blocking is effective in acute migraine attacks

The final proof of the importance of CGRP in migraine came from a therapeutic study.[9] Olcegepant as mentioned before is a highly selective and highly potent CGRP receptor antagonist. In a phase 2 study olcegepant dose-dependently alleviated symptoms of a migraine attack. An adaptive design was used whereby the dose was increased or decreased in each block of patients depending on the response in the previous block. The study identified doses of 2.5, 5, and 10 mg as highly effective and 2.5 mg was chosen as the preferred dose for future studies[9] (Figure 13.3). However, the development of the compound was stopped because of difficulties of absorption and no further treatment data are available. This remarkable proof of concept study has, however, stirred even more interest in CGRP and migraine than before. CGRP antagonists that are orally available are therefore awaited with great excitement and hopefully will turn out to become an important class of new migraine drugs.

Conclusions

The development of a non-peptide CGRP antagonist represents the first truly mechanism-based drug development for migraine. This development was based on almost two decades of basic and clinical research. Animal experiments and studies of human arteries demonstrated the location and effects of CGRP and its receptors as well as the effect of CGRP receptor blockade. The result suggested that CGRP is present in the sensory nervous system that is an area related to migraine and that it is a strong vasodilator. Crucial studies were then done in humans. First, increased release of CGRP during the migraine attack was suggested, although later studies found no such increase. Secondly, it was shown that CGRP infusion can induce vascular type headache in normal volunteers and in migraine subjects. Furthermore, in migraine subjects CGRP induced migraine attacks without aura. The final proof of the importance of CGRP in migraine came from a phase 2 study demonstrating that olcegepant, a non-peptide CGRP antagonist, had a highly significant effect in acute migraine attacks. It is extremely promising that mechanism-based drug development for migraine is now possible and more examples may soon follow the pioneering work on CGRP.

References

1. Edvinsson L, Ekman R, Jansen I, McCulloch J, Uddman R (1987) Calcitonin gene-related peptide and cerebral blood vessels: distribution and vasomotor effects. *J Cereb Blood Flow Metab* 7, 720–8.

2. Edvinsson L, Gulbenkian S, Barroso CP, Cunha e Sa M, Polak JM, Mortensen A, Jorgensen L, Jansen-Olesen I (1998) Innervation of the human middle meningeal artery: immunohistochemistry, ultrastructure, and role of endothelium for vasomotility. *Peptides* 19, 1213–25.

3. Jansen-Olesen I, Jorgensen L, Engel U, Edvinsson L (2003) In-depth characterization of CGRP receptors in human intracranial arteries. *Eur J Pharmacol* 481, 207–16.

4. Jansen-Olesen I, Mortensen A, Edvinsson L (1996) Calcitonin gene-related peptide is released from capsaicin-sensitive nerve fibres and induces vasodilatation of human cerebral arteries concomitant with activation of adenylyl cyclase. *Cephalalgia* 16, 310–16.

5. Uddman R, Edvinsson L, Ekblad E, Hakanson R, Sundler F (1986) Calcitonin gene-related peptide (CGRP): perivascular distribution and vasodilatory effects. *Regul Peptides* 15, 1–23.

6. Uddman R, Edvinsson L, Ekman R, Kingman T, McCulloch J (1985) Innervation of the feline cerebral vasculature by nerve fibers containing calcitonin gene-related peptide: trigeminal origin and co-existence with substance P. *Neurosci Lett* 62, 131–6.

7. Edvinsson L, Goadsby PJ (1994) Neuropeptides in migraine and cluster headache. *Cephalalgia* 14, 320–7.

8. Goadsby PJ, Edvinsson L, Ekman R (1990) Vasoactive peptide release in the extracerebral circulation of humans during migraine headache. *Ann Neurol* 28, 183–7.

9. Olesen J, Diener HC, Husstedt IW, Goadsby PJ, Hall D, Meier U, Pollentier S, Lesko LM (2004) Calcitonin gene-related peptide receptor antagonist BIBN 4096 BS for the acute treatment of migraine. *N Engl J Med* 350, 1104–10.

10. Amara SG, Jonas V, Rosenfeld MG, Ong ES, Evans RM (1982) Alternative RNA processing in calcitonin gene expression generates mRNAs encoding different polypeptide products. *Nature* 298, 240–4.

11. Morris HR, Panico M, Etienne T, Tippins J, Girgis SI, MacIntyre I (1984) Isolation and characterization of human calcitonin gene-related peptide. *Nature* 308, 746–8.

12. Amara SG, Arriza JL, Leff SE, Swanson LW, Evans RM, Rosenfeld MG (1985) Expression in brain of a messenger RNA encoding a novel neuropeptide homologous to calcitonin gene-related peptide. *Science* 229, 1094–107.

13. Skofitsch G, Jacobowitz DM (1985) Quantitative distribution of calcitonin gene-related peptide in the rat central nervous system. *Peptides* 6, 1069–73.

14. Mulderry PK, Ghatei MA, Spokes RA, *et al.* (1988) Differential expression of alpha-CGRP and beta-CGRP by primary sensory neurons and enteric autonomic neurons of the rat. *Neuroscience* 25, 195–205.

15. Gibson SJ, Polak JM, Bloom SR, *et al.* (1984) Calcitonin gene-related peptide immunoreactivity in the spinal cord of man and of eight other species. *J Neurosci* 4, 3101–11.

16. Mulderry PK, Ghatei MA, Rodrigo J, Allen JM, Rosenfeld MG, Polak JM, Bloom SR (1985) Calcitonin gene-related peptide in cardiovascular tissues of the rat. *Neuroscience* 14, 947–54.

17. Wharton J, Gulbenkian S, Mulderry PK, Ghatei MA, McGregor GP, Bloom SR, Polak JM (1986) Capsaicin induces a depletion of calcitonin gene-related peptide (CGRP)-immunoreactive nerves in the cardiovascular system of the guinea pig and rat. *J Auton Nerv Syst* 16, 289–309.

18. Ashina M, Bendtsen L, Jensen R, Schifter S, Jansen-Olesen I, Olesen J (2000) Plasma levels of calcitonin gene-related peptide in chronic tension-type headache. *Neurology* 55, 1335–40.

19. Goadsby PJ, Edvinsson L, Ekman R (1988) Release of vasoactive peptides in the extracerebral circulation of humans and the cat during activation of the trigeminovascular system. *Ann Neurol* 23, 193–6.

20. Tvedskov JF, Lipka K, Ashina M, Iversen HK, Schifter S, Olesen J (2005) No increase of calcitonin gene-related peptide in jugular blood during migraine. *Ann Neurol* 58, 561–8.

21. Franco-Cereceda A, Saria A, Lundberg JM (1989) Differential release of calcitonin gene-related peptide and neuropeptide Y from the isolated heart by capsaicin, ischaemia, nicotine, bradykinin and ouabain. *Acta Physiol Scand* 135, 173–87.

22. Geppetti P, Del Bianco E, Santicioli P, Lippe IT, Maggi CA, Sicuteri F (1990) Release of sensory neuropeptides from dural venous sinuses of guinea pig. *Brain Res* 510, 58–62.

23. Schwenger N, Dux M, de Col R, Carr R, Messlinger K (2007) Interaction of calcitonin gene-related peptide, nitric oxide and histamine release in neurogenic blood flow and afferent activation in the rat cranial dura mater. *Cephalalgia* 27, 481–91.

24. Holzer P, Jocic M, Peskar BA (1995) Mediation by prostaglandins of the nitric oxide-induced neurogenic vasodilatation in rat skin. *Br J Pharmacol* 116, 2365–70.

25. Dennis T, Fournier A, Cadieux A, Pomerleau F, Jolicoeur FB, St Pierre S, Quirion R (1990) hCGRP8-37, a calcitonin gene-related peptide antagonist revealing calcitonin gene-related peptide receptor heterogeneity in brain and periphery. *J Pharmacol Exp Ther* 254, 123–8.

26. Donoso MV, Fournier A, St-Pierre S, Huidobro-Toro JP (1990) Pharmacological characterization of CGRP1 receptor subtype in the vascular system of the rat: studies with hCGRP fragments and analogs. *Peptides* 11, 885–9.

27. Waugh DJ, Bockman CS, Smith DD, Abel PW (1999) Limitations in using peptide drugs to characterize calcitonin gene-related peptide receptors. *J Pharmacol Exp Ther* 289, 1419–26.

28. McLatchie LM, Fraser NJ, Main MJ, Wise A, Brown J, Thompson N, Solari R, Lee MG, Foord SM (1998) RAMPs regulate the transport and ligand specificity of the calcitonin-receptor-like receptor. *Nature* 393, 333–9.

29. Muff R, Leuthauser K, Buhlmann N, Foord SM, Fischer JA, Born W (1998) Receptor activity modifying proteins regulate the activity of a calcitonin gene-related peptide receptor in rabbit aortic endothelial cells. *FEBS Lett* 441, 366–8.

30. Fraser NJ, Wise A, Brown J, McLatchie LM, Main MJ, Foord SM (1999) The amino terminus of receptor activity modifying proteins is a critical determinant of glycosylation state and ligand binding of calcitonin receptor-like receptor. *Mol Pharmacol* 55, 1054–9.

31. Evans BN, Rosenblatt MI, Mnayer LO, Oliver KR, Dickerson IM (2000) CGRP-RCP, a novel protein required for signal transduction at calcitonin gene-related peptide and adrenomedullin receptors. *J Biol Chem* 275, 31438–43.

32. Struthers AD, Brown MJ, Macdonald DW, Beacham JL, Stevenson JC, Morris HR, MacIntyre I (1986) Human calcitonin gene related peptide: a potent endogenous vasodilator in man. *Clin Sci (Lond)* 70, 389–93.

33. Juul R, Aakhus S, Bjornstad K, Gisvold SE, Brubakk AO, Edvinsson L (1994) Calcitonin gene-related peptide (human alpha-CGRP) counteracts vasoconstriction in human subarachnoid haemorrhage. *Neurosci Lett* 170, 67–70.

34. Petersen KA, Lassen LH, Birk S, Lesko L, Olesen J (2005) BIBN4096BS antagonizes human alpha-calcitonin gene related peptide-induced headache and extracerebral artery dilatation. *Clin Pharmacol Ther* 77, 202–13.

35. Petersen KA, Birk S, Lassen LH, Kruuse C, Jonassen O, Lesko L, Olesen J (2005) The CGRP-antagonist, BIBN4096BS does not affect cerebral or systemic haemodynamics in healthy volunteers. *Cephalalgia* 25, 139–47.

36. Petersen KA, Birk S, Doods H, Edvinsson L, Olesen J (2004) Inhibitory effect of BIBN4096BS on cephalic vasodilatation induced by CGRP or transcranial electrical stimulation in the rat. *Br J Pharmacol* 143, 697–704.

37. Petersen KA, Nilsson E, Olesen J, Edvinsson L (2005) Presence and function of the calcitonin gene-related peptide receptor on rat pial arteries investigated in vitro and in vivo. *Cephalalgia* 25, 424–32.

38. Edvinsson L, Nilsson E, Jansen-Olesen I (2007) Inhibitory effect of BIBN4096BS, CGRP(8-37), a CGRP antibody and an RNA-Spiegelmer on CGRP induced vasodilatation in the perfused and non-perfused rat middle cerebral artery. *Br J Pharmacol* 150, 633–40.

39. Goadsby PJ, Edvinsson L (1993) The trigeminovascular system and migraine: studies characterizing cerebrovascular and neuropeptide changes seen in humans and cats. *Ann Neurol* 33, 48–56.

40. Sarchielli P, Alberti A, Codini M, Floridi A, Gallai V (2000) Nitric oxide metabolites, prostaglandins and trigeminal vasoactive peptides in internal jugular vein blood during spontaneous migraine attacks. *Cephalalgia* 20, 907–18.

41. Olesen J, Iversen HK, Thomsen LL (1993) Nitric oxide supersensitivity: a possible molecular mechanism of migraine pain. *Neuroreport* 4, 1027–30.

42. Offenhauser N, Zinck T, Hoffmann J, Schiemann K, Schuh-Hofer S, Rohde W, Arnold G, Dirnagl U, Jansen-Olesen I, Reuter U (2005) CGRP release and c-fos expression within trigeminal nucleus caudalis of the rat following glyceryltrinitrate infusion. *Cephalalgia* 25, 225–36.

43. Tidgren B, Theodorsson E, Hjemdahl P (1991) Renal and systemic plasma immunoreactive neuropeptide Y and calcitonin gene-related peptide responses to mental stress and adrenaline in humans. *Clin Physiol* 11, 9–19.

44. Pedersen-Bjergaard U, Nielsen LB, Jensen K, Edvinsson L, Jansen I, Olesen J (1991) Calcitonin gene-related peptide, neurokinin A and substance P: effects on nociception and neurogenic inflammation in human skin and temporal muscle. *Peptides* 12, 333–7.

45. Levy D, Burstein R, Strassman AM (2005) Calcitonin gene-related peptide does not excite or sensitize meningeal nociceptors: implications for the pathophysiology of migraine. *Ann Neurol* 58, 698–705.

46. Grant AD, Pinter E, Salmon AM, Brain SD (2005) An examination of neurogenic mechanisms involved in mustard oil-induced inflammation in the mouse. *Eur J Pharmacol* 507, 273–80.

47. Lassen LH, Haderslev PA, Jacobsen VB, Iversen HK, Sperling B, Olesen J (2002) CGRP may play a causative role in migraine. *Cephalalgia* 22, 54–61.

48. Hershey JC, Corcoran HA, Baskin EP, Salvatore CA, Mosser S, Williams TM, Koblan KS, Hargreaves RJ, Kane SA (2005) Investigation of the species selectivity of a nonpeptide CGRP receptor antagonist using a novel pharmacodynamic assay. *Regul Pept* 127, 71–7.

14

New 5-hydroxytryptamine-related drug targets

Pramod R. Saxena

Migraine is a complex familial neurovascular syndrome, which involves episodic brain dysfunction resulting in severe, debilitating, pulsatile, mostly unilateral headache associated with nausea, vomiting, photophobia, and/or phonophobia.[1,2] It is intimately related to 5-hydroxytryptamine (serotonin, 5-HT), but the exact role of this biogenic amine in migraine pathophysiology is still not fully delineated. There is evidence for high (trigger phase) as well as low (chronic phase) serotonergic activity in the brain[3] and plasma 5-HT concentrations may decrease during the headache phase, particularly in patients with migraine with aura.[3,4] The link between 5-HT and migraine is further strengthened by the fact that intravenous administration of 5-HT can alleviate migraine attack[5] and several drugs effective in migraine, both as acute and prophylactic treatments, are high affinity 5-HT receptor ligands.[6–8]

5-hydroxytryptamine receptors and antimigraine drugs

Based on operational (selective agonists and antagonists and ligand-binding affinities), transductional (intracellular transduction mechanisms), and structural (molecular structure) criteria, at least 14 members of the 5-HT receptor family, belonging to seven classes (5-HT_1 to 5-HT_7), have been identified (see Table 14.1).[9,10] The functional aspects of 5-HT_5 and 5-HT_6 receptors need still to be ascertained, but the other receptors are well characterized.

Ergotamine and dihydroergotamine interact with a variety of receptors, including 5-HT_{1A}, 5-HT_{1B}, 5-HT_{1D}, 5-HT_{2A}, 5-HT_{2B}, 5-HT_{5B}, adrenergic α_1, α_2, and dopamine D_2 receptors with affinity constants around 8–9, and 5-HT_{1F}, 5-HT_{2C}, 5-HT_{5A}, and 5-HT_7 receptors with affinity constants around 7. In addition, there is evidence that both ergotamine and dihydroergotamine can activate a novel, not yet characterized receptor.[6,11] Methysergide, a semisynthetic ergot derivative, is a potent 5-HT_2 receptor antagonist, not distinguishing between the 5-HT_{2A}, 5-HT_{2B}, and 5-HT_{2C} subtypes.[8] Perhaps less well known, methysergide is also an agonist at the 5-HT_{1B}[12] and an antagonist at the 5-HT_7 receptor mediating vasodilatation.[13–15] In contrast, sumatriptan is a much more selective drug, showing high affinity for 5-HT_{1B} and 5-HT_{1D} and 5-HT_{1F} receptors.[6,7]

Table 14.1 Classification of 5-hydroxytryptamine (5-HT) receptors

Receptor	Agonists	Antagonists	Transduction	Localization	Function
5-HT$_{1A}$	8-OH-DPAT	WAY 100635	↓ Adenylyl cyclase	Raphé nucleus	Central hypotension
5-HT$_{1B}$[a,b]	Sumatriptan	SB224289	↓ Adenylyl cyclase	Cranial blood vessels	Vasoconstriction
5-HT$_{1D}$[b]	PNU109291	BRL15572	↓ Adenylyl cyclase	Presynaptic neurons	Autoreceptor
5-HT$_{1E}$[c]	5-HT	Methiothepin	↓ Adenylyl cyclase	Cortex	Unknown
5-HT$_{1F}$[b]	LY344864	Methysergide	↓ Adenylyl cyclase	CNS	↓ Trigeminal system
5-HT$_{2A}$[d]	DOI	Ketanserin	↑ Phospholipase C	Smooth muscle, platelets	Contraction, aggregation
5-HT$_{2B}$[d]	BW723C86	SB204741	↑ Phospholipase C	Rat fundus, endothelium	Contraction, nitric oxide release
5-HT$_{2C}$[d]	Ro 60–0175	SB242084	↑ Phospholipase C	Choroid plexus	CSF production?
5-HT$_3$	2-Methyl-5-HT	Tropisetron	Na$^+$/K$^+$ channel	Peripheral nerves	↑ Neuronal activity
5-HT$_4$	Renzapride, BIMU8	GR113808	↑ Adenylyl cyclase	Gastrointestinal tract, pig, and human atrium	↑ Neuronal activity, tachycardia
5-HT$_{5A/5B}$	5-HT, ergotamine	LSD	?	CNS	Unknown
5-HT$_6$[e]	5-MeO-T ≥ 5-HT	Ro 04–6790	↑ Adenylyl cyclase	CNS	Unknown
5-HT$_7$[e]	5-CT >> 5-HT	SB258719	↑ Adenylyl cyclase	CNS, smooth muscles	Circadian rhythm, relaxation

CNS, central nervous system; CSF, cerebrospinal fluid; for compounds (see references 9 and 10).

[a] Sumatriptan as well as other triptans are agonists at 5-HT$_{1B/1D}$ receptors and some triptans also have an agonist action at the 5-HT$_{1F}$ receptor. [b]GR127935 is equipotent on 5-HT$_{1B/1D}$ receptors and displays a moderate affinity for the 5-HT$_{1F}$ receptor. [c]There are no selective agonists or antagonists thus far and very high doses of methiothepin are required to produce effective blockade at the 5-HT$_{1E}$ receptor. [d]DOI is an equipotent agonist at the three 5-HT$_2$ receptors. [e]Although there are no selective agonists yet and mesulergine is an antagonist showing 300-fold selectivity for the cloned 5-HT$_7$ receptor (pK$_D$ = 8.2) over the cloned 5-HT$_6$ receptor (pK$_D$ = 5.8).

Drug targets

With the above background in mind, the following drug targets based on 5-HT receptors will be discussed.

Cranioselective 5-hydroxytryptamine 1B receptor agonists

Ergotamine, dihydroergotamine,[6] and methysergide[8] as well as the triptans[7] have a selective vasoconstrictor action within the carotid arterial bed, causing an almost exclusive reduction of the arteriovenous anastomotic fraction. *In vitro* experiments show that these drugs cause a more potent contraction of cranial arteries than that of peripheral vessels. For example, sumatriptan and eletriptan more effectively contract the human middle meningeal artery than coronary artery or saphenous vein (see Figure 14.1).[16] The figure also shows that eletriptan may be less effective than sumatriptan on the coronary artery.[16] Thus, it may be possible to further improve the cranio-coronary selectivity by, for example, designing appropriate 5-HT$_{1B}$ receptor partial agonists, so that only cranial vasoconstriction manifests without any coronary contraction.

Combined 5-hydroxytryptamine 1B receptor and α_2-adrenoceptor agonists

Since 1906, ergot alkaloids have been described as α-adrenoceptor antagonists, but this property, a textbook knowledge,[17] is only observed with very high doses, bearing

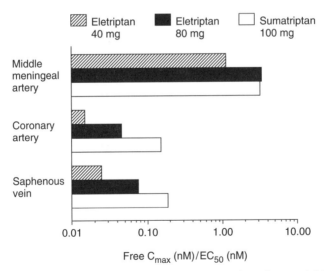

Fig. 14.1 Relationship between the reported C_{max} concentration in patients and EC_{50} values of eletriptan (40 mg and 80 mg) and sumatriptan (100 mg) in contracting human isolated middle meningeal artery, coronary artery, and saphenous vein (for details, see reference 16). Note that both eletriptan and sumatriptan are more potent at the middle meningeal artery than at the coronary artery or saphenous vein, but it appears that eletriptan is even less effective than sumatriptan on the coronary artery.

absolutely no relevance to therapeutic use. In therapeutic concentrations, ergot alkaloids behave as $5\text{-}HT_{1B/1D}$ as well as α-adrenoceptor agonists.[6] More recently, we have argued that, particularly, the α_{2C}-adrenoceptor is a target for novel antimigraine drugs.[12,18] Thus, it seems attractive to design compounds with agonist actions at both $5\text{-}HT_{1B}$ and α_{2C} receptors. This dual action may enhance therapeutic action and lower coronary and hypertensive side-effect potential, as the α_{2C}-adrenoceptor does not mediate peripheral vasoconstriction.[17]

Selective 5-hydroxytryptamine 1D receptor agonists

In contrast to our view that the main mechanism of the therapeutic action of triptans involves cranial vasoconstriction,[7] others feel that these drugs alleviate migraine mainly by affecting trigeminal pain pathway.[2,19] The main population of 5-HT receptors within the trigeminal pain pathway appears to be of the $5\text{-}HT_{1D}$ type.[20] Therefore, selective $5\text{-}HT_{1D}$ receptor agonists, which would lack vasoconstrictor properties,[9] are attractive to develop. However, one such compound, PNU 142633, proved ineffective in migraine.[21] It is argued that the ineffectiveness of PNU 142633 is related to its poor brain penetration and weak agonist effect on the human $5\text{-}HT_{1D}$ receptor; PNU 142633 was selected on the basis of its affinity to the gorilla $5\text{-}HT_{1D}$ receptor.[22] However, it has to be pointed out that many other selective, orally bioavailable, human $5\text{-}HT_{1D}$ receptor agonists have been described.[23,24] None of them has made it to the clinic.

5-Hydroxytryptamine 1F receptor agonists

The $5\text{-}HT_{1F}$ receptor agonist LY334370 was found effective in acute migraine,[25] but at plasma concentrations at which it can also interact with $5\text{-}HT_{1B/1D}$ receptors. The development of this compound was, however, discontinued due to animal toxicity. Thus, the $5\text{-}HT_{1F}$ receptor remains a putative target in migraine, but it must be realized that triptans having $5\text{-}HT_{1F}$ receptor affinity are clinically as effective as those without[7]. Moreover, the Pharmaceutical Company (Lilly) that championed this target seems to have given it up. This does not augur well for this target.

5-Hydroxytryptamine 2 receptor antagonists

The efficacy of methysergide had been ascribed to its $5\text{-}HT_2$ receptor antagonist property, but, as pointed out earlier,[8] this view is unsustainable because many potent $5\text{-}HT_2$ receptor antagonists (mianserin, sergolexole, ketanserin, ICI 169 369) have little or no prophylactic effect in migraine. Thus, this 5-HT receptor target is not to be fancied.

Selective 5-hydroxytryptamine 7 receptor antagonists

Methysergide has a high affinity for $5\text{-}HT_7$ receptors.[10] The drug antagonizes vasodilator responses in several vascular tissues, including the cranial arteries.[13–15] Thus, selective $5\text{-}HT_7$ receptor antagonists might be effective in migraine prophylaxis. Several novel compounds are already available,[26] but their central effects may or may not be an asset.

Selective agonists at 'ergot' receptor

There is evidence that a part of the vasoconstrictor effect of ergotamine and dihydroer-gotamine as well as 5-HT involves a novel, not yet characterized receptor.[27,28] It may be possible to clone this receptor and target it for new drug development.

Conclusions

5-HT is intimately related to migraine and several drugs effective in migraine are high affinity ligands at 5-HT receptors. The ergot alkaloids and triptans behave as potent agonists at $5\text{-HT}_{1B/1D}$ receptors, with some triptans also acting at the 5-HT_{1F} receptor. Methysergide is also a 5-HT_{1B} receptor agonist, but it is an antagonist at 5-HT_2 and 5-HT_7 receptors. In addition, the ergot alkaloids can elicit vasoconstriction via another, not yet characterized, receptor. Thus, the following avenues may be explored for new drug development: (1) cranioselective 5-HT_{1B} receptor agonists; (2) combined 5-HT_{1B} receptor and α_2-adrenoceptor agonists; (3) selective 5-HT_{1D} receptor agonists; (4) 5-HT_{1F} receptor agonists; (5) 5-HT_2 receptor antagonists; (6) selective 5-HT_7 receptor antagonists; and (7) selective agonist at 'ergot' receptor.

References

1. Silberstein S (2004) Migraine. *Lancet* 363, 381–91.
2. Goadsby PJ (2007) Recent advances in understanding migraine mechanisms, molecules and therapeutics. *Trends Mol Med* 13, 39–44.
3. Hamel E, Saxena PR (2006) 5-Hydroxytryptamine involvement in migraines. In: Olesen J, Goadsby PJ, Ramadan NM, Tfelt-Hansen P, Welch KMA (eds) *The Headaches*, 3rd edn, pp. 275–80. Lippincott, Williams & Wilkins, Philadelphia, PA.
4. Nagata E, Shibata M, Hamada J, *et al.* (2006) Plasma 5-hydroxytryptamine (5-HT) in migraine during an attack-free period. *Headache* 46, 592–6.
5. Kimball RW, Friedman AP, Vallejo E (1960) Effect of serotonin in migraine patients. *Neurology* 10, 107–11.
6. Tfelt-Hansen P, Saxena PR (2006) Ergot alkaloids in the acute treatment of migraines. In: Olesen J, Goadsby PJ, Ramadan NM, Tfelt-Hansen P, Welch KMA (eds) *The Headaches*, 3rd edn, pp. 459–67. Lippincott, Williams & Wilkins, Philadelphia, PA.
7. Saxena PR, Tfelt-Hansen P (2006) Triptans, $5\text{-HT}_{1B/1D}$ receptor agonists in the acute treatment of migraines. In: Olesen J, Goadsby PJ, Ramadan NM, Tfelt-Hansen P, Welch KMA (eds) *The Headaches*, 3rd edn, pp. 469–503. Lippincott, Williams & Wilkins, Philadelphia, PA.
8. Tfelt-Hansen P, Saxena PR (2006) Antiserotonin drugs in migraine prophylaxis. In: Olesen J, Goadsby PJ, Ramadan NM, Tfelt-Hansen P, Welch KMA (eds) *The Headaches*, 3rd edn, pp. 529–37. Lippincott, Williams & Wilkins, Philadelphia, PA.
9. Villalón CM, Centurión D, Valdivia LF, De Vries P, Saxena PR (2003) Migraine: pathophysiology, pharmacology, treatment and future trends. *Curr Vasc Pharmacol* 1, 71–84.
10. Hoyer D, Clarke DE, Fozard JR, *et al.* (1994) International Union of Pharmacology classification of receptors for 5-hydroxytryptamine (Serotonin). *Pharmacol Rev* 46, 157–203.
11. De Vries P, Villalón CM, Heiligers JPC, Saxena PR (1998) Characterization of 5-HT receptors mediating constriction of porcine carotid arteriovenous anastomoses; involvement of $5\text{-HT}_{1B/1D}$ and novel receptors. *Br J Pharmacol* 123, 1561–70.

12. Villalón CM, De Vries P, Rabelo G, Centurion D, Sanchez-Lopez A, Saxena PR (1999) Canine external carotid vasoconstriction to methysergide, ergotamine and dihydroergotamine: role of 5-HT$_{1B/1D}$ receptors and alpha$_2$-adrenoceptors. *Br J Pharmacol* 126, 585–94.

13. De Vries P, De Visser PA, Heiligers JPC, Villalón CM, Saxena PR (1999) Changes in systemic and regional haemodynamics during 5-HT$_7$ receptor-mediated depressor responses in rats. *Naunyn Schmiedebergs Arch Pharmacol* 359, 331–8.

14. Terrón JA, Falcon-Neri A (1999) Pharmacological evidence for the 5-HT$_7$ receptor mediating smooth muscle relaxation in canine cerebral arteries. *Br J Pharmacol* 127, 609–16.

15. Lambert GA, Donaldson C, Hoskin KL, Boers PM, Zagami AS (2004) Dilatation induced by 5-HT in the middle meningeal artery of the anaesthetised cat. *Naunyn Schmiedebergs Arch Pharmacol* 369, 591–601.

16. Maassen Van Den Brink A, Van den Broek RW, De Vries R, Bogers AJ, Avezaat CJ, Saxena PR (2000) Craniovascular selectivity of eletriptan and sumatriptan in human isolated blood vessels. *Neurology* 55, 1524–30.

17. Hoffman BB, Lefkowitz RJ (1996) Catecholamines, sympathomimetic drugs and adrenergic receptor antagonists. In: Hardman JG, Limbird LE, Molinoff PB, Ruddon RW, Goodman Gilman A (eds) *Goodman & Gilman's The Pharmacological Basis of Therapeutics*, 9th edn, pp. 199–248. McGraw-Hill Book Co., New York.

18. Willems EW, Valdivia LF, Villalón CM, Saxena PR (2003) Possible role of alpha-adrenoceptor subtypes in acute migraine therapy. *Cephalalgia* 23, 245–57.

19. Shields KG, Goadsby PJ (2006) Serotonin receptors modulate trigeminovascular responses in ventroposteromedial nucleus of thalamus: A migraine target? *Neurobiol Dis* 23, 491–501.

20. Longmore J, Shaw D, Smith D, *et al.* (1997) Differential distribution of 5HT$_{1D}$- and 5HT$_{1B}$-immunoreactivity within the human trigemino-cerebrovascular system: implications for the discovery of new antimigraine drugs. *Cephalalgia* 17, 833–42.

21. Gomez-Mancilla B, Cutler NR, Leibowitz MT, *et al.* (2001) Safety and efficacy of PNU-142633, a selective 5-HT$_{1D}$ agonist, in patients with acute migraine. *Cephalalgia* 21, 727–32.

22. Goadsby PJ (2007) Serotonin receptor ligands: treatments of acute migraine and cluster headache. *Handb Exp Pharmacol* 177, 129–43.

23. Chambers MS, Street LJ, Goodacre S, *et al.* (1999) 3-(Piperazinylpropyl)indoles: selective, orally bioavailable h5-HT$_{1D}$ receptor agonists as potential antimigraine agents. *J Med Chem* 42, 691–705.

24. Isaac M, Slassi A (2001) Recent advances in 5-HT$_{1D}$-selective agonists. *IDrugs* 4, 189–96.

25. Goldstein DJ, Roon KI, Offen WW, *et al.* (2001) Selective serotonin$_{1F}$ (5-HT$_{1F}$) receptor agonist in acute migraine: a randomised controlled trial. *Lancet* 358, 1230–4.

26. Pouzet B (2002) SB-258741: a 5-HT$_7$ receptor antagonist of potential clinical interest. *CNS Drug Rev* 8, 90–100.

27. Den Boer MO, Heiligers JPC, Saxena PR (1991) Carotid vascular effects of ergotamine and dihydroergotamine in the pig: no exclusive mediation via 5-HT$_1$-like receptors. *Br J Pharmacol* 104, 183–9.

28. De Vries P, Villalón CM, Heiligers JPC, Saxena PR (1998) Characterisation of 5-HT receptors mediating constriction of porcine carotid arteriovenous anastomoses; involvement of 5-HT$_{1B/1D}$ and novel receptors. *Br J Pharmacol* 123, 1561–70.

15

Effect of two novel calcitonin gene-related peptide-binding compounds in a closed cranial window rat model

Louise Juhl, Lars Edvinsson, Jes Olesen, and Inger Jansen-Olesen

Noxious stimulation of dural and cerebral arteries is known to elicit migraine pain.[1] Calcitonin gene-related peptide (CGRP) is the most abundant peptide in trigeminal perivascular nerve fibres that innervate various pain sensitive intracranial structures.[2,3] Two potential migraine therapeutic agents capable of tightly and specifically binding CGRP have been developed; a CGRP-binding RNA-Spiegelmer (NOX-C89) and a CGRP monoclonal antibody.[4] The NOX-C89 is highly resistant to degradation and able to inhibit the function of the target peptide.[5,6] When PEGylated, NOX-C89 has a half-life of 12 h.[5] The CGRP-binding antibody has been raised in rabbit for the use in CGRP-related disorders, such as migraine.[4] In the present study, the RNA-Spiegelmer (NOX-C89) and the CGRP antibody were examined in the *in vivo* genuine closed cranial window model[7,8] to investigate whether they were able to inhibit CGRP-induced and neurogenically induced vasodilatation of dural and pial artery.

Methods

Male Sprague–Dawley rats ($n = 12$) were anaesthetized and the trachea was intubated. Catheters were placed in the left and right femoral artery and vein for the continuous measurement of blood pressure, sampling of blood for gas tension analysis, infusion of anaesthetic, and infusion of the test substance. The bone was thinned with a drill and a bipolar stimulation electrode was placed above the cortical surface of the cranial window to induce neurogenically dilatation (25 V, 5 Hz, 1 ms pulse width and 10 s duration). For visualization of the middle meningeal artery and pial artery, a video-microscope was used and a video dimension analyser continuously measured the diameter of the arteries. During the entire experiment, changes in dimensions arising from vessel constriction or dilatation were automatically followed by rapid time resolution and displayed on a digital panel. Dilatation of the vessels and changes in blood pressure were calculated as the percentage change from baseline, which was defined as the average of the 60 s preceding the administration of test substance. Vessel diameter was measured at the peak response occurring 1–2 min after drug administration.

Results

There was no significant difference between first electrical stimulation and stimulation after infusion of NOX-C89 in any of the arteries (data not shown). Furthermore, there was no change in blood pressure after electrical stimulation (data not shown). The first infusion of CGRP induced a significant dilatation of the dural artery (38 ± 17%, Figure 15.1A) and of the pial artery (14 ± 1%, Figure 15.1B). After administration of NOX-C89, infusion of CGRP resulted in a significantly smaller increase of the dural artery ($P < 0.05$) compared with the first CGRP infusion. Also in pial arteries

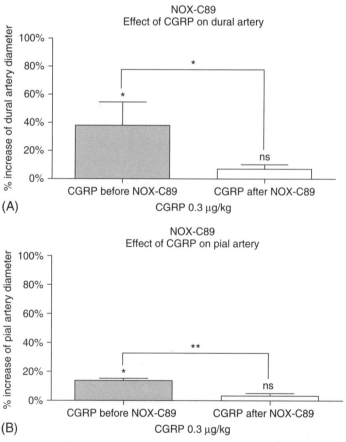

Fig. 15.1 Effect of PEGylated NOX-C89 on calcitonin gene-related peptide (CGRP)-induced vasodilatation of dural and pial artery ($n = 6$). *Indicates significantly different from baseline or significantly different from first administration ($P < 0.05$, **$P < 0.01$). ns indicates not significantly different from baseline values ($P > 0.05$).

CGRP caused a significantly smaller dilatation in the presence of NOX-C89 ($P < 0.01$, Figure 15.1B). PEGylated NOX-C89 infusion by itself had no effect on any of the investigated parameters.

The difference in response to electrical stimulation with and without the CGRP antibody was not significant ($P > 0.05$) (data not shown). Without antibody, the infusion of CGRP resulted in a dilatation of the dural artery diameter of $23 \pm 5\%$ compared with $12 \pm 3\%$ in the presence of the antibody ($P < 0.05$, Figure 15.2A). There was no significant inhibition of pial artery dilatation to CGRP infusion in the presence of the antibody ($P > 0.05$, Figure 15.2B).

Discussion

In the present study electrical stimulation evoked a reproducible dilatation of dural and pial vessels, mediated via CGRP release. The effect was not blocked by a 1 mg/kg

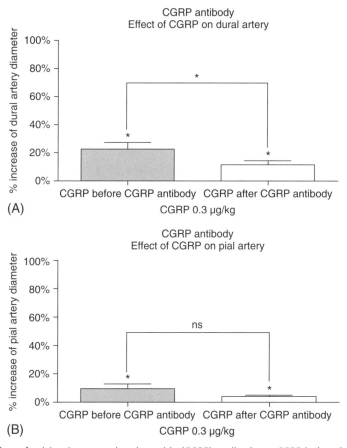

Fig. 15.2 Effect of calcitonin gene-related peptide (CGRP) antibody on CGRP-induced vasodilatation of dural and pial artery ($n = 6$). *Indicates significantly different from baseline or significantly different from first administration ($P < 0.05$). ns indicates not significantly different from first treatment (line between the two columns) ($P > 0.05$).

intravenous infusion of the PEGylated NOX-C89. However, previous studies with a continuous infusion of 5 mg/kg non-PEGylated NOX-C89 showed significant inhibition of the mean increase in meningeal artery blood flow after electrical stimulation.[9] NOX-C89 leaves the body extremely fast (half-life 10–30 min) when administered intravenously. Thus, the non-PEGylated NOX-C89 would not be effective for therapeutic use due to its rapid clearance. This situation can be addressed by attaching large molecules, e.g. polyethylene glycol (PEG) to the NOX-C89 to reduce its elimination and increase its presence in the circulation. During intravenous infusion of 0.3 µg/kg CGRP, PEGylated NOX-C89 significantly inhibited the dilatation in both cerebral and dural arteries. It is suggested that the intravenous administration of the PEGylated NOX-C89 is likely to bind to circulating CGRP thus preventing the neuropeptide from activating its receptors. In the concentrations used, PEGylated NOX-C89 is effective, but unlikely to penetrate the vessel wall and the blood–brain barrier because it could not inhibit dilatation of the pial artery evoked by electrical stimulation.

Administration of a CGRP antibody caused no significant inhibition of the vasodilatation brought about by electrical stimulation in any of the arteries. Similar results were found with another monoclonal CGRP antibody, rat monoclonal antibody C4.19 IgG (1–3 mg), which did not block skin blood flow response to antidromic nerve stimulation.[10] When given acutely, the CGRP antibody is unlikely to penetrate the tissue of the cranial vessels and thereby reach the synaptic cleft. Thus, it is unable to achieve blockade of perivascular CGRP, which is released upon electrical stimulation.

In the present study, the CGRP antibody did not show any effect on CGRP-induced dilatation of the pial artery. The evoked dilatation of the dural artery was, however, significantly blocked by the CGRP antibody. From previous studies we have concluded that the effect on pial arteries is mostly or completely autoregulatory and secondary to a drop in systemic blood pressure and thus not a direct effect of CGRP on the smooth muscle receptors in pial arteries.[11] However, in a novel *in vitro* study using myograph baths we have in rat middle cerebral arteries found that the CGRP antibody inhibited the CGRP-induced relaxation in a concentration-dependent manner.[4] Thus, the inhibition of dural but not pial artery dilatation suggests that the passage of the CGRP antibody over the blood–brain barrier is very slow.

In conclusion, we observed that neither the PEGylated NOX-C89 nor the CGRP antibody inhibited the dilatation caused by electrical stimulation of the dural and pial arteries. Both the PEGylated NOX-C89 and the CGRP antibody were, however, able to significantly inhibit CGRP-induced vasodilatation of the dural artery while the effect on the pial artery was inhibited only after administration of NOX-C89.

References

1. Ray B (1940) Experimental studies on headaches, pain sensitive structures of the head and their significance in headaches. *Arch Surg* 41, 813–56.
2. Uddman R, Edvinsson L (1989) Neuropeptides in the cerebral circulation. *Cerebrovasc Brain Metab Rev* 1, 230–52.

3. Edvinsson L, Gulbenkian S, Barroso CP, Cunha e Sa M, Polak JM, Mortensen A, Jorgensen L, Jansen-Olesen I (1998) Innervation of the human middle meningeal artery: immunohistochemistry, ultrastructure, and role of endothelium for vasomotility. *Peptides* 19, 1213–25.

4. Edvinsson L, Nilsson E, Jansen-Olesen I (2007) Inhibitory effect of BIBN4096BS, CGRP(8–37), a CGRP antibody and an RNA-Spiegelmer on CGRP induced vasodilatation in the perfused and non-perfused rat middle cerebral artery. *Br J Pharmacol* 150, 633–40.

5. Vater A, Klussmann S (2003) Toward third-generation aptamers: Spiegelmers and their therapeutic prospects. *Curr Opin Drug Discov Dev* 6, 253–61.

6. Helmling S, Maasch C, Eulberg D, Buchner K, Schroder W, Lange C, Vonhoff S, Wlotzka B, Tschop MH, Rosewicz S, Klussmann S (2004) Inhibition of ghrelin action in vitro and in vivo by an RNA-Spiegelmer. *Proc Natl Acad Sci USA* 101, 13174–9.

7. Williamson DJ, Hargreaves RJ, Hill RG, Shepheard SL (1997) Intravital microscope studies on the effects of neurokinin agonists and calcitonin gene-related peptide on dural vessel diameter in the anaesthetized rat. *Cephalalgia* 17, 518–24.

8. Petersen KA, Dyrby L, Williamson D, Edvinsson L, Olesen J (2005) Effect of hypotension and carbon dioxide changes in an improved genuine closed cranial window rat model. *Cephalalgia* 25, 23–9.

9. Denekas T, Troltzsch M, Vater A, Klussmann S, Messlinger K (2006) Inhibition of stimulated meningeal blood flow by a calcitonin gene-related peptide binding mirror-image RNA oligonucleotide. *Br J Pharmacol* 148, 536–43.

10. Tan KK, Brown MJ, Hargreaves RJ, Shepheard SL, Cook DA, Hill RG (1995) Calcitonin gene-related peptide as an endogenous vasodilator: immunoblockade studies in vivo with an anti-calcitonin gene-related peptide monoclonal antibody and its Fab′ fragment. *Clin Sci (Lond)* 89, 565–73.

11. Petersen KA, Lassen LH, Birk S, Lesko L, Olesen J (2005) BIBN4096BS antagonizes human alpha-calcitonin gene related peptide-induced headache and extracerebral artery dilatation. *Clin Pharmacol Ther* 77, 202–13.

16

Vasoactive intestinal polypeptide is unlikely to be a target for headache and migraine treatment

Jakob Møller Hansen, Alexandra Maria Rahmann, Jes Olesen, and Messoud Ashina

Introduction

For a long time, the parasympathetic nervous system has been implicated in the patho-genesis of migraine[1] and the last years have put increasing focus on the role of the parasympathetic system in migraine.[2–4] It has been suggested that the parasympathetic outflow to cephalic vasculature may trigger activation and sensitization of perivascular sensory afferents[4] and thereby migraine pain.

Parasympathetic efferent nerves release various neuropeptides including vasoactive intestinal polypeptide (VIP) to regulate haemodynamics of the brain.[5] Both *in vitro* and *in vivo* studies have demonstrated that VIP acts as a powerful vasodilator in various species, including humans,[6–8] and there is evidence that VIP level is increased in the jugular venous blood during migraine attacks in a subgroup of patients with migraine associated with marked autonomic symptoms[9] and in patients with cluster headache.[10]

The headache eliciting effect of VIP and its effect on brain haemodynamics have not been systematically studied in humans. We therefore conducted two studies to test the following hypotheses:

1. Infusion of VIP induces headache and arterial dilatation in healthy volunteers (study I).[11]

2. Infusion of VIP induces migraine and arterial dilatation in patients with migraine without aura (study II).[12]

Design and methods

In two randomized, double-blinded, placebo-controlled crossover studies, the subjects (12 healthy volunteers and 13 migraineurs) were allocated to receive 8 pmol/kg per min VIP or placebo (isotonic saline) over 25 min on 2 days separated by at least 1 week in two randomized, double-blinded, placebo-controlled crossover fashion. For statistical analy-sis the area under the curve (AUC) between VIP and placebo day was compared.[13]

The following variables were recorded:

* headache intensity on a verbal rating scale from 0 to 10;
* the middle cerebral artery (MCA) blood flow velocity ($V_{meanMCA}$) by transcranial Doppler;
* the diameter of the superficial temporal artery by a high-resolution ultrasonography unit.

In addition, plasma levels of VIP were measured by radioimmunoassay, and in study I we recorded the cerebral blood flow (CBF) by single-photon emission computed tomography (SPECT).

Results

Study I

Vasoactive intestinal polypeptide induced headache in healthy volunteers

During the immediate phase (0–30 min), five subjects reported headache on the VIP day and one subject on the placebo day (Table 16.1). The AUC from 0 to 30 min was significantly higher on the VIP day, 0 (0–23.8), than on the placebo day, 0 (0–0) ($P = 0.04$) (Figure 16.1). Six subjects reported delayed headache, three on each trial day. We found no difference in the $AUC_{delayed\ headache}$ recorded from 120 min to 12 h after infusion between VIP and placebo days ($P = 0.75$).

Middle cerebral artery blood flow velocity and cerebral blood flow

During the immediate phase ($AUC_{0-30min}$), $V_{meanMCA}$ decreased significantly on the VIP day compared with the placebo day ($P < 0.001$) with a mean difference in peak response between VIP and placebo at T_{20} of –11.3% (–16% to –6.6%, 95% CI). There were no changes after VIP for global CBF ($AUC_{0-60min}$, $P = 0.10$) or for regional CBF_{MCA} ($AUC_{0-60min}$, $P = 0.10$) when compared with placebo. The mean changes in MCA diameter were calculated to be 8.4% (SD 6.2) between baseline and T_{20} for VIP and

Table 16.1 Number of controls and patients reporting headache and migraine headache.

	VIP	Placebo	P
Study I			
Immediate phase (0–30 min)	5/12	1/12	0.13
Post-infusion phase (30–120 min)	3/12	2/12	1.00
Delayed headache (3–11 h)	3/12	3/12	1.00
Migraine-like headache	1/12	0/12	1.00
Study II			
Immediate phase (0–30 min)	10/13	0/13	0.002
Post-infusion phase (30–120 min)	7/13	4/13	0.51
Delayed headache (3–11 h)	3/13	2/13	1.00
Migraine-like headache	0/13	1/13	1.00

Groups compared and tested with the McNemar test.

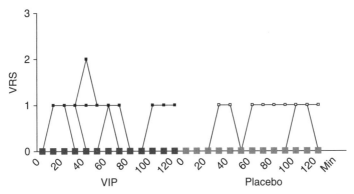

Fig. 16.1 Headache response for healthy volunteers. Individual and median headache scores on a verbal rating scale (VRS). There was no difference in the number of subjects who reported headache in the immediate phase (0–30 min) after vasoactive intestinal polypeptide (VIP; five subjects) and after placebo (one subject) ($P = 0.13$). During the post-infusion period (30–120 min), three subjects reported headache on the VIP day and three on the placebo day.

4.6% (SD 9.3) between baseline and T_{20} for placebo, without significant difference between VIP and placebo ($P = 0.29$). During the post-infusion period ($AUC_{30-120min}$), there was no difference between VIP and placebo days ($P = 0.17$).

Superficial temporal artery (STA)

During the immediate phase ($AUC_{0-30min}$), the diameter of STA increased significantly on the VIP day compared with the placebo day ($P = 0.04$). The mean peak increase in STA diameter was 27.8% (SD 12.1) at T_{20} compared with baseline.

Plasma vasoactive intestinal polypeptide

Plasma VIP was significantly higher on VIP days compared with placebo ($AUC_{0-80min}$, $P < 0.001$). Peak plasma concentration of VIP was measured at the end of the infusion ($T_{25\ min}$) on the VIP day and was 111.4 (SD 47.8) pmol/l.

Study II

Vasoactive intestinal polypeptide induced headache in migraine without aura

None of the patients reported migraine after VIP infusion. One subject developed a migraine attack after placebo infusion.

During the immediate phase (0–30 min), ten patients reported a mild headache on the VIP day but none of the patients reported headache on the placebo day (Table 16.1). The $AUC_{0-30\ min}$ on the VIP day, 23 (6–25), was significantly larger than on the placebo day, 5 (0–40) ($P = 0.005$) (Figure 16.2). Three patients reported delayed headache on the VIP day (3–11 h after start of infusion) and two patients on the placebo day (3–11 h after start of infusion). We found no difference in the $AUC_{delayed}$ headache recorded from 120 min to 12 h after start of infusion between VIP, 0 (0–3) and placebo days, 0 (0–0) ($P = 0.89$).

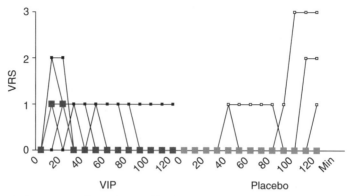

Fig. 16.2 Headache response for patients with migraine without aura. More patients reported headache in the immediate phase (0–30 min) after vasoactive intestinal polypeptide (VIP; 10 patients) than after placebo (0 patients) ($P = 0.002$). During the post-infusion period (30–120 min), seven patients reported headache on the VIP day and four patients on the placebo day.

Middle cerebral artery blood flow velocity

During the immediate phase ($AUC_{0-30min}$), $V_{meanMCA}$ decreased significantly on the VIP day compared with the placebo ($P = 0.001$). The peak response was 16.3% (SD 5.9) on the VIP day and 0.01% (SD 4.3) on the placebo day at T_{20}, compared with baseline.

Superficial temporal artery

During immediate phase ($AUC_{0-30min}$), the diameter of STA increased significantly on the VIP day compared with the placebo day ($P < 0.001$). Peak increase in STA diameter occurred 20 min after start of VIP infusion and was 46.0% (SD 13.9) compared to baseline.

Plasma vasoactive intestinal polypeptide

The $AUC_{plasmaVIP\ 0-30min}$ was significantly higher on the VIP day compared with the placebo day ($P < 0.001$), but there was no significant difference in the postinfusion period 30–120 min ($P = 0.07$).

Discussion

The major outcome of the present studies is that systemic administration of the powerful vasodilator VIP induces only a very mild and short-lasting headache, and no migraine attacks.

Can vasoactive intestinal polypeptide induce headache?

Experimental vasodilatation of the internal carotid artery and MCA was able to induce focal head pain in humans,[14] and in migraine attacks associated with MCA dilatation, both pain and dilatation could be reversed by sumatriptan.[15] Although VIP induced a marked dilatation of cranial arteries, it caused only a very mild and short-lasting headache.

This mild headache response is probably not due to an insufficient dosage of VIP. Compared with the endogenous VIP level, we found a very high plasma concentration during VIP infusion (mean 111.4 pmol/l). The effects of exogenous VIP are mediated through $VPAC_1$ and $VPAC_2$ receptors, which have a binding affinity (IC_{50}) of 1 to 4 nM.[16] The high prevalence of systemic adverse effects, such as a substantial increase in heart rate on the VIP day, facial flushing (92%), palpitations (67%), and feeling of warmth (75%) during infusion in healthy volunteers, indicates that the VIP dosage was high enough to activate the VIP receptors and induce marked haemodynamic effects.

Slow passage of VIP across the blood–brain barrier (BBB) is another possibility. We observed a mild and short decrease in V_{MCA} and no change in CBF, while the dilatation of the STA was more pronounced and longer lasting. This difference in response between two vascular beds could be caused by the BBB as the STA has no barrier. If the BBB is bypassed and VIP injected intracisternally in dogs, a persistent vasodilatation (120 min) was reported in the basilar artery.[17] In mice, only 0.15% of the injected VIP could be found in the brain 10 min after intravenous administration[18] but if a VIP-analogue is coupled to a transport vector, more of the perfusate can be found in the brain after 10 min.[19] If the BBB is bypassed, VIP is able to increase CBF in rats[20] and baboons.[21] Collectively, these data indicate that the BBB is very tight in arterioles, but less tight in the MCA. Dilatation of STA seems without headache inducing effect as previously described,[22,23] while the mild and short-lasting effect on MCA corresponds to a mild and short-lasting headache. In conclusion, despite a marked vasodilator effect in the extracranial vessels and increased plasma VIP, healthy subjects developed only a very mild headache after VIP.

Why did vasoactive intestinal polypeptide fail to induce migraine?

Migraine patients show increased sensitivity to a range of vasodilators,[15,24] but even a marked VIP-induced vasodilatation of cranial arteries was not sufficient to trigger migraine attacks in patients with migraine without aura.

A model has been proposed in which migraine is the result of activation of postganglionic parasympathetic neurons in the sphenopalatine ganglion, resulting in vasodilatation and local release of inflammatory molecules that activate meningeal nociceptors.[25] Based on this, we speculated that systemic administration of VIP might cause headache by inducing vasodilatation and activation or sensitization of nociceptors.

Exogenous VIP, like in our study, reaches a high concentration on the endothelial VIP-receptor, VPAC1, which has been found on the endothelium in pigs.[26] Vasodilatation caused by activation of these receptors is likely co-mediated by nitric oxide release from parasympathetic efferents.[26] In that case, one would expect the same response after intravenous VIP as after infusion of the nitric oxide donor, glyceryl trinitrate, i.e. initial vasodilatation and induction of a delayed migraine attack.[24] Nitric oxide and VIP act predominantly synergistically in respect to vessel tone, but the two transmitters may act as antagonists in inflammatory processes.[27,28] This may explain why VIP failed to induce migraine attacks.

The binding of VIP to its receptors activates the adenylate cyclase, increases cellular cAMP,[29] and causes vasodilatation.[30] Other compounds increasing the cAMP levels, such as calcitonin gene-related peptide[31] and cilostazol[32] have been found to have a headache-inducing effect in healthy volunteers and a migraine eliciting effect in migraine patients.

Another possible headache mechanism is direct activation and sensitization of sensory afferents around cerebral blood vessels by exogenous VIP. Slow passage of VIP across the BBB[18,21] may have prevented migraine, if VIP receptors on perivascular nerve terminals are relevant for migraine induction. This may explain why VIP failed to induce migraine attacks.

Experimental vasodilatation and delayed migraine attack

Spontaneous migraine attacks are accompanied by dilatation of the MCA[33] and experimental headache and migraine induced by glyceryl trinitrate, histamine, calcitonin gene-related peptide and dipyridamole are associated with initial vasodilatation,[24,31,34–36] which could imply that vasodilatation may play a major part in triggering migraine attacks.

So far, all cerebral vasodilators that have been tested are able to induce headache in healthy subjects and migraine in migraine sufferers. VIP is the first substance that markedly dilates intra- and extracranial arteries but nevertheless does not induce migraine. It has been demonstrated that sildenafil (a PDE 5 inhibitor) triggers migraine attacks without changes in the MCA diameter.[37] Thus, migraine induction can occur without arterial dilatation. In summary, these results further weaken the hypothesis of a purely vascular origin of migraine.

Conclusions

Intravenous infusion of VIP induces only a very mild and short-lasting headache in both healthy controls and in patients with migraine without aura. Thus, our initial hypothesis, that the powerful vasodilator VIP might be a trigger factor for headache and migraine, and ability to induce migraine attacks could not be confirmed.

We suggest that VIP is not critically involved in migraine pathogenesis, and in contrast to calcitonin gene-related peptide,[38] antagonism to VIP is unlikely to be a beneficial migraine treatment.

Acknowledgements

The authors would like to acknowledge the important contribution to the original papers from our co-authors: Troels Wienecke MD, John Sitarz MD, Steffen Birk PhD, Peter Sandor Oturai PhD, and Jan Fahrenkrug PhD.

References

1. Möllendorff W (1867) Über hemikranie. *Arch Pathol Anat Klin Med* 41, 385–95.
2. Avnon Y, Nitzan M, Sprecher E, Rogowski Z, Yarnitsky D (2003) Different patterns of parasympathetic activation in uni- and bilateral migraineurs. *Brain* 126, 1660–70.

3. Janig W (2003) Relationship between pain and autonomic phenomena in headache and other pain conditions. *Cephalalgia* 23 (Suppl 1), 43–8.

4. Yarnitsky D, Goor-Aryeh I, Bajwa ZH, Ransil BI, Cutrer FM, Sottile A, Burstein R (2003) Wolff Award: Possible parasympathetic contributions to peripheral and central sensitization during migraine. *Headache* 43(7), 704–14.

5. Gulbenkian S, Uddman R, Edvinsson L (2001) Neuronal messengers in the human cerebral circulation. *Peptides* 22, 995–1007.

6. White RP (1987) Responses of human basilar arteries to vasoactive intestinal polypeptide. *Life Sci* 41, 1155–63.

7. Suzuki Y, McMaster D, Lederis K, Rorstad OP (1984) Characterization of the relaxant effects of vasoactive intestinal peptide (VIP) and PHI on isolated brain arteries. *Brain Res* 322, 9–16.

8. Edvinsson L, Ekman R, Jansen I, Ottosson A, Uddman R (1987) Peptide-containing nerve fibers in human cerebral arteries: immunocytochemistry, radioimmunoassay, and in vitro pharmacology. *Ann Neurol* 21, 431–7.

9. Goadsby PJ, Edvinsson L, Ekman R (1990) Vasoactive peptide release in the extracerebral circulation of humans during migraine headache. *Ann Neurol* 28, 183–7.

10. Edvinsson L, Goadsby PJ (1994) Neuropeptides in migraine and cluster headache. *Cephalalgia* 14, 320–7.

11. Hansen J, Sitarz J, Birk S, Rahmann Oturai P, Fahrenkrug, *et al.* (2006) Vasoactive intestinal polypeptide evokes only a minimal headache in healthy volunteers. *Cephalalgia* 26(8), 992–1003.

12. Rahmann A, Wienecke T, Hansen JM, Fahrenkrug J, Olesen J, Ashina M (2008) Vasoactive intestinal peptide causes marked cephalic vasodilation but does not induce migraine. *Cephalalgia* 28(3), 226–36.

13. Matthews JN, Altman DG, Campbell MJ, Royston P (1990) Analysis of serial measurements in medical research. *BMJ* 300, 230–5.

14. Nichols FT, 3rd, Mawad M, Mohr JP, Stein B, Hilal S, Michelsen WJ (1990) Focal headache during balloon inflation in the internal carotid and middle cerebral arteries. *Stroke* 21(4), 555–9.

15. Friberg L, Olesen J, Iversen HK, Sperling B (1991) Migraine pain associated with middle cerebral artery dilatation: reversal by sumatriptan. *Lancet* 338, 13–17.

16. Harmar AJ, Arimura A, Gozes I, Journot L, Laburthe M, Pisegna JR, *et al.* (1998) International Union of Pharmacology. XVIII. Nomenclature of receptors for vasoactive intestinal peptide and pituitary adenylate cyclase-activating polypeptide. *Pharmacol Rev* 50(2), 265–70.

17. Seki Y, Suzuki Y, Baskaya MK, Kano T, Saito K, Takayasu M, *et al.* (1995) The effects of pituitary adenylate cyclase-activating polypeptide on cerebral arteries and vertebral artery blood flow in anesthetized dogs. *Eur J Pharmacol* 275, 259–66.

18. Dogrukol-Ak D, Banks WA, Tuncel N, Tuncel M (2003) Passage of vasoactive intestinal peptide across the blood-brain barrier. *Peptides* 24, 437–44.

19. Bickel U, Yoshikawa T, Landaw EM, Faull KF, Pardridge WM (1993) Pharmacologic effects in vivo in brain by vector-mediated peptide drug delivery. *Proc Natl Acad Sci USA* 90, 2618–22.

20. Wu D, Pardridge WM (1996) Central nervous system pharmacologic effect in conscious rats after intravenous injection of a biotinylated vasoactive intestinal peptide analog coupled to a blood-brain barrier drug delivery system. *J Pharmacol Exp Ther* 279, 77–83.

21. McCulloch J, Edvinsson L (1980) Cerebral circulatory and metabolic effects of vasoactive intestinal polypeptide. *Am J Physiol* 238, H449–56.

22. Drummond PD, Lance JW (1983) Extracranial vascular changes and the source of pain in migraine headache. *Ann Neurol* 13, 32–7.

23. Myers DE, Boone SC, Gregg JM (1982) Superficial temporal arterial dilation without headache in extracranial-intracranial bypass patients. *Headache* 22, 118–21.

24. Thomsen LL, Kruuse C, Iversen HK, Olesen J (1994) A nitric oxide donor (nitroglycerin) triggers genuine migraine attacks. *Eur J Neurol* 1, 73–80.

25. Burstein R, Jakubowski M (2005) Unitary hypothesis for multiple triggers of the pain and strain of migraine. *J Comp Neurol* 493, 9–14.

26. Grant S, Lutz EM, McPhaden AR, Wadsworth RM (2006) Location and function of VPAC1, VPAC2 and NPR-C receptors in VIP-induced vasodilation of porcine basilar arteries. *J Cereb Blood Flow Metab* 26, 58–67.

27. Delgado M, Munoz-Elias EJ, Gomariz RP, Ganea D (1999) Vasoactive intestinal peptide and pituitary adenylate cyclase-activating polypeptide prevent inducible nitric oxide synthase transcription in macrophages by inhibiting NF-kappa B and IFN regulatory factor 1 activation. *J Immunol* 162, 4685–96.

28. Bandyopadhyay A, Chakder S, Rattan S (1997) Regulation of inducible and neuronal nitric oxide synthase gene expression by interferon-gamma and VIP. *Am J Physiol* 272, C1790–7.

29. McCulloch DA, Mackenzie CJ, Johnson MS, Robertson DN, Holland PJ, Ronaldson E, *et al.* (2002) Additional signals from VPAC/PAC family receptors. *Biochem Soc Trans* 30(4), 441–6.

30. Paterno R, Faraci FM, Heistad DD (1996) Role of Ca(2+)-dependent K+ channels in cerebral vasodilatation induced by increases in cyclic GMP and cyclic AMP in the rat. *Stroke* 27, 1603–7; Discussion 1607–8.

31. Lassen LH, Haderslev PA, Jacobsen VB, Iversen HK, Sperling B, Olesen J (2002) CGRP may play a causative role in migraine. *Cephalalgia* 22, 54–61.

32. Birk S, Kruuse C, Petersen KA, Tfelt-Hansen P, Olesen J (2006) The headache-inducing effect of cilostazol in human volunteers. *Cephalalgia* 26, 1304–9.

33. Thomsen LL, Iversen HK, Olesen J (1995) Cerebral blood flow velocities are reduced during attacks of unilateral migraine without aura. *Cephalalgia* 15, 109–16.

34. Kruuse C, Jacobsen TB, Lassen LH, Thomsen LL, Hasselbalch SG, Dige-Petersen H, Olesen J, (2000) Dipyridamole dilates large cerebral arteries concomitant to headache induction in healthy subjects. *J Cereb Blood Flow Metab* 20(9), 1372–9.

35. Kruuse C, Lassen LH, Iversen HK, Oestergaard S, Olesen J (2006) Dipyridamole may induce migraine in patients with migraine without aura. *Cephalalgia* 26, 925–33.

36. Lassen LH, Christiansen I, Iversen HK, Jansen-Olesen I, Olesen J (2003) The effect of nitric oxide synthase inhibition on histamine induced headache and arterial dilatation in migraineurs. *Cephalalgia* 23, 877–86.

37. Kruuse C, Thomsen LL, Birk S, Olesen J (2003) Migraine can be induced by sildenafil without changes in middle cerebral artery diameter. *Brain* 126, 241–7.

38. Olesen J, Diener HC, Husstedt IW, Goadsby PJ, Hall D, Meier U, *et al.* (2004) Calcitonin gene-related peptide receptor antagonist BIBN 4096 BS for the acute treatment of migraine. *N Engl J Med* 350(11), 1104–10.

17

Discussion summary: Calcitonin gene-related peptide and 5-hydroxytryptamine modulators

Rigmor Jensen

The potential role in the acute and prophylactic treatment of migraine by means of calcitonin gene-related peptide antagonists were debated. The initiating question was raised by Lars-Jacob Stovner, Trondheim, Norway about the stable blood pressure after the use of calcitonin gene-related peptide (CGRP) antagonists when CGRP is known as a potent vasodilator.

Several questions were also directed to Stephanie Kane about MK 0974, which is known to have a very high affinity of 1.4 nM for the rhesus CGRP receptor. However, very high plasma levels between 120 and 1000 nM are required to block CGRP-mediated skin dilatation in rhesus monkeys. How can one explain the high plasma levels required? Likewise there were several questions regarding the mode of action of MK 974. Does it function via a central mode of action and is it a selective central effect or can a peripheral action be excluded?

It was replied that only a small percentage of MK 974 crosses the blood–brain barrier and that may be the primary reason for the very few central nervous system side-effects noted in the clinical trials and the fairly high plasma levels required. Whether the mode of action is central or peripheral remains yet to be clarified.

Likewise Professor Doeds and Stephanie Kane debated the supplementary questions: can MK 974 also inhibit secondary hyperalgesia in the capsaicin model/rhesus model and does MK 974 influence CGRP levels following the capsaicin administration? The underlying pathophysiological role of CGRP in migraine was also debated; is the release of CGRP a stress response and secondary to the pain or is it released as an initiator of the migraine attack itself, an early mediator of the entire migraine cascade? The role of CGRP in other neurovascular diseases such as stroke and subarachnoidal haemorrhage are still under investigation.

The mechanisms of action of triptans was discussed by Professor Saxena in relation to the development of medication overuse headache. Triptans can fairly easily lead to the development of medication overuse headache but apparently also to fairly short-lasting rebound headache as compared with ergotamins or simple analgesics. As in epilepsy, 20–25% of migraine patients have absolutely no response to a given treatment, and are quite often listed as refractory patients. In this case, 20–25% of migraine patients are also refractive to the triptans independent of mode of administration. On a clinical basis, we cannot separate these patients via their phenotype but is it possible to characterize their reaction by other modalities? Saxena had no clear answer to that but the question gave rise to a lively discussion about acute migraine medications and their susceptibility to develop medication overuse headache. Should these refractory patients be treated with a combination therapy of a neuronal nitric oxide synthase inhibitor and a triptan or should their dosage be completely different? It could be highly interesting to characterize these patients on a molecular as well as on a clinical basis.

A question was addressed to Professor Saxena about the concentration of 5-hydroxy-tryptamine (5-HT) in perivascular nerves and the role of a peripheral versus a central mode of action of 5-HT receptor agonists was debated again. Alison Pilgrim replied to this discussion that 5-HT_{1F} are effective in the animal models but a very high dose is needed so far, and the potential role of toxicity is still under investigation.

A 5-HT_7 receptor antagonist could also be of interest but it should be made clear whether there are some central nervous system side-effects and crossing of the blood–brain barriers.

The poster sessions about vasoactive intestinal peptide and CGRP antibodies were presented by Louise Juhl and then discussed by the panel. In general, a caution about treatment with CGRP antibodies was emphasized as a more constant and stable CGRP blockade may provoke a rebound effect and cause other vascular health problems. It was concluded that the primary role of CGRPs in the central nervous system needs additional clarification before the role of CGRP antibodies in migraine can be established.

Session V

Ion channel modulators and antiepileptics

18

Migraine: from genes to pathophysiology – transgenic mouse models of migraine

Arn M.J.M. van den Maagdenberg

Migraine is a common, disabling, multifactorial, episodic neurovascular disorder of unknown aetiology.[1,2] The disease is typically characterized by recurrent attacks of severe throbbing unilateral headache that are accompanied by nausea and vomiting, and sensitivity to light and sound.[3] Attacks last from hours to several days. This type of migraine is called migraine without aura. In about one-third of patients the migraine attack is accompanied or preceded by transient focal neurological symptoms, known as the 'aura' (migraine with aura). Aura symptoms usually last less than 1 h and nearly always include visual symptoms. Less often sensory or aphasic symptoms are experienced, and rarely, motor ones. Up to one-third of migraineurs have both types of attacks during their lifetime. Some patients may have attacks of migraine aura without headache.[1,2] Migraine patients may experience premonitory symptoms such as retaining fluid, feeling tired, or having difficulty concentrating, which occur hours to a day or two before a migraine attack.[4]

Current treatment options for migraine patients are not optimal as not all patients respond to acute therapies and headache recurrence is a common problem. The choice of acute medication depends on severity and frequency of the headache and associated symptoms, the preferences of, the contraindications for, and the history of the patient (for review see reference 5). Mild attacks may be managed with analgesics or non-steroidal anti-inflammatory drugs while triptans may be used for more disabling attacks and for attacks that do not adequately respond to analgesics.[1,6] The prophylactic drugs in migraine with the best-documented effectiveness are the β-blockers, sodium valproate and topiramate and flunarizine. However, in general, the efficacy of migraine prophylactic drugs is limited: at most 55% will have a 50% reduction of the attack frequency.[7] In addition, currently available prophylactic drugs have a large risk of adverse effects. Clearly, better, especially prophylactic, well tolerated treatment options are needed. To identify novel treatment targets, it is important to unravel the molecular biological mechanisms in migraine. Most likely, migraineurs have a genetically determined reduced trigger threshold for migraine triggers. Therefore, the identification of 'threshold genes' and deciphering their function will help to unravel the triggering mechanisms for migraine attacks.

Genetic studies in hemiplegic migraine

Genetic factors play an important part in migraine pathophysiology by lowering the trigger threshold for migraine attacks. Genetic research in migraine has mainly focused on the identification of genes involved in familial hemiplegic migraine (FHM).[8] FHM is a rare, severe, monogenic subtype of migraine with aura, characterized by at least some degree of hemiparesis during the aura.[3] The hemiparesis may last from minutes to several hours or even days. Patients are frequently initially misdiagnosed with epilepsy. Apart from the hemiparesis, the other headache and aura features of the FHM attack are identical to those of attacks of the common types of migraine. In addition to attacks with hemiparesis, the majority of FHM patients also experience attacks of 'normal' migraine with or without aura. As in the common forms of migraine, attacks of FHM may be triggered by mild head trauma. Thus, from a clinical point of view, FHM seems a valid model for the common forms of migraine (for review see reference 9). Major clinical differences, apart from the hemiparesis, include that FHM in about 20% of the cases may also be associated with cerebellar ataxia and other neurological symptoms such as epilepsy, mental retardation, brain oedema, and (fatal) coma.

Familial hemiplegic migraine genes and functional consequences

Thus far, three genes for FHM have been identified: *CACNA1A* (FHM1; chromosome 19p13),[10] encoding the pore-forming α_1-subunit of voltage-gated neuronal $Ca_v2.1$ (P/Q-type) calcium channels; *ATP1A2* (FHM2; 1q23),[11] encoding the α_2-subunit of glial cell Na^+,K^+ pumps; and *SCN1A* (FHM3; 2q24),[12] encoding the pore-forming α_1-subunit of voltage-gated neuronal $Na_v1.1$ sodium channels. Mutations in FHM genes are associated with a wide range of clinical phenotypes, including pure forms of FHM, or combinations of FHM with various degrees of cerebellar ataxia, various forms of epilepsy, or in rare cases fatal coma due to excessive cerebral oedema.[13,14] Specific for FHM1, mutations can also be associated with episodic ataxia type 2 or spinocerebellar ataxia type 6.[10,15] With the identification of these genes, the concept of FHM, and likely also common types of migraine, as ionopathies, i.e. disorders of disturbed ion transport,[9] has gained increasing acceptance. With the identification of these molecular targets, new opportunities have become available to perform neurobiological experiments to study the triggering mechanisms of migraine attacks.

Functional cellular studies on FHM mutations suggest that migraine is caused by disturbed cellular ion transport.[8] FHM1 mutations affect the function of $Ca_v2.1$ calcium channels, which are expressed in neurons throughout the brain as well as at neuromuscular junctions in the peripheral nervous system, and are involved in neurotransmitter release. Depolarization of synaptic cell membranes results in influx of Ca^{2+} through these calcium channels at presynaptic terminals. Subsequently, neurotransmitters are released into the synaptic cleft. At the single channel level, FHM1 mutations were shown to open at more negative voltages compared with normal channels and have an enhanced channel open probability.[16,17] This *gain-of-function* effect results in increased Ca^{2+} influx, which would predict increased neurotransmission.

FHM2 mutations in the *ATP1A2* gene affect Na^+/K^+ pumps that are primarily expressed in glial cells in the adult brain. Astrocytic Na^+/K^+ pumps transport Na^+ ions out and K^+ ions into the cell and are essential for the clearance of neurotransmitters and K^+ from the synaptic cleft. All FHM2 mutations studied thus far result in a *loss-of-function* or a kinetically altered Na^+/K^+ pump.[11,19] Such a defect may result in a reduced uptake of ions and neurotransmitters from the synaptic cleft.

Finally, FHM3 mutations in the *SCN1A* gene seem to predict a more rapid recovery from fast inactivation of neuronal $Na_v1.1$ sodium channels following depolarization.[12] Considering the role of $Na_v1.1$ channels in the generation and propagation of action potentials, the overall effect of FHM3 mutations most likely is enhanced neuronal excitability and neurotransmitter release.

Therefore, from the cellular studies it can be hypothesized that the net result of the mutations in the three FHM genes is the same: a disturbed ionic balance and concomitantly increased release of the excitatory neurotransmitter glutamate at cortical neurons[20] (Figure 18.1). These functional studies have clearly increased our knowledge on mechanisms of migraine at the *cellular* (i.e. neuronal and glial) level. However, it is important to integrate this knowledge with our current understanding of migraine pathophysiology as a disease of the *brain*.

Current views on migraine pathophysiology

In the last decade it has become generally accepted that migraine is a disorder of the brain, with vascular changes being secondary to brain deregulation. Much is known about the pathophysiology of migraine once the attack has started, but it is largely unknown why and how migraine attacks begin. Most progress in elucidating migraine mechanisms was made for the aura phase of migraine attacks (for review see reference 21). The current view is that the migraine aura is caused by a phenomenon called 'cortical spreading depression' (CSD); a wave of intense neuronal activity that slowly progresses over the cortex and is followed by a period of neuronal inactivity. Elevated extracellular levels of K^+ and glutamate are crucial to the initiation and propagation of CSD. Less is known about the headache phase, but activation of the trigeminovascular system (TGVS) seems to play an important part. Meningeal and superficial cortical blood vessels are innervated by the trigeminal nerve and project to the trigeminal nucleus caudalis within the brainstem, which in turn projects to higher order pain centres. Studies in rats have provided evidence that CSDs can activate the TGVS, thus linking the mechanisms for aura and headache.[22] Genetically sensitized animal models—that is transgenic mice with human pathogenic migraine mutations—will be instrumental to test whether they have an increased susceptibility for CSD, and perhaps activation of the TGVS. In other words, it can be tested whether these mice have inherited a propensity to develop migraine attacks because of the presence of an FHM mutation.

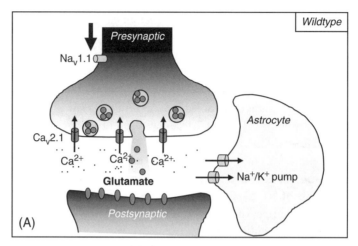

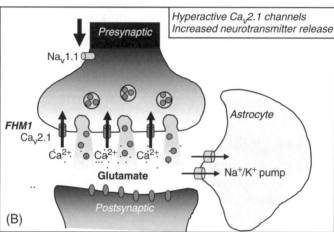

Fig. 18.1 Schematic representation of functional consequences of FHM1, FHM2, and FHM3 mutations in cortical synapse predicting increased extracellular glutamate neurotransmitter levels. (A) In a wild type situation, influx of Ca^{2+} (small black dots) through $Ca_V2.1$ channels (–) at presynaptic terminal occurs after an action potential (thick arrow), involving the activation of $Na_V1.1$ channels (–). Synaptic vesicles fuse with the plasma membrane and neurotransmitters (larger spheres) are released into the synaptic cleft. Neurotransmitters can bind to receptors (–) on the postsynaptic membrane or are cleared from the synaptic cleft by sodium gradient-driven glutamate transporters indirectly regulated by ATP-driven Na^+/K^+ pumps (–) of the astrocyte, as indicated by the horizontal arrows. (B) FHM1 mutations produce mutant $Ca_V2.1$ calcium channels resulting in an increased influx of Ca^{2+} and subsequent increase in neurotransmitter release.

Transgenic mouse models for migraine

The main advantage of knockin mouse models, carrying human mutations, is that they express the mutant gene in its most natural environment, including all transcriptional and post-translational variations. Using a gene-targeting approach, the FHM1 R192Q mutation, previously identified in patients with pure FHM (without additional

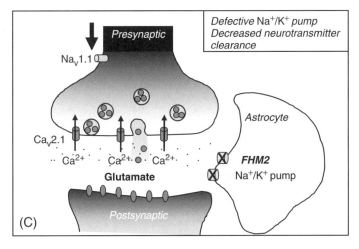

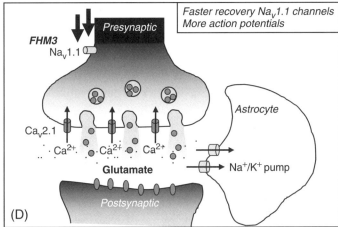

Fig. 18.1 (*Continued*) (C) FHM2 mutations result in a reduced activity of the ATP-driven Na^+/K^+ pump, disturbing the Na^+ gradient required for glutamate transporter function and increased neurotransmitter levels. (D) FHM3 mutations result in a faster recovery from $Na_v1.1$ channel inactivation. As a result, neuronal firing rate is increased and consequently neurotransmitter levels.

symptoms),[10] was introduced into the endogenous *Cacna1a* mouse gene.[23] FHM1 R192Q mice do not show any overt behavioural or anatomical abnormalities. However, we did observe gain-of-function effects on several important parameters: (1) an increased calcium current was measured in cerebellar granule cells isolated from R192Q FHM1; (2) at the neuromuscular junction, this translates to an increased evoked and spontaneous neurotransmitter release under conditions that also occur during CSD (e.g. at low extracellular Ca^{2+} and high K^+ levels). Additional studies of the neuromuscular junction showed a gene-dosage effect (i.e. the abnormalities in heterozygous mice are intermediate between wild type and homozygous mice).[24] (3) Most relevant for migraine pathophysiology, the FHM1 R192Q mice revealed a reduced threshold and an increased propagation velocity of CSD. These observations indicate that the FHM1 mice are useful models to study migraine pathophysiology *in vivo*. Recently, a second FHM1 knockin mouse strain was generated by us (van den Maagdenberg, unpublished), carrying the clinically more severe S218L mutation, previously identified in patients with FHM associated with ataxia and fatal cerebral oedema and coma.[25] FHM1 S218L knockin mice exhibit ataxia similar to what can be found in patients carrying this mutation. Effects on calcium influx, neurotransmitter release, and CSD were similar to what was observed for the FHM1 R192Q mice, but the changes were even more prominent, in line with the severity of the phenotype in patients with this mutation.

FHM2 and FHM3 knockin mouse models are not yet available, but will be of great interest too. Knockout mice that completely lack the Na^+/K^+ pump have been generated and exhibit a severe phenotype: homozygous animals die at birth due to respiratory problems.[26,27]

Relevance of transgenic FHM1 knockin mice for drug development

The recently generated FHM1 knockin mice will prove valuable tools to study migraine mechanisms in animal models that are genetically sensitized (i.e. because of the presence of an FHM mutation they should have a higher propensity to have attacks). Because $Ca_v2.1$ channels are expressed in all structures that have been implicated in migraine pathophysiology, including cerebral cortex, trigeminal ganglia, and brainstem nuclei involved in nociception, it is feasible to use the FHM1 knockin mice and study *how* these brain structures cause migraine. For instance, it can be tested whether possible migraine drugs can normalize the function in these brain structures of FHM1 knockin mice.

Gain-of-function effects observed in FHM1 knockin mice on calcium influx, neurotransmitter release, and decreased threshold for CSD suggest that $Ca_v2.1$ channel blockers might be useful drugs for this form of migraine—and perhaps—common migraine. In more detail, FHM1 mutations seem to result in a shift of the activation voltage range to more hyperpolarized lower voltages, thereby increasing their open probability, leading to a rise in intracellular calcium. Therefore a drug that shifts the activation range of $Ca_v2.1$ channels to more depolarized voltages might interfere with subsequent actions and thus ultimately prevent or stop a migraine attack. Interestingly, some of the currently used antimigraine drugs are blockers of L-type calcium channels. A drug that has shown a potent inhibitory effect on presynaptic $Ca_v2.1$ channels and reduces plasma extravasation is α-eudesmol. This drug reduces the release of vasoactive neuropeptides such as substance P and CGRP.[28] Notably, in migraine patients CGRP levels are elevated, CGRP infusion can trigger a migraine attack and triptans block the release of CGRP.[29] Therefore, CGRP antagonists and drugs affecting the release of CGRP might be effective in the treatment of acute migraine. Future studies will have to indicate whether CGRP release is different in the FHM1 knockin mice.

Genetic models of migraine will facilitate research of increased sensitivity to migraine triggers and metabolic homeostasis. Thus, we can better understand how a migraine attack is triggered. Central to the pathology of the FHM1 knockin mice is the decreased threshold for CSD, but it still has to be determined whether activation of the trigemino-vascular system is facilitated in the transgenic mice. In this respect it is important to realize that in cortical neurons $Ca_v2.1$ calcium channels are the main channel type involved in the release of glutamate and that glutamate can facilitate CSD.[30] The fact that ketamine, an NMDA receptor antagonist, reduces the severity and duration of aura symptoms in FHM patients[31] and AMPA/GluR5 receptor antagonist LY293558 was effective in preclinical models of migraine,[32] reinforces the important role glutamate has in migraine pathophysiology.

A recent publication by Ayata, et al.[33] provides compelling evidence that FHM1 knockin mice are relevant models for migraine. The researchers asked the intriguing question whether migraine prophylactic drugs with known efficacy have anti-CSD activity. Prophylactic drugs were tested from various pharmacological classes: β-adrenergic receptor blocker propanolol, tricyclic antidepressant amitriptyline, anticonvulsants topiramate and valproate, and serotonergic drug methysergide, to investigate whether they can increase the threshold for CSD. It was shown that chronic daily, but not acute administration of migraine prophylactic drugs in rats, in a dose- and duration-dependent manner, suppressed KCl-induced CSD frequency by 40–80% and decreased the triggering threshold for inducing CSD. Importantly, D-propanolol, a clinically ineffective drug, did not show these effects.

Although CSD can activate ipsilateral trigeminal nucleus caudalis neurons and causes a long-lasting blood flow increase in the rat middle meningeal artery and a dural plasma protein leakage that can be inhibited by ipsilateral trigeminal nerve section,[22] it is still controversial whether CSD can initiate the migraine headache cascade in *patients*. The majority of migraine patients do not experience auras, the headache may occur at the same side of the aura, instead of the expected opposite side if CSD would have triggered the trigeminovascular system, and the aura may sometimes occur after the headache has started. Clearly the exact role of CSD in triggering migraine headache mechanisms in humans remains unclear and needs further investigation. A relevant question is whether FHM1 knockin mice have increased susceptibility for *headache pain* and whether the threshold for activation of the TGVS in these mice is lowered, for instance after CSD. Studies currently performed in the FHM1 knockin mice will have to answer these questions.

In conclusion, the identification of genes that increase the susceptibility for migraine attacks and the generation and detailed characterization of transgenic mouse models with human pathogenic mutations will prove not only valuable to obtain more insight in to the pathophysiology, but also valuable for testing drugs for migraine.

Acknowledgements

This work was supported by grants from EUROHEAD (LSHM-CT-2004-504837), The Netherlands Organization for Scientific Research (NWO) (Vici 918.56.602), and The Center of Medical System Biology (CMSB) established by the Netherlands Genomic Initiative/Netherlands Organization for Scientific Research (NGI/NWO).

References

1. Ferrari MD (1998) Migraine. *Lancet* 351, 1043–51.

2. Goadsby PJ, Lipton RB, Ferrari MD (2000) Migraine–current understanding and treatment. *N Engl J Med* 346, 257–70.

3. Headache Classification Subcommittee of the International Headache Society (2004) The International Classification of Headache Disorders, 2nd Edition. *Cephalalgia* 24, 1–160.

4. Giffin NJ, Ruggiero L, Lipton RB, *et al.* (2003) Premonitory symptoms in migraine: an electronic diary study. *Neurology* 60, 935–40.

5. Stam AH, Haan J, Frants RR, Ferrari MD, van den Maagdenberg AM (2005) Migraine: new treatment options from molecular biology. *Expert Rev Neurother* 5, 653–61.

6. Silberstein SD (2004) Migraine. *Lancet* 363, 381–91.

7. Ramadan NM, Schultz LL, Gilkey SJ (1997) Migraine prophylactic drugs: proof of efficacy, utilization and cost. *Cephalalgia* 17, 73–80.

8. Van den Maagdenberg AM, Haan J, Terwindt GM, Ferrari MD (2007) Migraine: gene mutations and functional consequences. *Curr Opin Neurol* 20, 299–305.

9. Ferrari MD, Goadsby PJ (2006) Migraine as a cerebral ionopathy with abnormal central sensory processing. In: Gilman S (ed.) *Neurobiology of Disease*, Elsevier.

10. Ophoff RA, Terwindt GM, Vergouwe MN, *et al.* (1996) Familial hemiplegic migraine and episodic ataxia type-2 are caused by mutations in the Ca^{2+} channel gene CACNL1A4. *Cell* 87, 543–52.

11. De Fusco M, Marconi R, Silvestri L, *et al* (2003) Haploinsufficiency of ATP1A2 encoding the Na^+/K^+ pump alpha2 subunit associated with familial hemiplegic migraine type 2. *Nat Genet* 33, 192–6.

12. Dichgans M, Freilinger T, Eckstein G, *et al.* (2005) Mutation in the neuronal voltage-gated sodium channel SCN1A in familial hemiplegic migraine. *Lancet* 366, 371–7.

13. Ducros A, Denier C, Joutel A, *et al.* (2001) The clinical spectrum of familial hemiplegic migraine associated with mutations in a neuronal calcium channel. *N Engl J Med* 345, 17–24.

14. Kors EE, Vanmolkot KR, Haan J, Frants RR, Van den Maagdenberg AM, Ferrari MD (2004) Recent findings in headache genetics. *Curr Opin Neurol* 17, 283–8.

15. Zhuchenko O, Bailey J, Donnen P, *et al.* (1997) Autosomal dominant cerebellar ataxia (SCA6) associated with small polyglutamine expansions in the a1A-voltage-dependent calcium channel. *Nat Genet* 15, 62–9.

16. Hans M, Luvisetto S, Williams ME, *et al.* (1999) Functional consequences of mutations in the human alpha(1A) calcium channel subunit linked to familial hemiplegic migraine. *J Neurosci* 19, 1610–19.

17. Tottene A, Fellin T, Pagnutti S, *et al.* (2002) Familial hemiplegic migraine mutations increase Ca2+ influx through single human CaV2.1 channels and decrease maximal CaV2.1 current density in neurons. *Proc Natl Acad Sci USA* 99, 13284–9.

18. Tottene A, Pivotto F, Fellin T, Cesetti T, van den Maagdenberg AM, Pietrobon D (2005) Specific kinetic alterations of human CaV2.1 calcium channels produced by mutation S218L causing familial hemiplegic migraine and delayed cerebral edema and coma after minor head trauma. *J Biol Chem* 280, 17678–86.

19. Segall L, Mezzetti A, Scanzano R, Gargus JJ, Purisima E, Blostein R (2005) Alterations in the alpha2 isoform of Na,K-ATPase associated with familial hemiplegic migraine type 2. *Proc Natl Acad Sci USA* 102, 11106–11.

20. Moskowitz MA, Bolay H, Dalkara T (2004) Deciphering migraine mechanisms: clues from familial hemiplegic migraine genotypes. *Ann Neurol* 55, 276–80.

21. Pietrobon D, Striessnig J (2003) Neurobiology of migraine. *Nat Rev Neurosci* 4, 386–98.

22. Bolay H, Reuter U, Dunn AK, Huang Z, Boas DA, Moskowitz MA (2002) Intrinsic brain activity triggers trigeminal meningeal afferents in a migraine model. *Nat Med* 8, 136–42.

23. Van den Maagdenberg AM, Pietrobon D, Pizzorusso T, *et al.* (2004) A Cacna1a knockin migraine mouse model with increased susceptibility to cortical spreading depression. *Neuron* 41, 701–10.

24. Kaja S, van de Ven RC, Broos LA, *et al.* (2005) Gene dosage-dependent transmitter release changes at neuromuscular synapses of CACNA1A R192Q knockin mice are non-progressive and do not lead to morphological changes or muscle weakness. *Neuroscience* 135, 81–95.

25. Kors EE, Terwindt GM, Vermeulen FL, *et al.* (2001) Delayed cerebral edema and fatal coma after minor head trauma: role of CACNA1A calcium channel subunit gene and relationship with familial hemiplegic migraine. *Ann Neurol* 49, 753–60.

26. James PF, Grupp IL, Grupp G, *et al.* (1999) Identification of a specific role for the Na,K-ATPase alpha 2 isoform as a regulator of calcium in the heart. *Mol Cell* 3, 555–63.

27. Ikeda K, Onaka T, Yamakado M, *et al.* (2003) Degeneration of the amygdala/piriform cortex and enhanced fear/anxiety behaviors in sodium pump alpha2 subunit (Atp1a2)-deficient mice. *J Neurosci* 23, 4667–76.

28. Asakura K, Kanemasa T, Minagawa K, *et al.* (2000) α-Eudesmol, a P/Q-type Ca^{2+} channel blocker, inhibits neurogenic vasodilation and extravasation following electrical stimulation of trigeminal ganglion. *Brain Res* 873, 94–101.

29. Knight YE, Edvinsson L, Goadsby PJ (1999) Blockade of calcitonin gene-related peptide release after superior sagittal sinus stimulation in cat: a comparison of avitrptan and CP122,288. *Neuropeptides* 33, 41–6.

30. Waeber C, Moskowitz MA (2003) Therapeutic implications of central and peripheral neurologic mechanisms in migraine. *Neurology* 61 (Suppl. 4), S9–20.

31. Kaube H, Herzog J, Kaufer T, Dichgans M, Diener HC (2000) Aura in some patients with familial hemiplegic migraine can be stopped by intranasal ketamine. *Neurology* 55, 139–41.

32. Sang CN, Ramadan NM, Wallihan RG, *et al.* (2004) LY293558, a novel AMPA/GluR5 antagonist, is efficacious and well-tolerated in acute migraine. *Cephalalgia* 24, 596–602.

33. Ayata C, Jin H, Kudo C, Dalkara T, Moskowitz MA (2006) Suppression of cortical spreading depression in migraine prophylaxis. *Ann Neurol* 59, 652–61.

19

K$_{ATP}$ channels and migraine

Inger Jansen-Olesen and Kenneth Beri Ploug

Adenosine 5´-triphosphate-sensitive K⁺ (K$_{ATP}$) channels

Adenosine 5´-triphosphate (ATP) sensitive K⁺ (K$_{ATP}$) channels respond to changes in the cellular metabolic state as well as to a number of endogenous vasodilators.[1] Dissociation of ATP and thus activation of K$_{ATP}$ channels causes hyperpolarization of smooth muscle cells[2] and endothelial cells.[3,4] In vascular smooth muscle cells hyperpolarization prevents opening of depolarization-activated Ca^{2+} channels, thus blocking calcium entry to the cell which results in vasodilatation.[5] In some, but not all, endothelial cells, the hyperpolarization elevates the concentration of intracellular calcium and thereby promotes Ca^{2+}-dependent formation of nitric oxide (NO).[3,4,6]

Distribution of K$_{ATP}$ channels

The K$_{ATP}$ channels have been described in diverse cell types, including cardiomyocytes,[7] pancreatic b cells,[8] neurons,[9] skeletal muscle cells,[10] and vascular smooth muscle cells,[11,12] where they play important physiological and pathophysiological roles.

Composition of K$_{ATP}$ channels

The molecular structure of K$_{ATP}$ channels is thought to be a heteromultimeric (tetrameric) complex of two subunits. One of them is the poreforming inward-rectifying K⁺ channel type 6.x (Kir6.x) in which 6.x can be either 6.1 or 6.2 and the other subunit is a sulphonylurea receptor (SUR) that belongs to the ATP-binding cassette superfamily. Two different SURs have been identified in rodents and humans, SUR1 and SUR2 that are encoded by two genes containing 39 and 38 exons respectively. In addition, the SUR2 gene has been shown to undergo alternative splicing at exon 38 to generate the two splice variants SUR2A and SUR2B.[13] Expression of the SURs with Kir6.1 or Kir6.2 subunits has revealed K$_{ATP}$ channels with distinct biophysical and pharmacological properties (Figure 19.1, Table 19.1).

Why are K$_{ATP}$ channels interesting in relation to migraine?

The K$_{ATP}$ channel openers pinacidil and levcromakalim have been used in clinical trials. Pinacidil was studied for the treatment of essential hypertension.[14–19] In these studies headache was the most prominent side-effect being reported in between 7% and 22% of the patients. The clinical trials with pinacidil were followed by trials using levcromakalim

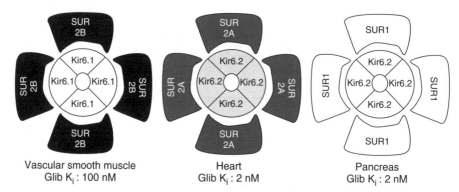

Fig. 19.1 Schematic drawing of K$_{ATP}$ channel conformation in different tissues. The half inhibition values of whole-cell K$_{ATP}$ channel currents by glibenclamide (Glib) in the different tissues are given.

for treatment of asthma and essential hypertension.[20–23] Between 29% and 76% of the patients reported headache as a side-effect and the project on K$_{ATP}$ channel openers for the use in treatment of essential hypertension and/or asthma was closed (Table 19.2).

As these compounds cause significant headache in a high proportion of normal subjects, it appears likely that they can also provoke migraine in migraine sufferers. This opens the possibility that a K$_{ATP}$ channel blocker might be effective in the treatment of migraine. However, as K$_{ATP}$ channels are present and of high physiological importance in many tissues around the body, a potential K$_{ATP}$ channel blocker for migraine treatment must be as subtype specific as possible in order to avoid possible side-effects.

Characterization of K$_{ATP}$ channels in intracranial arteries

Effect of K$_{ATP}$ channel openers

K$_{ATP}$ channel openers increase the open-state probability of the smooth muscle cell by 10–100-fold depending on the concentration of ATP.[2] Several studies using synthetic

Table 19.1 Diversity of K$_{ATP}$ channels.

	Conductance	Tissue expression	Inhibition by ATP (IC$_{50}$)	Pharmacology
Kir6.2 + SUR1	~75 pS	Pancreas, brain	~10 μM	Activated by diazoxide; high-affinity glibenclamide inhibition
Kir6.2 + SUR2A	~80 pS	Cardiac myocytes, skeletal muscle	~100 μM	Activated by cromakalim, pinacidil but not diazoxide; low-affinity glibenclamide inhibition
Kir6.1 + SUR2B	~33 pS	Smooth muscle (various)	~1–3 mM	Activated by cromakalim, pinacidil, and diazoxide; low-affinity glibenclamide inhibition

Data in the table are adapted from references 13 and 63.

Table 19.2 Incidence of headache in clinical trials with levcromakalim.

Dose (daily)	Indication	No. of patients	No. of patients with headache (% of patients)	Drop outs due to headache (No.)	References
1.5 mg	Essential hypertension	8	4 (50%)	Single dose	Singer et al.[21]
1.5 mg	Asthma	16	10 (62%)	–	Williams et al.[23]
0.5–1.0 mg	Essential hypertension	14	4 (29%)	1 (7%)	Suzuki et al.[22]
0.125–0.5 mg	Asthma	25	19 (76%)	–	Kidney et al.[20]

K$_{ATP}$ channel openers and sulphonylurea inhibitors suggest that K$_{ATP}$ channels are functional in cerebral blood vessels from several species, including humans[24–31] (Figure 19.2). *In situ* application of direct activators of K$_{ATP}$ channels causes dilatory effects in rat basilar arteries[32,33] and cerebral arterioles.[34] Functionality of K$_{ATP}$ channels has also been shown *in vitro* and *in vivo* in rat dural arteries[35] (Figure 19.3).

In contrast to these findings, some studies failed to obtain functional evidence supporting the presence of K$_{ATP}$ channels in middle cerebral arteries.[36, 37] Other studies showed a less potent response in rat middle cerebral arteries as compared with basilar and middle meningeal/dural arteries *in vitro* as well as *in vivo*[31,35] (Figure 19.3). The reason for these differences is not clear. The smaller size of the middle cerebral artery increases the probability of the endothelium becoming damaged during mounting in the small vessel myograph. However, in perfusion studies the K$_{ATP}$ channel openers were inefficient when administered intraluminally.[38]

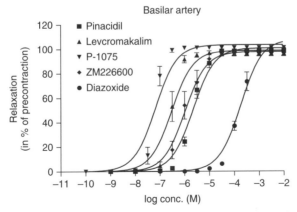

Fig. 19.2 Relaxation induced by cumulative concentrations of the K$_{ATP}$ channel openers pinacidil, levcromakalim, P-1075, ZM226600, and diazoxide in rat basilar artery. Reproduced from *European Journal of Pharmacology*, 523 (1–3), Jansen-Olesen, Mortenson CH, El-Bariaki N, Ploug KB, Characterization of K(ATP)-channels in rat basilar and middle cerebral arteries: studies of vasomoter responses and mRNA expression (2005), pp. 109–18, with permission from Elsevier.

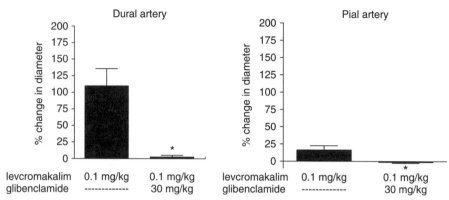

Fig. 19.3 Effect of levcromakalim on dural and pial artery diameter in absence and presence of glibenclamide 30 mg/kg. Values given as mean ± SEM, $n = 9$. Statistical analysis performed by Student's t-test *$P < 0.05$. Reproduced from *Cephalalgia* 25(4), Gozalov A, Peterson KA, Mortensen C, *et al.* Role of KATP channels in the regulation of rat dura and pia artery diameter (2005), pp. 249–60, with permission from Blackwell Publishing.

In order to characterize the composition of cerebrovascular K_{ATP} channel SUR subtypes from functional studies, a correlation study was performed. The relaxant potency of four K_{ATP} channel openers in rat basilar and middle cerebral arteries were correlated to the affinity of the same four K_{ATP} channel openers obtained in COS-7 cell lines expressing either human SUR2B, rat SUR2A, or hamster SUR1.[39] A significant correlation between vasodilator potency and binding affinity to SUR2B and SUR2A subunits was found.[31] Thus, rat basilar and middle cerebral artery vasodilatation by K_{ATP} channel openers is likely to be mediated via binding to either the SUR2B or SUR2A subunit.

K_{ATP} channel blockers

A number of agents have been shown to block K_{ATP} channels *in vitro*. Those in clinical use do so by affinity to SUR1 (tolbutamide and glicazide) or SUR1 and SUR2 (glibenclamide, glimepiride, repaglinide, and meglitinide).[40] In vascular studies glibenclamide has been the blocker of choice. Glibenclamide inhibits whole-cell K_{ATP} currents with a half-inhibition value (K_i) at 100 nM. This is an approximately 50 times higher K_i value than found in pancreas and heart (approximately 2 nM)[41] (Figure 19.1). Several *in vitro* studies have been performed showing the antagonistic effect of glibenclamide on K_{ATP} channel opener induced relaxation in dog middle cerebral arteries,[42] rat basilar arteries,[30,31] rabbit cerebral arteries,[43] and rat middle meningeal arteries.[35] In rat middle cerebral arteries, only a weak antagonistic effect of glibenclamide was observed.[31] In addition, glibenclamide has been shown to inhibit levcromakalim and pinacidil induced dilatation of rat dural and pial arteries *in vivo*[35] (Figure 19.3).

The morpholinoguanidine antagonist PNU-37883A is selective for vascular K_{ATP} channels[44–46] and channels containing Kir6.1.[47,48] We have in a still unpublished study shown that PNU37883A is an efficient non-competitive blocker of P-1075-induced relaxation of the rat basilar artery *in vitro*. Furthermore, PNU37883A is an efficient blocker of levcromakalim induced dilatation of rat dural arteries *in vivo* (unpublished).

Modulation of K$_{ATP}$ channels by endogenous transmitters

A number of endogenous vasodilators act partly through membrane hyperpolarization caused by K$_{ATP}$ channel activation.[12,49] In arteries, relaxations due to calcitonin gene-related peptide (CGRP) appear to involve activation of cyclic adenosine 3′,5′-monophosphate (cAMP) and subsequent protein kinase A (PKA) activation of K$_{ATP}$ channels.[12,49–51] This mechanism of action has also been disclosed in rat basilar arteries *in situ*[52] and rat pial and dural arteries *in vivo*[53] (Figure 19.4). Other relaxant agents that have been suggested to activate K$_{ATP}$ channels via PKA are adenosine,[54] prostacyclin,[55] and vasoactive intestinal polypeptide.[11] NO derived from the endothelium relaxes vascular smooth muscle cells partly through activation of K$^+$ channels. Most studies point towards an opening of calcium activated potassium channels but opening of K$_{ATP}$ channels following cross-activation of PKA has also been suggested.[56] The *in vitro* and *in vivo* relaxation of rat pial and dural arteries after administration of the NO-donor glyceryltrinitrate (GTN) was not inhibited by glibenclamide.[53] Thus, there is no evidence for this mechanism to exist in cranial arteries.

The vasoconstrictors serotonin and histamine inhibit pinacidil-induced currents in cerebral artery smooth muscle cells.[43] Part of the mechanism of action of vasoconstrictors may involve inhibition of K$_{ATP}$ channels via increase in PKC activity or decrease in PKA activity.[57] Also endothelin,[58] angiotensin II,[59] and vasopressin[60] may act this way.

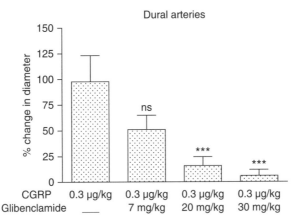

Fig. 19.4 Effect of calcitonin gene-related peptide (CGRP; 0.3 μg/kg) on dural artery diameter in the presence or absence of glibenclamide 7 mg/kg, 20 mg/kg, and 30 mg/kg. Values given as mean ± SEM, n = 6. Statistical analysis comparing responses in presence and in absence of glibenclamide performed by Dunnett's test: ns (P > 0.05); ***(P < 0.005). Reproduced from *The Journal of Pharmacology*, 553(1–3), Ploug KB, Edvinsson L, Olesen J, *et al.*, Pharmacological and molecular comparison of K(ATP) channels in rat basilar and middle cerebral arteries (2006), pp. 254–62, with permission from Elsevier.

Molecular characterization of K_{ATP} channels in intracranial arteries

Messenger RNA expression of K_{ATP} channel subunits

By conventional reverse transcription–polymerase chain reaction, molecular expression of Kir6.1, Kir6.2, SUR1, SUR2A, and SUR2B was shown in rat basilar and middle cerebral arteries.[31] These findings are consistent with other reports showing the presence of Kir6.1 in combination with SUR2B in cultured and fresh smooth muscle cells from rat basilar arteries.[61,62] In the same tissues quantitative real-time polymerase chain reaction revealed that Kir6.1 and SUR2B mRNAs are the predominant transcripts. Also a lower amount of SUR1 mRNA is present, while SUR2A mRNA is barely detected[38] (Figure 19.5). The data also indicated that Kir6.1 mRNA levels are higher than SUR2B mRNA levels, especially in the middle cerebral arteries. Though fluctuations in mRNA number may be stochastic, this discrepancy does not account for the 4:4 Kir6.x/SUR stochiometry found in assembled K_{ATP} channels at the plasma membrane.[38]

Protein expression of K_{ATP} channel subunits

Together with the mRNA expression studies, the protein expression studies strongly suggest that rat basilar and middle cerebral arteries are primarily composed of the Kir6.1/SUR2B combination of K_{ATP} channels[38] (Figure 19.6). In addition, there is a possibility for a small population of SUR1 subunits to assemble with Kir6.1 subunits to form functional K_{ATP} channels together with the major vascular Kir6.1/SUR2B complex.

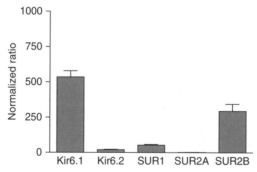

Fig. 19.5 Graphic representation of the quantitative real-time polymerase chain reaction results (mRNA expression studies). A total of three different cDNA batches were prepared from rat cerebral arteries and analysed by each set of primers indicated under the columns. For further details please see reference 38. Reproduced from *The Journal of Pharmacology*, 553(1–3), Ploug KB, Edvinsson L, Olesen J, *et al.*, Pharmacological and molecular comparison of K(ATP) channels in rat basilar and middle cerebral arteries (2006), pp.254–62, with permission from Elsevier.

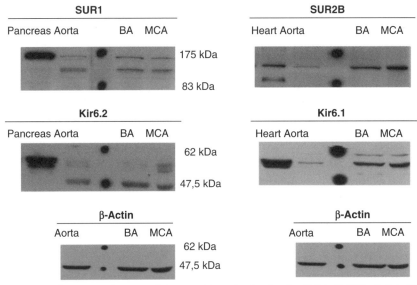

Fig. 19.6 Chemifluorescent images of Western blots. Antibodies for SUR1, SUR2B, Kir6.1, Kir6.2, and β-actin were tested with positive control lysates along with the basilar (BA) and middle cerebral artery (MCA) samples. A pre-stained protein marker was run along with the samples. For further details please see reference 38. Reproduced from *The Journal of Pharmacology*, 553(1–3), Ploug KB, Edvinsson L, Olesen J, *et al.*, Pharmacological and molecular comparison of K(ATP) channels in rat basilar and middle cerebral arteries (2006), pp. 254–62, with permission from Elsevier.

Conclusions

In clinical trials with K_{ATP} channel openers headache has been the primary side-effect. The opening of K_{ATP} channels causes dilatation of pial and dural arteries *in vitro* and *in vivo*. Pharmacological and molecular data show that the K_{ATP} channels mediating these effects are comprised mainly of the Kir6.1/SUR2B subunit combination. The Kir6.1/SUR2B complex is different from the composition of the K_{ATP} channel in heart and pancreas. This raises the possibility that a Kir6.1/SUR2B selective K_{ATP} channel blocker may be efficient in the treatment of migraine and that such a blocker may not have unwanted effects on heart and pancreas (no hypoglycaemia).

References

1. Nelson MT, Brayden JE (1993) Regulation of arterial tone by calcium-dependent K+ channels and ATP-sensitive K+ channels. *Cardiovasc Drugs Ther* 7 (Suppl. 3), 605–10.
2. Brayden JE (2002) Functional roles of KATP channels in vascular smooth muscle. *Clin Exp Pharmacol Physiol* 29, 312–16.
3. Luckhoff A, Busse R (1990) Activators of potassium channels enhance calcium influx into endothelial cells as a consequence of potassium currents. *Naunyn Schmiedebergs Arch Pharmacol* 342, 94–9.
4. Luckhoff A, Busse R (1990) Calcium influx into endothelial cells and formation of endothelium-derived relaxing factor is controlled by the membrane potential. *Pflugers Arch* 416, 305–11.

5. Quast U (1996) ATP-sensitive K+ channels in the kidney. *Naunyn Schmiedebergs Arch Pharmacol* 354, 213–25.

6. Gasser R, Koppel H, Brussee H, Grisold M, Holzmann S, Klein W (1998) EDRF does not mediate coronary vasodilation secondary to simulated ischemia: a study on KATP channels and N omega-nitro-L-arginine on coronary perfusion pressure in isolated Langendorff-perfused guinea-pig hearts. *Cardiovasc Drugs Ther* 12, 279–84.

7. Noma A (1983) ATP-regulated K+ channels in cardiac muscle. *Nature* 305, 147–8.

8. Ashcroft FM, Harrison DE, Ashcroft SJ (1984) Glucose induces closure of single potassium channels in isolated rat pancreatic beta-cells. *Nature* 312, 446–8.

9. Ashford ML, Sturgess NC, Trout NJ, Gardner NJ, Hales CN (1988) Adenosine-5'-triphosphate-sensitive ion channels in neonatal rat cultured central neurones. *Pflugers Arch* 412, 297–304.

10. Spruce AE, Standen NB, Stanfield PR (1985) Voltage-dependent ATP-sensitive potassium channels of skeletal muscle membrane. *Nature* 316, 736–8.

11. Standen NB, Quayle JM, Davies NW, Brayden JE, Huang Y, Nelson MT (1989) Hyperpolarizing vasodilators activate ATP-sensitive K+ channels in arterial smooth muscle. *Science* 245, 177–80.

12. Nelson MT, Patlak JB, Worley JF, Standen NB (1990) Calcium channels, potassium channels, and voltage dependence of arterial smooth muscle tone. *Am J Physiol* 259, 3–18.

13. Yokoshiki H, Sunagawa M, Seki T, Sperelakis N (1998) ATP-sensitive K+ channels in pancreatic, cardiac, and vascular smooth muscle cells. *Am J Physiol* 274, 25–37.

14. D'Arcy V, Laher M, McCoy D, Sullivan P, Walsh CH, Hickey MP (1985) Pinacidil, a new vasodilator, in the treatment of mild to moderate essential hypertension. *Eur J Clin Pharmacol* 28, 347–9.

15. Goldberg MR (1988) Clinical pharmacology of pinacidil, a prototype for drugs that affect potassium channels. *J Cardiovasc Pharmacol* 12 (Suppl. 2), S41–7.

16. Laher MS, Hickey MP (1985) Pharmacokinetics and bioavailability of pinacidil capsules in human volunteers. *J Int Med Res* 13, 159–62.

17. Muiesan G, Fariello R, Muiesan ML, Christensen OE (1985) Effect of pinacidil on blood pressure, plasma catecholamines and plasma renin activity in essential hypertension. *Eur J Clin Pharmacol* 28, 495–9.

18. Sterndorff B, Johansen P (1988) The antihypertensive effect of pinacidil versus prazosin in mild to moderate hypertensive patients seen in general practice. *Acta Med Scand* 224, 329–36.

19. Zachariah PK, Sheps SG, Schirger A, *et al.* (1986) Antihypertensive efficacy of pinacidil–automatic ambulatory blood pressure monitoring. *Eur J Clin Pharmacol* 31, 133–41.

20. Kidney JC, Fuller RW, Worsdell YM, Lavender EA, Chung KF, Barnes PJ (1993) Effect of an oral potassium channel activator, BRL 38227, on airway function and responsiveness in asthmatic patients: comparison with oral salbutamol. *Thorax* 48, 130–3.

21. Singer DR, Markandu ND, Miller MA, Sugden AL, MacGregor GA (1989) Potassium channel stimulation in normal subjects and in patients with essential hypertension: an acute study with cromakalim (BRL 34915) *J Hypertens* Suppl. 7, S294–5.

22. Suzuki S, Yano K, Kusano S, Hashimoto T (1995) Antihypertensive effect of levcromakalim in patients with essential hypertension. Study by 24-h ambulatory blood pressure monitoring. *Arzneimittelforschung* 45, 859–64.

23. Williams AJ, Lee TH, Cochrane GM, *et al.* (1990) Attenuation of nocturnal asthma by cromakalim. *Lancet* 336, 334–6.

24. Kitazono T, Faraci FM, Taguchi H, Heistad DD (1995) Role of potassium channels in cerebral blood vessels. *Stroke* 26, 1713–23.

25. Hempelmann RG, Barth HL, Mehdorn HM, Pradel RH, Ziegler A (1995) Effects of potassium channel openers in isolated human cerebral arteries. *Neurosurgery* 37, 1146–53.

26. Nagao T, Ibayashi S, Sadoshima S, *et al.* (1996) Distribution and physiological roles of ATP-sensitive K+ channels in the vertebrobasilar system of the rabbit. *Circ Res* 78, 238–43.

27. Iwamoto T, Nishimura N, Morita T, Sukamoto T (1993) Differential vasorelaxant effects of K(+)-channel openers and Ca(2+)-channel blockers on canine isolated arteries. *J Pharm Pharmacol* 45, 292–7.

28. Zhang H, Stockbridge N, Weir B, Vollrath B, Cook D (1992) Vasodilatation of canine cerebral arteries by nicorandil, pinacidil and lemakalim. *Gen Pharmacol* 23, 197–201.

29. Parsons AA, Ksoll E, Mackert JR, Schilling L, Wahl M (1991) Comparison of cromakalim-induced relaxation of potassium precontracted rabbit, cat, and rat isolated cerebral arteries. *Naunyn Schmiedebergs Arch Pharmacol* 343, 384–92.

30. Ksoll E, Parsons AA, Mackert JR, Schilling L, Wahl M (1991) Analysis of cromakalim-, pinacidil-, and nicorandil-induced relaxation of the 5-hydroxytryptamine precontracted rat isolated basilar artery. *Naunyn Schmiedebergs Arch Pharmacol* 343, 377–83.

31. Jansen-Olesen I, Mortensen CH, El-Bariaki N, Ploug KB (2005) Characterization of K(ATP)-channels in rat basilar and middle cerebral arteries: studies of vasomotor responses and mRNA expression. *Eur J Pharmacol* 523, 109–18.

32. Faraci FM, Heistad DD (1993) Role of ATP-sensitive potassium channels in the basilar artery. *Am J Physiol* 264, 8–13.

33. Toyoda K, Fujii K, Ibayashi S, Kitazono T, Nagao T, Fujishima M (1997) Role of ATP-sensitive potassium channels in brain stem circulation during hypotension. *Am J Physiol* 273, H1342–6.

34. Wahl M, Parsons AA, Schilling L (1994) Dilating effect of perivascularly applied potassium channel openers cromakalim and pinacidil in rat and cat pial arteries in situ. *Cardiovasc Res* 28, 1803–7.

35. Gozalov A, Petersen KA, Mortensen C, Jansen-Olesen I, Klaerke D, Olesen J (2005) Role of KATP channels in the regulation of rat dura and pia artery diameter. *Cephalalgia* 25, 249–60.

36. McCarron JG, Quayle JM, Halpern W, Nelson MT (1991) Cromakalim and pinacidil dilate small mesenteric arteries but not small cerebral arteries. *Am J Physiol* 261, H287–91.

37. McPherson GA, Stork AP (1992) The resistance of some rat cerebral arteries to the vasorelaxant effect of cromakalim and other K+ channel openers. *Br J Pharmacol* 105, 51–8.

38. Ploug KB, Edvinsson L, Olesen J, Jansen-Olesen I (2006) Pharmacological and molecular comparison of K(ATP) channels in rat basilar and middle cerebral arteries. *Eur J Pharmacol* 553, 254–62.

39. Schwanstecher M, Sieverding C, Dorschner H, Gross I, Aguilar-Bryan L, Schwanstecher C, *et al.* (1998) Potassium channel openers require ATP to bind to and act through sulfonylurea receptors. *Embo J* 17, 5529–35.

40. Ashcroft FM, Gribble FM (1999) ATP-sensitive K+ channels and insulin secretion: their role in health and disease. *Diabetologia* 42, 903–19.

41. Wellman GC, Nelson MT (2002) Ion channels in cerebral arteries. In: Edvinsson L, Krause DN (eds) *Cerebral Blood Flow and Metabolism*, 2nd edn, pp. 71–87. Lippincott Williams & Wilkins, Philadelphia, PA.

42. Masuzawa K, Asano M, Matsuda T, Imaizumi Y, Watanabe M (1990) Possible involvement of ATP-sensitive K+ channels in the relaxant response of dog middle cerebral artery to cromakalim. *J Pharmacol Exp Ther* 255, 818–25.

43. Kleppisch T, Nelson MT (1995) ATP-sensitive K+ currents in cerebral arterial smooth muscle: pharmacological and hormonal modulation. *Am J Physiol* 269, H1634–40.

44. Guillemare E, Honore E, De Weille J, Fosset M, Lazdunski M, Meisheri K (1994) Functional receptors in Xenopus oocytes for U-37883A, a novel ATP-sensitive K+ channel blocker: comparison with rat insulinoma cells. *Mol Pharmacol* 46, 139–45.

45. Meisheri KD, Humphrey SJ, Khan SA, Cipkus-Dubray LA, Smith MP, Jones AW (1993) 4-morpholinecarboximidine-N-1-adamantyl-N'-cyclohexylhydrochloride (U-37883A): pharmacological characterization of a novel antagonist of vascular ATP-sensitive K+ channel openers. *J Pharmacol Exp Ther* 266, 655–65.

46. Wellman GC, Barrett-Jolley R, Koppel H, Everitt D, Quayle JM (1999) Inhibition of vascular K(ATP) channels by U-37883A: a comparison with cardiac and skeletal muscle. *Br J Pharmacol* 128, 909–16.

47. Kovalev H, Quayle JM, Kamishima T, Lodwick D (2004) Molecular analysis of the subtype-selective inhibition of cloned KATP channels by PNU-37883A. *Br J Pharmacol* 141, 867–73.

48. Surah-Narwal S, Xu SZ, McHugh D, *et al.* (1999) Block of human aorta Kir6.1 by the vascular KATP channel inhibitor U37883A. *Br J Pharmacol* 128, 667–72.

49. Nelson MT, Huang Y, Brayden JE, Hescheler J, Standen NB (1990) Arterial dilations in response to calcitonin gene-related peptide involve activation of K+ channels. *Nature* 344, 770–3.

50. Miyoshi H, Nakaya Y (1995) Calcitonin gene-related peptide activates the K+ channels of vascular smooth muscle cells via adenylate cyclase. *Basic Res Cardiol* 90, 332–6.

51. Quayle JM, Bonev AD, Brayden JE, Nelson MT (1994) Calcitonin gene-related peptide activated ATP-sensitive K+ currents in rabbit arterial smooth muscle via protein kinase A. *J Physiol* 475, 9–13.

52. Kitazono T, Heistad DD, Faraci FM (1993) Role of ATP-sensitive K+ channels in CGRP-induced dilatation of basilar artery in vivo. *Am J Physiol* 265, 581–5.

53. Gozalov A, Jansen-Olesen I, Klaerke D, Olesen J (In press) Role of KATP channels in cephalic vasodilatation induced by CGRP, NO and transcranial electrical stimulation in the rat. *Cephalalgia*

54. Belloni FL, Hintze TH (1991) Glibenclamide attenuates adenosine-induced bradycardia and coronary vasodilatation. *Am J Physiol* 261, 720–7.

55. Jackson WF, Konig A, Dambacher T, Busse R (1993) Prostacyclin-induced vasodilation in rabbit heart is mediated by ATP-sensitive potassium channels. *Am J Physiol* 264, 238–43.

56. Murphy ME, Brayden JE (1995) Nitric oxide hyperpolarizes rabbit mesenteric arteries via ATP-sensitive potassium channels. *J Physiol* 486 (Pt 1), 47–58.

57. Hayabuchi Y, Davies NW, Standen NB (2001) Angiotensin II inhibits rat arterial KATP channels by inhibiting steady-state protein kinase A activity and activating protein kinase Ce. *J Physiol* 530, 193–205.

58. Miyoshi Y, Nakaya Y, Wakatsuki T, *et al.* (1992) Endothelin blocks ATP-sensitive K+ channels and depolarizes smooth muscle cells of porcine coronary artery. *Circ Res* 70, 612–16.

59. Miyoshi Y, Nakaya Y (1991) Angiotensin II blocks ATP-sensitive K+ channels in porcine coronary artery smooth muscle cells. *Biochem Biophys Res Commun* 181, 700–6.

60. Wakatsuki T, Nakaya Y, Inoue I (1992) Vasopressin modulates K(+)-channel activities of cultured smooth muscle cells from porcine coronary artery. *Am J Physiol* 263, 491–6.

61. Li L, Wu J, Jiang C (2003) Differential expression of Kir6.1 and SUR2B mRNAs in the vasculature of various tissues in rats. *J Membr Biol* 196, 61–9.

62. Santa N, Kitazono T, Ago T, *et al.* (2003) ATP-sensitive potassium channels mediate dilatation of basilar artery in response to intracellular acidification in vivo. *Stroke* 34, 1276–80.

63. Coghlan MJ, Carroll WA, Gopalakrishnan M (2001) Recent developments in the biology and medicinal chemistry of potassium channel modulators: update from a decade of progress. *J Med Chem* 44, 1627–53.

20

Antiepileptic drugs and migraine

Michael A. Rogawski

Introduction

Antiepileptic drugs (AEDs) have broad utility in neurology and psychiatry. Apart from epilepsy, they are commonly used for the treatment of pain syndromes, mood disorders, and various neuromuscular conditions.[1] Among the pain syndromes for which AEDs are used, migraine headache is a common application. In the USA, the AEDs approved for use in the prophylaxis of migraine are divalproex sodium (valproate) and topiramate. There is extensive evidence from randomized controlled clinical trials that valproate is effective in preventing migraine attacks or reducing their frequency, severity, and duration.[2–6] Various open-label observational studies and small randomized controlled trials of topiramate and two large multicentre randomized controlled trials have established the effectiveness of topiramate in migraine prevention.[7,8] The US Food and Drug Administration approved valproate for migraine in 1996 and topiramate in 2004. The British Association for the Study of Headache (BASH) considers valproate and topiramate to be second-line prophylactic agents after the first-line beta-blockers and amitriptyline. Evidence from double-blind randomized placebo-controlled studies also support the effectiveness of gabapentin in migraine prophylaxis[9,10] and it is considered a third-line agent by BASH. Less robust clinical studies have indicated that carbamazepine,[11] lamotrigine,[12–15] zonisamide,[16,17] and levetiracetam[18] may also be effective in the treatment of migraine. A meta-analysis by the Cochrane Collaboration confirmed that as a class AEDs reduce migraine frequency and are relatively well tolerated.[5]

AEDs are generally useful for the treatment of disorders of excessive, synchronous cellular excitability.[19] They are broadly effective in suppressing excessive or ectopic activity in neural cells and in some instances in muscle.[1] A key characteristic of AEDs is that they are able to suppress pathological patterns of excitation with only minimal interference with normal cellular activity. In this chapter, I describe current concepts in the pathophysiology of migraine, which posit that a reduced threshold for activation in the migraineur leads to excessive neural activity. This, in turn, induces cortical spreading depression (CSD) that is the precursor to migraine pain. With this general theoretical schema as a backdrop, I then consider how diverse AEDs useful in migraine prophylaxis protect against the appearance of pathological neural discharges. Much of the information on AED mechanisms is derived from studies aiming to define the action of the AEDs in epilepsy. However, given the similarities between the triggering mechanisms in epilepsy and migraine, the mechanistic studies are likely applicable to an understanding of migraine as well. Remarkably, each of the agents acts through a unique molecular target and reduces hyperexcitability in a distinctive way. However, the end result is a reduction in the frequency of migraine attacks.

Migraine as an episodic disorder

The syndromes for which AEDs are used are characteristically episodic in nature. Episodic phenomena are common symptoms of disease.[20,21] They include seizures, headaches, cardiac arrhythmias, episodic movement disorders, and periodic paralyses. Although they affect diverse organ systems and have different outward manifestation, the disorders that exhibit episodic symptoms have a number of common features. They are chronic disorders that often occur in otherwise normal individuals and the attacks may be precipitated by factors such as stress, fatigue, or diet. Disorders exhibiting episodic symptoms often have a genetic component and are first experienced in infancy, child-hood, or adolescence. As the genetic bases of the syndromes have been identified, it has become clear that many episodic disorders are due to defects in membrane ion channels, or, more broadly, ion (or neurotransmitter) transport molecules. Disorders associated with defects in ion channels have become known as 'channelopathies.' As ion channels are the principal mediators of cellular excitability properties, it can be presumed that the underlying pathophysiological basis of diverse channelopathies is altered cellular excitability. For some episodic disorders—for example, some genetic epilepsies, long QT syndromes, and periodic paralyses—it has been possible to define the specific nature of the change in cellular excitability that results from the mutations that cause the disorders. Often this is a gain-of-function increase in excitability, but in some instances there may be a reduction in excitability in a specific cell population (for example, in inhibitory interneurons) that leads to a net increase in circuit excitability (as in severe myoclonic epilepsy in infancy[22]). Additional evidence for a common pathophysiological basis among the episodic disorders is that they may occur together. In particular, there is strong evidence of comorbidity between migraine and epilepsy.[23,24] As discussed by Ottman and Lipton,[25] this comorbidity may not be due to a common genetic susceptibility. Rather, it may be the case that a state of altered brain excitability from whatever cause—environmental as well as genetic—might increase the risk of both migraine and epilepsy. (Alternative explanations of comorbidity that were considered less likely given the available evidence are that migraine attacks or seizures cause brain injury leading to the other disorder, or that there are shared environmental risk factors.)

Migraine is an episodic disorder that shares many clinical characteristics with other episodic disorders known to be channelopathies. Importantly, migraine aggregates in families, so that the risk of migraine is 50% greater in relatives of migraineurs than in relatives of controls.[26,27] This suggests that complex genetic factors contribute to the risk for migraine, as is the case for epilepsy.[28] Many epilepsy syndromes that are inherited in a Mendelian fashion have been found to be due to mutations in ion channels and there is reason to believe that epilepsy susceptibility may be broadly due, at least in part, to variations in ion channels that predispose to altered neuronal excitability. The commonality of migraine and epilepsy is supported by the identification of ion channel mutations in some types of familial hemiplegic migraine (FHM), a subtype of migraine with aura. These various considerations provide a basis to speculate that migraine generally, like epilepsy, may be a disorder of excessive cellular excitability. If this is the case, it is not surprising that AEDs have found utility in migraine treatment.

Familial hemiplegic migraine

FHM is a rare subtype of migraine with aura that is inherited in a Mendelian autosomal dominant fashion. Three different genes cosegregate with FHM. The first to be described was *CACNA1A*, which encodes the pore-forming subunit $Ca_v2.1$ of neuronal P/Q-type calcium channels.[29] Mutations in *CACNA1A* account for about one-half of all cases of FHM. FHM mutations in *CACNA1A* cause an increase in the calcium flux of single channels but there is paradoxically a decrease in the maximal $Ca_v2.1$ current density in neurons.[30] Thus, precisely how the FHM mutations influence cellular excitability is obscure. Interestingly, mutations in *CACNA1A* are also associated with the episodic ataxia syndrome EA-2, the spinocerebellar ataxia syndrome SCA-6, and also idiopathic generalized epilepsy.[31] Moreover, mutations in homologues of the gene can cause absence-like seizures in rodents.[32]

The second FHM gene to be described was *ATP1A2*, which encodes the α2 subunit of Na^+-K^+-ATPase.[33] One family has been described in which a mutation in the *ATP1A2* gene was not only associated with FHM, but also with benign familial infantile convulsions.[34] Other allelic conditions include alternating hemiplegia of childhood, basilar-type migraine, and migraine without aura.[35] FHM mutations in ATP1A2 lead to complete inactivation of the protein.[36] Seizures can be produced by inhibition of Na^+-K^+-ATPase,[37,38] presumably because neuronal resting membrane potential is less well maintained at a hyperpolarized level so that neurons can be more easily brought to threshold and excited. A similar increased excitability mechanism is likely to account for the FHM attacks.

The third FHM gene is *SCN1A*, which encodes the pore-forming α1-subunit of neuronal voltage-gated sodium channel $Na_v1.1$.[39] Mutations in this gene have been associated with generalized epilepsy with febrile seizures plus (GEFS+) and severe myoclonic epilepsy of infancy (SMEI). The FHM mutation in *SCN1A* is believed to accelerate recovery from sodium channel fast inactivation, which would be expected to cause an increased tendency toward repetitive action potential firing.[40] Many AEDs reduce repetitive action potential firing and conversely sodium channel toxins that promote repetitive action potential firing (such as pyrethroids and veratradine) induce seizures. Therefore, it is believed that repetitive firing is critical to at least some types of seizures, including those occurring in GEFS+.[41] In the case of FHM associated with *SCN1A* mutations, it can be presumed that enhanced repetitive spike firing may also underlie the occurrence of migraine.

FHM is distinguished from typical migraine by its Mendelian inheritance and association with hemiparesis. Nevertheless, there are sufficient similarities in headache characteristics and triggers to suggest that an understanding of the pathophysiological basis of FHM can shed light on the underlying mechanisms of the far more frequently encountered non-hemiplegic migraine syndromes. It is remarkable that mutations in FHM genes can cause either migraine or epilepsy, or in some cases both, clearly demonstrating a commonality between FHM and epilepsy, and supporting the notion that migraine generally, like epilepsy, is a disorder of neuronal hyperexcitability. This concept is supported by the observation that the known FHM genes encode protein complexes that play a direct role in neuronal excitability mechanisms. Thus, they are either ion channels, or in the case of *ATP1A2*, a molecule that regulates the level of membrane potential and thus indirectly influences ion channel gating and function.

Cortical spreading depression

CSD is becoming increasingly accepted as the basis for the aura in migraine and the trigger for the subsequent headache pain. The phenomenon was first described by Leão[42] who found that weak electrical or mechanical stimulation of the exposed cerebral cortex in the rabbit elicited a decrease in the spontaneous activity (depression of the EEG signal) at the stimulated region that slowly spread in all directions at 3–5 mm/min. Recovery of the initial pattern of spontaneous activity occurred over 5–10 min. Although Leão focused on the suppression of neuronal activity in CSD, Grafstein's subsequent work demonstrated that the depression is actually preceded by neural activation[43,44]. Recording from small isolated slabs of cortex in cerveau isolé (midbrain transected) cats, Grafstein was able to confirm Leão's observation that spreading depression is associated with a slow negative DC shift and depressed neural activity. However, she observed that there is a brief (2–3 s) burst of action potential activity at the initiation of the DC negativity and she hypothesized that the intense neuronal activity caused potassium elevations in the interstitial space that led to the depolarization and excitation of adjacent neurons, which in turn are 'thrown into intense activity and liberate more K^+.' Spreading depression is thus a slowly propagating wave of neuronal depolarization that travels across the cortex and is followed by long-lasting suppression of neuronal activity.

The initial suggestion that spreading depression is responsible for the migraine aura was based on a comparison between the rates of progression of the aura and of spreading depression. Migraine aura is any transient neurological disturbance that appears shortly before or during the development of a migraine headache. Most commonly, the aura arises in the primary visual cortex and typically involves spreading scintillating scotomas with a characteristic distribution of fortification figures. The disturbance usually starts at the centre of the visual field and propagates to peripheral zones within 10–15 min. Function returns to normal within another 10–15 min.[45] The rate of development of the visual symptoms suggests that there is a front of hyperactivation in the visual cortex that moves at a speed of approximately 3 mm/min. Milner[46] noted that the speed of propagation of the visual symptoms was the same as that of spreading depression, leading to the hypothesis that spreading depression is the physiological basis for the aura. Interestingly, in subjects experiencing somatosensory symptoms, the rate of spread of symptoms along the sensory homunculus occurs at a similar rate.

Numerous neuroimaging studies in humans have supported the concept that spreading depression-like phenomena in neocortex occur with migraine aura.[47,48] In particular, using functional magnetic resonance imaging, it has been possible to demonstrate slowly propagating neurovascular changes in visual cortex that occur together with visual symptoms of patients experiencing visual aura.[49]

Given these various lines of evidence, there is general consensus that spreading depression accounts for migraine aura. However, as there are no pain fibres in the brain parenchyma, it has been difficult to understand how the alterations in brain tissue excitability of spreading depression induce the intense pain that follows. A recent study of blood flow in the rat cortex following the induction of spreading depression has been interpreted as providing the link.[50] These studies have shown that CSD in the rat is associated with changes in extracerebral cephalic blood flow as a result of vasodilation within the middle meningeal artery. It is hypothesized that the intrinsic neurophysiological events occurring in the brain during spreading depression irritate axon collateral nociceptors in pia and dura mater leading to trigeminal and parasympathetic activation. Trigeminal pain afferents originating in the meningeal vessels pass through the trigeminal ganglion and synapse on second order neurons in the trigeminocervical complex. These nociceptive neurons, in turn, project through the trigeminal nucleus, and after decussating in the brainstem, form synapses with neurons in the thalamus. Hippocampal spreading depression is also able to activate the trigeminal nucleus,[51] but the role of the hippocampus in migraine has not been well characterized. It is conceivable that spreading depression in areas such as the hippocampus or other regions of the limbic system could be a cause of migraine without aura, especially as these headaches can be associated with disturbances in memory, abnormal perceptual experiences (olfactory or gustatory hallucinations and distortions of body image), or changes in mood.[52]

Following on the work of Leão and Grafstein, there have been numerous investigations into the physiological basis of spreading depression. It has been found that in addition to the classical triggers, the phenomenon can be induced by elevated extracellular potassium, glutamate, and inhibition of Na^+/K^+-ATPase.[53] Although Grafstein proposed that intense neural activation and elevations in extracellular potassium are responsible for the propagation of CSD, this has recently been questioned by Herraras,[54] at least as far as its central role in the spread of the depressed neural activity. Indeed, tetrodotoxin blockade of neuron firing fails to interfere with spreading depression in some situations, so intense neuronal activity does not seem to be required. Seconds before the neuronal activity is recorded and millimetres ahead of it, subthreshold pacemaker field oscillations can be detected that are resistant to synaptic transmission blockade. Thus, as an alternative to the potassium hypothesis, Herraras has suggested that neuronal synchronization and field oscillations that precede the front of depolarization play a critical role in extending the zone of depressed activity. The synchronization has been hypothesized to be due to non-synaptic interactions between neurons possibly mediated by the excitatory neurotransmitter glutamate or through gap junctional interactions. Recently, glia have been implicated as the source of glutamate.[55] These ideas are intriguing given the recent demonstration that calcium signalling in astrocytes may lead to the induction of epileptiform hypersynchronous activity in adjacent neuronal networks as a result of glutamate released from the astrocytes.[56] Several AEDs, including valproate and gabapentin, with demonstrated activity in migraine prophylaxis, effectively suppress calcium signalling in astrocytes. The activity of valproate and gabapentin is more robust than that of phenytoin, which has not been demonstrated to have activity in migraine. Thus, it seems plausible that astrocytes are an important target for AEDs in migraine prophylaxis. However, it is noteworthy that spreading depression can occur even when intracellular calcium waves are eliminated.[57] At present, the contribution of astrocytes to spreading depression is incompletely defined; additional evidence is needed to characterize how and when they play a part, if any. Therefore, notwithstanding the interesting possibility that astrocytes could be a target for AEDs in migraine, in this chapter I focus on neurons where the actions of these agents are much better understood. Even if neuronal hyperactivity is not *required* for CSD, this does not eliminate the fact that such activity can trigger CSD and very likely plays a part in migraine. It is probably too simplistic to presume that suppression of the high frequency firing noted by Grafstein[43] to be associated with the onset of spreading depression accounts for the activity of AEDs in protecting against migraine attacks. Rather, those AEDs that are effective in migraine may suppress the synchronizing mechanisms that Herraras has proposed are critical to CSD. Interference with synchronizing mechanisms may similarly be responsible for the effectiveness of AEDs in epilepsy, although how this might occur is still largely a matter of speculation.

Enhanced cortical responsiveness in migraine

As is the case for many episodic disorders, the precise trigger for the migraine attack is enigmatic. Many clinical factors such as diet, alterations in sleep, or stress are known to predispose to attacks. How these factors bring on a migraine attack is not known. However, there is evidence for enhanced cortical responsiveness to diverse stimuli in migraineurs.[58,59] The techniques that have been used include psychophysical studies; visual, auditory, and somatosensory evoked potentials; magnetoencephalography; and transcranial magnetic stimulation (TMS) of the motor cortex. In all cases, there is evidence of heightened reactivity between migraine attacks. Results from TMS of the occipital (visual) cortex have been particularly compelling. Most but not all studies have observed a reduced threshold for induction of phosphenes in migraineurs compared with controls. This phenomenon appears to be equally present in subjects that experience migraine without aura as those with migraine with aura.

In the remainder of this chapter, I consider the current understanding of the mechanisms of AEDs that are used for migraine prophylaxis or for which there is some supportive clinical evidence of efficacy. While many AEDs have activity in migraine, it is certainly not the case that all AEDs have such activity. Therefore, I close with some selected examples of AEDs that are not likely to be effective in migraine. Consideration of the mechanisms of these agents can be useful in narrowing the set of targets to be considered in the development of antimigraine therapies and may provide insight into the neurobiological similarities and differences between migraine and epilepsy.

Cellular mechanism of antiepileptic drugs widely used for migraine prophylaxis

Valproate

Valproate has many pharmacological actions, none of which by itself can completely account for its clinical activity in epilepsy and the other conditions for which it is used, including migraine.[60] It has therefore been proposed that valproate acts through a combination of actions. Among these various actions, Löscher[61,62] has concluded that increases in GABA turnover that are produced in specific brain regions is of particular importance in the ability of valproate to control seizure generation and propagation. However, agents that act on GABA systems have not in general been found to influence spreading depression or to be effective in the treatment of migraine. Therefore, it seems likely that other known or unknown actions of valproate might account for the clinical efficacy in migraine prophylaxis. There is limited evidence that valproate may inhibit N-methyl-D-aspartate or kainate receptor-mediated synaptic transmission;[63,64] whether these actions could contribute to the efficacy of valproate in migraine prophylaxis is not known. As noted previously, valproate seems to potently inhibit astrocytic calcium signalling. It will be of interest to determine the underlying basis of this action and whether it has relevance for the antimigraine activity of valproate.

Acute treatment with valproate has generally not been found to influence spreading depression.[65,66] However, recently Ayata et al.[66] found that prolonged treatment with valproate along with many other drugs useful in migraine prophylaxis, including beta-blockers, topiramate, methysergide, and amitriptyline, reduced the number of potassium-induced CSD events and increased the electrical stimulation threshold for CSD in rats. These results suggest that all of the effective drugs could be acting in a common fashion to induce a plastic change in brain excitability mechanisms that lead to resistance to spreading depression.

Topiramate

Several studies have shown that topiramate can suppress CSD in rats and cats at doses comparable with those that protect against seizures.[66,67] In addition, topiramate is able to inhibit evoked activity in dorsal horn neurons in the cervical spinal cord (C2) that are believed to mediate headache pain.[68] Pain in migraine is hypothesized to be due to activation of trigeminal nerve axons (presumably by CSD), which then release calcitonin gene-related peptide (CGRP) and other peptide mediators from terminals near the meningeal vessels to cause vasodilation. Whether or not the vasodilation is responsible for the pain, it is a useful marker of activation of the trigeminal system. Topiramate inhibited neurogenic dural vasodilation but did not inhibit vasodilation induced by CGRP, leading to the conclusion that topiramate might act presynaptically on trigeminal nerve terminals to inhibit the release of CGRP.[69] Thus, topiramate appears to have a dual mechanism in migraine. The drug may inhibit activation of the attacks by raising the threshold for CSD and could also specifically interfere with pain mechanisms through effects on the trigeminovascular system.

Several cellular mechanisms have been proposed to underlie the therapeutic activity of topiramate: (1) activity-dependent attenuation of voltage-dependent sodium currents; (2) inhibition of high voltage-activated calcium channels; (3) potentiation of $GABA_A$ receptor-mediated currents; (4) inhibition of AMPA/kainate receptors; (5) inhibition of types II and IV carbonic anhydrase isoenzymes; and (6) activation of a steady potassium current.[60,70] The effects on sodium channels, high voltage-activated calcium channels, and $GABA_A$ receptors are unlikely to contribute in a substantial way to the antimigraine action because there is little evidence that drugs that target these mechanisms are effective in migraine prophylaxis.[71] Similarly, the carbonic anhydrase inhibition is not likely to be relevant to the antimigraine activity of topiramate.[72] However, the report that topiramate can activate a potassium current is intriguing inasmuch as potassium channel openers with activity on KCNQ channels have shown modest activity in an experimental model of spreading depression (see section on retigabine below).

Among the diverse pharmacological actions of topiramate, the interaction with ionotropic glutamate receptors is perhaps the most likely action to be relevant to its antimigraine activity. Topiramate is not a simple receptor antagonist, although there is considerable evidence that it can influence the functional activity of AMPA/kainate-type glutamate receptors; there is no evidence that topiramate blocks N-methyl-D-aspartate receptors.[73] Thus, in cultured neurons, topiramate was found to inhibit responses to kainate, an agonist of AMPA and kainate receptors.[73] More recently, topiramate was reported to be a more potent and efficacious inhibitor of GluR5 kainate receptor currents in basolateral amygdala principal neurons than of AMPA receptor currents.[74] AMPA receptors are crucial for excitatory synaptic transmission throughout the central nervous system, and drugs that substantially block AMPA receptors are expected to produce dramatic neurobehavioural impairment. Thus, the finding that topiramate is weak and has low efficacy as an AMPA receptor antagonist corresponds with the clinical observation that the drug is reasonably well tolerated. Blockade of GluR5 kainate receptors is not expected to have the side effects associated with blockade of AMPA receptors. In fact, mice genetically engineered to lack GluR5 are grossly normal neurologically. However, GluR5 kainate receptors represent an interesting target for migraine therapy. GluR5 kainate receptors regulate pain transmission in the spinal cord[75,76] and GluR5 kainate receptor subunits and functional GluR5 kainate receptors are expressed in trigeminal neurons.[77] Moreover, GluR5 antagonists are active in migraine models[78,79] and intravenous LY293558 (tezampanel), an antagonist of AMPA and GluR5 kainate receptors, was found to dramatically improve headache in a small controlled clinical trial in acute migraine.[80] Although the response rate for LY293558 (69%) was somewhat less than for subcutaneous sumatriptan (86%), LY293558 was better tolerated. In normal volunteers, LY293558 was found to cause 'hazy vision,' a reversible side-effect that is believed to be mechanism-related and due to effects in the retina.[81] This concerning side-effect was not spontaneously reported by the migraineurs, possibly because they had already experienced various visual symptoms in the setting of the acute migraine attack. The clinical trial results with LY293558 are compatible with the concept that GluR5 kainate receptors are an attractive target in migraine. However, because LY293558 is not selective for AMPA receptors, additional studies with more selective antagonists are required. An additional phase II clinical trial of subcutaneous LY293558 for the abortive treatment of migraine is currently ongoing under the sponsorship of Torrey Pines Therapeutics. An oral prodrug form of LY293558 is also under investigation for migraine.

The inhibitory action of topiramate on GluR5 kainate receptors develops slowly, suggesting that it acts indirectly.[74] The effects on ion channels are complex and are unlikely to occur through direct effects on channel gating, but are more likely to be mediated indirectly, possibly through inhibition of channel phosphorylation. Recently, it has been found that topiramate inhibits phosphorylation of serine 845 of the AMPA receptor GluR1 subunit,[82] suggesting that the effect of the drug on AMPA and perhaps also kainate receptors could be due to an alteration in the phosphorylation state of the protein. The ability of topiramate to functionally inhibit GluR5 kainate receptors *in vivo* was confirmed in experiments in mice with selective glutamate receptor antagonists, where anticonvulsant doses of topiramate blocked clonic seizures induced by a selective GluR5 kainate receptor agonist but not by an agonist of AMPA receptors.[83] Taken together, the results with LY293558 and topiramate provide a compelling justification for further studies to investigate GluR5 kainate receptors as targets for migraine therapy.

Antiepileptic drugs that are possibly effective for migraine prophylaxis

Gabapentin and pregabalin

In the USA, gabapentin and its analogue pregabalin are not approved for use in migraine, although gabapentin is indicated for postherpetic neuralgia and pregabalin is indicated for this pain condition as well as for diabetic neuropathy. Gabapentin, the lipophilic 3-cyclohexyl analogue of GABA, was originally synthesized in an attempt to develop a brain-penetrant GABA agonist. Although both gabapentin and pregabalin [(R)-3-isobutyl-GABA] are based on a GABA backbone, bulky aliphatic substituents in the molecules preclude binding to the GABA recognition site on $GABA_A$ receptors. The drugs also do not interact with other sites on $GABA_A$ receptors, including the benzodiazepine recognition site.[84] High-affinity binding sites for gabapentin and pregabalin in brain have been identified as $\alpha_2\delta$ proteins, which are believed to be auxiliary subunits of voltage-activated calcium channels.[85] The binding affinities of gabapentin, pregabalin, and related structures to $\alpha_2\delta$ subunits correlates in a stereoselective fashion with their analgesic activity.[86] In addition, knock in of a mutation (R217A) in the $\alpha_2\delta$-1 subunit in mice, which results in markedly reduced binding of gabapentin and pregabalin, eliminates their analgesic activity without influencing the analgesic activity of morphine.[87,88] Thus, there is strong support for the notion that the analgesic activity of gabapentin and pregabalin is mediated through the interaction with α2δ. Whether this accounts for the prophylactic activity in migraine remains to be determined. In this regard it is noteworthy that as yet there is no evidence that gabapentin or pregabalin can influence the neural mechanisms that trigger migraine (spreading depression).

The α2δ subunits are highly glycosylated proteins of molecular mass approximately 150 kDa (997–1150 amino acid residues). There are four homologous forms, but only subtypes 1 and 2 bind gabapentin and pregabalin with high affinity.[89] α2δ-1 and α2δ-2 subunits are believed to form complexes with many voltage-dependent calcium channel types.[90] It is not yet clear which calcium channels are important for the therapeutic activity of gabapentin and pregabalin, nor is the functional role of the α2δ subunit complex fully understood. However, for some calcium channel types, α2δ subunit complex has been shown to allosterically enhance current amplitude and also promote channel trafficking to the membrane.[85] Functional studies of the effects of gabapentin on calcium channel activity have yielded divergent results; however, there is a general consensus that gabapentin and pregabalin reduce the release of neurotransmitters from neural tissue, with effects on CGRP, substance P, and glutamate release being of particular relevance to migraine prophylaxis.[91-94] It is noteworthy that the effect of gabapentin and pregabalin on these mediators is generally only observed in the presence of nerve injury associated with inflammation and hyperalgesia. Thus, α2δ ligands have minimal effects on physiological neuro transmitter release but significantly inhibit sensitized or abnormal release. Although the mechanism underlying this selectivity is not understood, it may explain the relatively benign side-effect profiles of gabapentin and pregabalin as neuro transmitter release under normal conditions is maintained.

Recent studies indicate that the ability of gabapentin and pregabalin to influence release of neuroactive substances may not be dependent upon calcium entry through voltage-sensitive calcium channels.[85] Rather, α2δ subunit proteins might influence synaptic release directly, possibly through interactions with the release machinery that are independent of the main pore-forming α1 calcium channel subunits. It has been speculated that binding of the drugs to α2δ subunits directly influences the release machinery, possibly by affecting physical interactions between presynaptic calcium channels and proteins mediating exocytosis.[88] A recent report has provided evidence that the action of gabapentin is not to directly reduce calcium channel activity, but rather to inhibit the trafficking of calcium channels to the plasma membrane.[95]

Gabapentin and pregabalin are absorbed in the gut and pass across the blood–brain barrier via the system L transporter, which is specialized for the transport of large neutral amino acids.[96] The fact that these drugs are substrates for this transporter is essential to their therapeutic activity because it allows them to gain access to the central nervous system.[97] However, because the transporter can be saturated, the ability to achieve high blood and brain levels is limited. A gabapentin prodrug, XP13512 [(±)-1-([(α-isobutanoyloxyethoxy)carbonyl] aminomethyl)-1-cyclohexane acetic acid], is under development that may avoid these problems.[98] XP12512 is absorbed by high-capacity nutrient transporters and then rapidly converted to gabapentin, so the rate limiting absorption by the system L is circumvented.

Zonisamide

There is limited information, largely from open label clinical trials, suggesting that zonisamide may be effective in migraine prophylaxis in adults and children.[16,17,99–102] Taken together with the available base of information on zonisamide, a case can be made that further study of the drug in controlled trials is warranted. Zonisamide has a unique chemical structure consisting of an aromatic fused benzene-isoxazole ring and a sulphonamide side chain. Topiramate also contains a sulphur atom in an O-sulphamate moiety that is structurally similar to the sulphonamide in zonisamide. Thus, zonisamide and topiramate are the only sulphur-containing AEDs. Carbonic anhydrase inhibitors such as acetazolamide also have a sulphonamide side chain, and indeed, both AEDs inhibit carbonic anhydrase.[103] There are intriguing similarities between zonisamide and topiramate in addition to their shared chemistry. Both drugs are associated with weight loss rather than the weight gain commonly observed with AEDs, and both drugs have been linked to nephrolithiasis and hypohidrosis, which could be due to their common action as carbonic anhydrase inhibitors. As zonisamide has so many similarities to topiramate, it would not be surprising if zonisamide, like topiramate, has efficacy in migraine prophylaxis.

In animal seizure models, zonisamide has a profile of activity similar to that of sodium channel modulating AEDs, such as phenytoin, carbamazepine, and lamotrigine.[60] Indeed, there is evidence that zonisamide can interact with voltage-activated sodium channels at low, therapeutically relevant concentrations and that the effect on sodium channels is similar to that of other sodium channel modulating AEDs. However, zonisamide has several additional pharmacological actions that could contribute to its anticonvulsant activity including effects on T-type voltage-dependent calcium channels, presynaptic effects to inhibit or facilitate neurotransmitter release, and effects on neurotransmitter turnover and metabolism. As noted, zonisamide is also an inhibitor of carbonic anhydrase, although this alone is unlikely to be relevant to its putative efficacy in migraine as there is no compelling evidence that more potent carbonic anhydrase inhibitors such as acetazolamide have antimigraine activity. It is noteworthy that there is pharmacological evidence that carbonic anhydrase inhibition is not responsible for the anticonvulsant activity of zonisamide.

As is the case for other sodium channel modulating AEDs, the ability of zonisamide to modulate voltage-dependent sodium channels is expected to reduce action potential evoked release of glutamate through a presynaptic action. In fact, recordings from hippocampal neurons in rat brain slices have confirmed this action.[104] Studies with microdialysis in freely moving rats have indicated that zonisamide has complex effects on the release of various neurotransmitters including GABA, dopamine, serotonin, and acetylcholine. How these effects could contribute to the activity of zonisamide in migraine is uncertain. Overall, the known pharmacological actions of zonisamide on voltage-dependent ion channels and other well-characterized targets may not fully explain the putative efficacy in migraine, raising the possibility that the drug could have actions on one or more as yet undefined targets.

Levetiracetam

Limited information from retrospective and open label trials suggests that levetiracetam may have utility in migraine prophylaxis.[18,105–110] Levetiracetam has been marketed for epilepsy therapy since 2000, but its molecular target in brain was only recently identified.[111] The discovery of this target—the synaptic vesicle protein SV2A— represents a milestone in AED research for two reasons. First, because SV2 is a component of the synaptic release machinery, it focuses attention on the presynaptic nerve terminal as a site of action of AEDs. Second, the knowledge of the molecular target of levetiracetam has made it possible to screen for follow-on compounds with improved properties. Using this approach, two structural analogues of levetiracetam with 10-fold greater SV2A binding activity have been identified and advanced to clinical trials. These compounds are seletracetam (ucb 44212) and brivaracetam (ucb 34714). Brivaracetam has been studied in epilepsy and neuropathic pain; phase II clinical trials in refractory partial seizures were promising and phase III clinical trials are ongoing. The mechanism whereby binding to SV2A results in anticonvulsant activity is unknown. SV2A is an abundant protein component of synaptic vesicles that is structurally similar to 12-transmembrane domain transporters, although a transporter activity for SV2A has not yet been identified. SV2A is not essential for synaptic transmission, but a recent study proposed that SV2A is a positive modulator of low-frequency synaptic transmission that may act by preparing vesicles for fusion.[112] Mice in which the protein has been deleted by gene targeting exhibit seizures.[113] It seems reasonable that the SV2A ligands could protect against states of excessive cellular excitability through effects on synaptic release mechanisms, although experimental support has not as yet been forthcoming.

Antiepileptic drugs in development with potential utility in migraine

Valproate-like agents

Valproate has a unique place in epilepsy therapy because of its broad spectrum of efficacy. In addition valproate is useful in the treatment of acute mania and, of course, migraine. However, valproate has several undesirable side-effects, including teratogenicity, weight gain, and reproductive dysfunction, and it occasionally causes hepatic and pancreatic toxicity.[114] Therefore, much attention has been focused on the development of agents that have the same broad spectrum of clinical efficacy as valproate without these undesirable characteristics. Because the precise mechanism of action of valproate is unknown, it is difficult to predict—based on preclinical studies—whether an analogue will have the same clinical efficacy. Nevertheless, several valproate-like compounds have been demonstrated to have a valproate-like profile in animal seizure and other behavioural models so that they have been advanced to clinical development.[115,116] In all cases, the compounds are amides, because it is believed that the acid forms predispose to teratogenicity. Indeed, the amide form of valproate, valpromide, is more potent as an anticonvulsant than valproate and it is not teratogenic in mice susceptible to neural tube defects. However, in humans valpromide is biotransformed to valproate, so it does not offer advantages to valproate. The focus has been on obtaining compounds with reduced or no conversion to valproate or the corresponding acid. It is unknown whether these compounds have activity in preclinical models relevant to migraine. However, they do appear to have activity in models of neuropathic pain, which in some cases is greater than for valproate.[117,118]

Three valproate-like compounds (two existing in more than one stereoisomeric form) that were discovered or extensively studied in the laboratory of Meir Bialer at the Hebrew University of Jerusalem are under active clinical development. The first to undergo human clinical trials was valrocemide (valproyl glycinamide; SPD493), which is now entering phase II development.[119] Valrocemide is more potent than valproate in animal seizure models, possibly due to its increased accumulation in brain. In rats and dogs, valrocemide is converted to minimal amounts of valproate, and embryotoxicity has not been observed in rats and rabbits. However, in humans, biotransformation of valrocemide to valproate is substantial. Therefore, although valrocemide could be safer than valproate, the risk of teratogenicity is not eliminated. Because of its relatively short half-life, three times daily dosing will be required, unless a controlled release formulation is developed.

The resolved isomers of valnoctamide (2-ethyl-3-methylpentanamide) and diisopropyl acetamide (PID) are also under active development. Like valrocemide, these isomers exhibit greater anticonvulsant activity and valnoctamide has been shown to have greater anti-allodynic potency than valproate.[116–118] However, they are not converted to valproate, which could be an advantage from the perspective of teratogenicity and the other idiosyncratic toxicities of valproate. Valnoctamide has two stereogenic carbons, so that the molecule exists in four stereoisomeric forms. Only small differences were found between the anticonvulsant potencies and pharmacokinetic properties of the (2S,3S) and (2R,3S) isomers.[120] The mixture of all four isomers was at one time marketed as an anxiolytic and sedative in Europe, but is not available at present. It appears that one or more of the isomers will be taken through a full development programme for central nervous system indications that could include migraine. Despite the fact that it was marketed as a sedative, anecdotal evidence indicates that valnoctamide is well tolerated and not strongly sedative.[115] Valnoctamide does not induce embryotoxicity in mice that are susceptible to valproate-induced spina bifida aperta.[121] However, the validity of this model as a predictor of risk for human spina bifida is uncertain.

PID, which is also expected to enter clinical development, has a single stereocentre. As in the case of valnoctamide, only small differences were found in the relative anticonvulsant potencies and pharmacokinetic properties of the enantiomers, with the (R)-enantiomer possibly being slightly more potent.[122–124] PID was also free of teratogenicity in susceptible mice.

Isovaleramide (3-methylbutanamide; NPS-1776) has a similar profile of activity to valproate in animal seizure models, but is weaker in potency.[125] Phase I clinical trials indicated that the compound is safe and well tolerated, but it is not currently being developed.

Retigabine

Retigabine [N-(2-amino-4-[fluorobenzylamino]-phenyl)carbamic acid; D-23129], the desaza-analogue of flupirtine (a non-opiate analgesic approved in Europe for general nociceptive pain), is an effective inhibitor of CSD[126] and therefore has potential in migraine therapy. Retigabine has activity in a broad spectrum of animal epilepsy models.[127–129] Clinical testing in several phase II clinical trials, largely in patients with partial seizures with or without secondary generalization who were refractory to available therapies, suggested that the compound is efficacious for the treatment of epilepsy. Several phase II studies have demonstrated efficacy in the treatment of partial seizures, including a dose-ranging study in 399 patients.[130] Two phase III trails (RESTORE 1 and 2) have confirmed the results of the phase II studies. As yet, retigabine has not been evaluated in migraine.

There has been considerable interest in the molecular pharmacology of retigabine, which is the first in a new class of KCNQ (Kv7) potassium channel openers. Retigabine causes a specific enhancement of M-type potassium current, which is carried by KCNQ-type potassium channels.[131–133] M-current is a slowly activating current whose threshold is near resting potential. The principal action of retigabine is to shift the activation of KCNQ channels underlying the M-current to more hyperpolarized membrane potentials, and also to slow their deactivation and accelerate their activation.[134,135] The critical action of the drug is to increase potassium current near resting potential, which reduces the excitability of neurons that express KCNQ2–5 subunits (Kv7.2–7.5). The cardiac-specific isoform KCNQ1 (KvLQT or Kv7.1) is not affected by retigabine. In addition to their localization in brain regions relevant to epilepsy, KCNQ/M channels are also present in elements of nociceptive sensory systems, including dorsal root ganglia neurons, and retigabine inhibits responses in chronic pain models.[136] Retigabine could therefore have efficacy in migraine as a result of its novel analgesic activity on sensory systems in addition to the effects on CSD. Indeed, there is evidence that KCNQ2 channels are expressed in the trigeminal ganglia and the trigeminal nucleus caudalis and it has been proposed that sensitization of this pathway could be a factor in migraine.[126]

Although most attention has been focused on the unique ability of retigabine to activate KCNQ channels, the drug also acts as a positive modulator of $GABA_A$ receptors.[137] Thus, retigabine enhances GABA-activated chloride current responses and GABAergic IPSCs at concentrations that are only modestly higher than those that influence KCNQ channels.[138,139] It has been suggested that the effects of retigabine on $GABA_A$ receptors could contribute to its efficacy in epilepsy and also to side-effects.[115] However, as $GABA_A$ receptor positive modulating activity is not associated with efficacy in migraine prophylaxis, KCNQ openers that lack activity on $GABA_A$ receptors could potentially have better tolerability.[140] Several novel compounds, including acrylamides, have been identified to have KNCQ opening activity and to inhibit CSD.[141–144] Some of these compounds are more than two orders of magnitude more potent than retigabine, but equally efficacious. ICA-105665, a compound reported to have specific KCNQ opening activity, has entered phase I trials for epilepsy but also may be developed for neuropathic pain.

Lacosamide

Lacosamide [(R)-2-acetamido-N-benzyl-3-methoxypropionamide; SPM 927; harkoseride], is a functionalized amino acid currently in phase III clinical trials for the treatment of partial epilepsy and diabetic neuropathic pain. Additionally, lacosamide is under investigation for migraine prophylaxis, fibromyalgia, and osteoarthritis. Lacosamide has activity in a broad spectrum of acute seizure models, but is inactive in the pentylenetetrazol model.[145] It also has demonstrated antihyperalgesic activity in a variety of acute and chronic inflammatory pain and neuropathic pain models, but does not have acute antinociceptive activity.[146] Its mechanism of action is not well understood.[115] Recently, however, it has been proposed that a novel action on voltage-gated sodium channels could underlie its therapeutic efficacy.[145] Unlike conventional sodium channel modulating AEDs, lacosamide does not have actions on fast inactivation. Rather, it seems to selectively promote slow inactivation, a distinct and less well-understood form of sodium channel inactivation that occurs on a time-scale of seconds to minutes, in contrast to fast inactivation, which occurs on a millisecond time-scale. The enhancement of slow inactivation could theoretically lead to selective inhibition of epileptiform activity, as epileptic depolarization of neurons is more prolonged than ordinary synaptic depolarization and is typically of the order of tens of seconds, the time-scale where slow inactivation is pertinent. It is not known whether this mechanism would be relevant to neuropathic pain or migraine. Lacosamide has also been found to bind to collapsin response mediator protein-2 (CRMP-2), a cytosolic phosphoprotein mainly expressed in the nervous system that promotes neurite extension and is involved in the signalling of growth inhibitory cues. Whether and how the interaction with CRMP-2 relates to the therapeutic activity of lacosamide remains to be determined.

Tonabersat

Tonabersat [SB-220453; cis-(−)-6-acetyl-4S-(3-chloro-4-fluorobenzoylamino)-3, 4-dihydro-2,2-dimethyl-2H-1-benzopyran-3S-ol] is a benzopyran with anticonvulsant properties that is a potent and effective blocker of CSD.[147–149] It has similar pharmacological properties to carabersat (SB-204269), which demonstrated efficacy in a phase II clinical trial for epilepsy, but whose development was not continued because of concerns about the possible cardiotoxicity of a metabolite. Tonabersat was not effective as an abortive agent in migraine (N. Upton, personal communication). However, a phase IIa clinical trial in migraine prophylaxis demonstrated a significant reduction in migraine frequency and in rescue medication days, with good tolerability. Although the mechanism of action of tonabersat in migraine is not known, the fact that it is an effective inhibitor of CSD is intriguing. The clinical trial results with tonabersat may reflect the fact that inhibition of CSD can prevent migraine from being triggered, but once migraine is established and downstream mechanisms come into play, CSD is no longer a factor. There is evidence that tonabersat is a selective blocker of gap junctions (N. Upton, personal communication). The extent to which this action contributes to the effect on CSD is uncertain. While gap junction inhibitors have been observed to modify spreading depression,[150] gap junction blockers do not eliminate CSD in all instances.[151,152] Therefore, although it is clear that tonabersat inhibits spreading depression, whether this is due to the effect of the drug on gap junctions remains to be demonstrated. However, it does raise the intriguing possibility that gap junctions could be drug targets for migraine therapy.

Antiepileptic drugs unlikely to be of utility in migraine

Carbamazepine and oxcarbazepine

Carbamazepine was the first AED studied in migraine, but there is only very limited clinical evidence of efficacy.[11,153] Carbamazepine is active itself and also serves as a prodrug for the active metabolite carbamazepine-10,11-epoxide. Oxcarbazepine, the 10-keto analogue of carbamazepine, also is biotransformed to active metabolites, $S(+)$-licarbazepine and $R(-)$-licarbazepine. The parent and its metabolites probably act mechanistically in a similar fashion to carbamazepine[19]. Interestingly, there is essentially no positive data in the literature on oxcarbazepine in migraine,[153] suggesting that neither carbamazepine nor oxcarbazepine are clinically effective. Moreover, neither drug seems to be effective in blocking CSD. Carbamazepine and oxcarbazepine are believed to protect against seizures largely through effects on voltage-gated sodium channels, which lead to the suppression of high-frequency repetitive action potential firing. While this action confers protection against partial and primary generalized tonic-clonic seizures, it is apparently not capable of preventing migraine. Clearly, not all AEDs are effective in migraine prophylaxis. It is tempting to suggest that antimigraine activity is a feature of 'broad-spectrum' AEDs (effective in partial and at least one type of primary generalized seizures other than primary generalized tonic-clonic seizures). This may be the case; however, gabapentin and pregabalin, which are not known to be broad-spectrum agents, would seem to contradict the rule. (Perhaps the efficacy of gabapentin and pregabalin relates to their analgesic activity rather than an ability to influence the hyperexcitability that triggers migraine.) In any case, sodium channel blockade is not likely to be a promising strategy for the development of migraine prophylactic agents.

Carisbamate

Carisbamate (RWJ333369; S-2-O-carbamoyl-1-ochlorophenyl-ethanol) is a monocarbamate with a broad spectrum of activity in a wide range of rodent epilepsy models. A phase IIb clinical trial for the treatment of partial onset seizures was recently completed demonstrating efficacy and good tolerability.[154] However, one phase III study demonstrated efficacy at only a single dose and the second failed to reach significance. A trial in migraine demonstrated that carisbamate does not have activity for migraine prophylaxis.

Ganaxolone

Ganaxolone (3α-hydroxy-3β-methyl-5α-pregnan-20-one) is the 3α-methyl synthetic analogue of the endogenous neurosteroid allopregnanolone (3α,5α-P), a metabolite of progesterone. Ganaxolone, like 3α,5α-P, does not have classical steroid hormone activity. Whereas it is believed that 3α,5α-P can be converted to metabolites with hormonal activity, ganaxolone cannot. Ganaxolone is a powerful positive allosteric modulator of $GABA_A$ receptors with potency and efficacy comparable with its endogenous congener 3α,5α-P.[155] Neurosteroid actions on $GABA_A$ receptors occur at sites distinct from the benzodiazepine modulatory site[156] and neurosteroids fail to demonstrate tolerance (at least with respect to anticonvulsant activity) that limits the clinical utility of benzodiazepines.[157] Ganaxolone is currently undergoing clinical trials for partial seizures in adults and infantile spasms in children aged 4–24 months.[158] In a rat migraine model (neurogenic plasma extravasation in dura mater), ganaxolone had activity at low doses (ED_{50}, 0.2 mg/kg) raising the possibility that it could be clinically effective in migraine. In the 1990s, ganaxolone was extensively investigated as an abortive migraine agent in single dose studies but was never evaluated for migraine prophylaxis. The first study (1042-0112) was a double-blind, placebo-controlled dose-ranging trial (20–500 mg) in 252 premenopausal women ages 18–55, 203 of whom received active drug within 8 h of the onset of moderate or severe migraine with or without aura. There was a suggestion that pain relief was correlated with plasma concentration. In the second study (1042-0116), an open-label trial of eight men and 22 women (three of whom were included in the 1042-0112 study) in which ganaxolone (500–1000 mg) was also administered within 8 h of the onset of moderate or severe migraine, there was minimal correlation of pain relief at 2 h with ganaxolone plasma concentration. In the final study (1042-0117), the allowable time from moderate to severe migraine headache onset to dosing was reduced to 2 h. Groups of 163 subjects ages 18–65 (132 women and 31 men in each group) received active drug (750 mg) or placebo. There was no statistically significant difference between treatment groups in migraine pain relief at 2 or 4 h postdose. A subgroup analysis of the menstruating women (25 receiving ganaxolone and 20 receiving placebo) demonstrated a statistically significant reduction in migraine pain ($P = 0.046$) in the drug-treated subjects. Overall, the clinical trials provided little evidence to support further studies of ganaxolone in acute migraine therapy in an unselected population and development for this indication has not progressed. The conclusion that ganaxolone lacks efficacy in migraine must be tempered by the fact that dosing in all studies occurred after pain onset. It cannot be concluded that the outcome would have been similarly unimpressive had the drug been administered on a prophylactic basis. In any case, however, the conclusion that ganaxolone lacks efficacy is consistent with the notion that the $GABA_A$ receptor is not an appropriate target for migraine therapy. The suggestion of utility in hormonally dependent migraine warrants attention. Given the potential of ganaxolone in the treatment of hormonally-sensitive epilepsy,[159,160] the intriguing possibility exists that the drug would be useful as a prophylactic agent specifically in menstrual migraine.

Acknowledgements

Portions of this chapter are based on the invited review 'Common pathophysiologic mechanisms in migraine and epilepsy'.[161]

References

1. Rogawski MA, Löscher W (2004) The neurobiology of antiepileptic drugs for the treatment of nonepileptic conditions. *Nat Med* 10, 685–92.
2. Rothrock JF (1997) Clinical studies of valproate for migraine prophylaxis. *Cephalalgia* 17, 81–3.
3. Hering R, Kuritzky A (1992) Sodium valproate in the prophylactic treatment of migraine: a double-blind study versus placebo. *Cephalalgia* 12, 81–4.
4. Freitag FG, Collins SD, Carlson HA, Goldstein J, Saper J, Silberstein S, Mathew N, Winner PK, Deaton R, Sommerville K; Depakote ER Migraine Study Group (2002) A randomized trial of divalproex sodium extended-release tablets in migraine prophylaxis. *Neurology* 58, 1652–9.
5. Chronicle E, Mulleners W (2004) Anticonvulsant drugs for migraine prophylaxis. *Cochrane Database Syst Rev* 3, CD003226.
6. Buchanan TM, Ramadan NM (2006) Prophylactic pharmacotherapy for migraine headaches. *Semin Neurol* 26, 188–98.
7. Brandes JL, Saper JR, Diamond M, Couch JR, Lewis DW, Schmitt J, Neto W, Schwabe S, Jacobs D; MIGR-002 Study Group (2004) Topiramate for migraine prevention: a randomized controlled trial. *JAMA* 291, 965–73.
8. Silberstein SD, Neto W, Schmitt J, Jacobs D; MIGR-001 Study Group (2004) Topiramate in migraine prevention: results of a large controlled trial. *Arch Neurol* 61, 490–5.
9. Di Trapani G, Mei D, Marra C, Mazza S, Capuano A (2000) Gabapentin in the prophylaxis of migraine: a double-blind randomized placebo-controlled study. *Clin Ter* 151, 145–8.
10. Mathew NT, Rapoport A, Saper J, Magnus L, Klapper J, Ramadan N, Stacey B, Tepper S (2001) Efficacy of gabapentin in migraine prophylaxis. *Headache* 41, 119–28.
11. Rompel H, Bauermeister PW (1970) Aetiology of migraine and prevention with carbamazepine (Tegretol): results of a double-blind, cross-over study. *South African Med J* 44, 75–80.
12. Steiner TJ, Findley LJ, Yuen AWC (1997) Lamotrigine versus placebo in the prophylaxis of migraine with and without aura. *Cephalalgia* 17, 109–12.
13. D'Andrea G, Granella F, Cadalini M, Manzoni GC (1999) Effectiveness of lamotrigine in the prophylaxis of migraine with aura: an open pilot study. *Cephalalgia* 19, 64–6.
14. Lampl C, Katsarava Z, Diener HC, Limmroth V (2005) Lamotrigine reduces migraine aura and migraine attacks in patients with migraine with aura. *J Neurol Neurosurg Psychiatry* 76, 1730–2.
15. Gupta P, Singh S, Goyal V, Shukla G, Behari M (2007) Low-dose topiramate versus lamotrigine in migraine prophylaxis (the lotolamp study). *Headache* 47, 402–12.
16. Drake ME Jr, Greathouse NI, Renner JB, Armentbright AD (2004) Open-label zonisamide for refractory migraine. *Clin Neuropharmacol* 27, 278–80.
17. Pakalnis A, Kring D (2006) Zonisamide prophylaxis in refractory pediatric headache. *Headache* 46, 804–7.
18. Brighina F, Palermo A, Aloisio A, Francolini M, Giglia G, Fierro B (2006) Levetiracetam in the prophylaxis of migraine with aura: a 6-month open-label study. *Clin Neuropharmacol* 29, 338–42.

19. Rogawski MA, Löscher W (2004) The neurobiology of antiepileptic drugs. *Nat Rev Neurosci* 5, 553–64.

20. Ptácek LJ (1998) The place of migraine as a channelopathy. *Curr Opin Neurol* 11, 217–26.

21. Haut SR, Bigal ME, Lipton RB (2006) Chronic disorders with episodic manifestations: focus on epilepsy and migraine. *Lancet Neurol* 5, 148–57.

22. Yu FH, Mantegazza M, Westenbroek RE, Robbins CA, Kalume F, Burton KA, Spain WJ, McKnight GS, Scheuer T, Catterall WA (2006) Reduced sodium current in GABAergic interneurons in a mouse model of severe myoclonic epilepsy in infancy. *Nat Neurosci* 9, 1142–9.

23. Ottman R, Lipton RB (1994) Comorbidity of migraine and epilepsy. *Neurology* 44, 2105–10.

24. Ludvigsson P, Hesdorffer D, Olafsson E, Kjartansson O, Hauser WA (2006) Migraine with aura is a risk factor for unprovoked seizures in children. *Ann Neurol* 59, 210–13.

25. Ottman R, Lipton RB (1996) Is the comorbidity of epilepsy and migraine due to a shared genetic susceptibility? *Neurology* 47, 918–24.

26. Stewart WF, Staffa J, Lipton RB, Ottman R (1997) Familial risk of migraine: a population-based study. *Ann Neurol* 41, 166–72.

27. Stewart WF, Bigal ME, Kolodner K, Dowson A, Liberman JN, Lipton RB (2006) Familial risk of migraine: variation by proband age at onset and headache severity. *Neurology* 66, 344–8.

28. Ferraro TN, Buono RJ (2006) Polygenic epilepsy. *Adv Neurol* 97, 389–98.

29. Ophoff RA, Terwindt GM, Vergouwe MN, van Eijk R, Oefner PJ, Hoffman SM, Lamerdin JE, Mohrenweiser HW, Bulman DE, Ferrari M, Haan J, Lindhout D, van Ommen GJ, Hofker MH, Ferrari MD, Frants RR (1996) Familial hemiplegic migraine and episodic ataxia type-2 are caused by mutations in the Ca^{2+} channel gene CACNL1A4. *Cell* 87, 543–52.

30. Tottene A, Fellin T, Pagnutti S, Luvisetto S, Striessnig J, Fletcher C, Pietrobon D (2002) Familial hemiplegic migraine mutations increase Ca^{2+} influx through single human $Ca_V2.1$ channels and decrease maximal $Ca_V2.1$ current density in neurons. *Proc Natl Acad Sci USA* 99, 13284–9.

31. Chioza B, Wilkie H, Nashef L, Blower J, McCormick D, Sham P, Asherson P, Makoff AJ (2001) Association between the α_{1a} calcium channel gene CACNA1A and idiopathic generalized epilepsy. *Neurology* 56, 1245–6.

32. Tokuda S, Kuramoto T, Tanaka K, Kaneko S, Takeuchi IK, Sasa M, Serikawa T (2007) The ataxic groggy rat has a missense mutation in the P/Q-type voltage-gated Ca^{2+} channel aα1A subunit gene and exhibits absence seizures. *Brain Res* 1133, 168–77.

33. De Fusco M, Marconi R, Silvestri L, Atorino L, Rampoldi L, Morgante L, Ballabio A, Aridon P, Casari G (2003) Haploinsufficiency of ATP1A2 encoding the Na^+/K^+ pump $\alpha2$ subunit associated with familial hemiplegic migraine type 2. *Nat Genet* 33, 192–6.

34. Vanmolkot KR, Kors EE, Hottenga JJ, Terwindt GM, Haan J, Hoefnagels WA, Black DF, Sandkuijl LA, Frants RR, Ferrari MD, van den Maagdenberg AM (2003) Novel mutations in the Na^+,K^+-ATPase pump gene ATP1A2 associated with familial hemiplegic migraine and benign familial infantile convulsions. *Ann Neurol* 54, 360–6.

35. De Vries B, Haan J, Frants RR, Van den Maagdenberg AM, Ferrari MD (2006) Genetic biomarkers for migraine. *Headache* 46, 1059–68.

36. Koenderink JB, Zifarelli G, Qiu LY, Schwarz W, De Pont JJ, Bamberg E, Friedrich T (2005) Na, K-ATPase mutations in familial hemiplegic migraine lead to functional inactivation. *Biochim Biophys Acta* 1669, 61–8.

37. Pedley TA, Zuckermann EC, Glaser GH (1969) Epileptogenic effects of localized ventricular perfusion of ouabain on dorsal hippocampus. *Exp Neurol* 25, 207–19.

38. Stone WE, Javid MJ (1982) Interactions of phenytoin with ouabain and other chemical convulsants. *Arch Int Pharmacodyn Ther* 260, 28–35.

39. Dichgans M, Freilinger T, Eckstein G, Babini E, Lorenz-Depiereux B, Biskup S, Ferrari MD, Herzog J, van den Maagdenberg AM, Pusch M, Strom TM (2005) Mutation in the neuronal voltage-gated sodium channel SCN1A in familial hemiplegic migraine. *Lancet* 366, 371–7.

40. Torkkeli PH, French AS (2002) Simulation of different firing patterns in paired spider mechanore-ceptor neurons: the role of Na⁺ channel inactivation. *J Neurophysiol* 87, 1363–8.

41. Spampanato J, Aradi I, Soltesz I, Goldin AL (2004) Increased neuronal firing in computer simula-tions of sodium channel mutations that cause generalized epilepsy with febrile seizures plus. *J Neurophysiol* 91, 2040–50.

42. Leão AAP (1944) Spreading depression of activity in the cerebral cortex. *J Neurophysiol* 7, 359–90.

43. Grafstein B (1956) Mechanism of spreading cortical depression. *J Neurophysiol* 19, 154–71.

44. Strong AJ (2005) Dr Bernice Grafstein's paper on the mechanism of spreading depression. *J Neurophysiol* 94, 5–7.

45. Lauritzen M (2001) Cortical spreading depression in migraine. *Cephalalgia* 21, 757–60.

46. Milner PM (1959) Note on a possible correspondence between the scotomas of migraine and spreading depression of Leão. *Electroencephalogr Clin Neurophysiol* 10, 705.

47. Olesen J, Larsen B, Lauritzen M (1981) Focal hyperemia followed by spreading oligemia and impaired activation of rCBF in classic migraine. *Ann Neurol* 9, 344–52.

48. Olesen J, Friberg L, Skyhøj Olsen T, Iversen HK, Lassen NA, Andersen AR, Karle A (1990) Timing and topography of cerebral blood flow aura, and headache during migraine attacks. *Ann Neurol* 28, 791–8.

49. Hadjikhani N, Sanchez Del Rio M, Wu O, Schwartz D, Bakker D, Fischl B, Kwong KK, Cutrer FM, Rosen BR, Tootell RB, Sorensen AG, Moskowitz MA (2001) Mechanisms of migraine aura revealed by functional MRI in human visual cortex. *Proc Natl Acad Sci USA* 98, 4687–92.

50. Bolay H, Reuter U, Dunn AK, Huang Z, Boas DA, Moskowitz MA (2002) Intrinsic brain activity triggers trigeminal meningeal afferents in a migraine model. *Nat Med* 8, 136–42.

51. Kunkler PE, Kraig RP (2003) Hippocampal spreading depression bilaterally activates the caudal trigeminal nucleus in rodents. *Hippocampus* 13, 835–44.

52. Morrison DP (1990) Abnormal perceptual experiences in migraine. *Cephalalgia* 10, 273–7.

53. Sanchez-Del-Rio M, Reuter U, Moskowitz MA (2006) New insights into migraine pathophysiology. *Curr Opin Neurol* 19, 294–8.

54. Herreras O (2005) Electrical prodromals of spreading depression void Grafstein's potassium hypothesis. *J Neurophysiol* 94, 3656.

55. Larrosa B, Pastor J, Lopez-Aguado L, Herreras O (2006) A role for glutamate and glia in the fast network oscillations preceding spreading depression. *Neuroscience* 141, 1057–68.

56. Tian GF, Azmi H, Takano T, Xu Q, Peng W, Lin J, Oberheim N, Lou N, Wang X, Zielke HR, Kang J, Nedergaard M (2005) An astrocytic basis of epilepsy. *Nature Med* 11, 973–81.

57. Basarsky TA, Duffy SN, Andrew RD, MacVicar BA (1998) Imaging spreading depression and associated intracellular calcium waves in brain slices. *J Neurosci* 18, 7189–99.

58. Palmer JE, Chronicle EP, Rolan P, Mulleners (2000) Cortical hyperexcitability is cortical under-inhibition: evidence from a novel functional test of migraine patients. *Cephalalgia* 20, 525–32.

59. Mulleners WM, Chronicle EP, Palmer JE, Koehler PJ, Vredeveld JW (2001) Visual cortex excitability in migraine with and without aura. *Headache* 41, 565–72.

60. Macdonald RL, Rogawski MA (2008) Cellular effects of antiepileptic drugs. In: Engel J Jr, Pedley TA (eds) *Epilepsy A Comprehensive Textbook*, 2nd edn, pp. 1433–45. Lippincott Williams & Wilkins, Philadelphia, PA.

61. Löscher W (2002) Basic pharmacology of valproate: a review after 35 years of clinical use for the treatment of epilepsy. *CNS Drugs* 16, 669–94.

62. Löscher W (2002) Valproic acid. Mechanisms of action. In: Levy RH, Mattson RH, Meldrum BS, Perucca E (eds) *Antiepileptic Drugs*, pp. 768–79. Lippincott-Raven, Philadelphia, PA.

63. Gean PW, Huang CC, Hung CR, Tsai JJ (1994) Valproic acid suppresses the synaptic response mediated by the NMDA receptors in rat amygdalar slices. *Brain Res Bull* 33, 333–6.

64. Gobbi G, Janiri L (2006) Sodium- and magnesium-valproate in vivo modulate glutamatergic and GABAergic synapses in the medial prefrontal cortex. *Psychopharmacology (Berl)* 185, 255–62.

65. Kaube H, Goadsby PJ (1994) Anti-migraine compounds fail to modulate the propagation of cortical spreading depression in the cat. *Eur Neurol* 34, 30–5.

66. Ayata C, Jin H, Kudo C, Dalkara T, Moskowitz MA (2006) Suppression of cortical spreading depression in migraine prophylaxis. *Ann Neurol* 59, 652–61.

67. Akerman S, Goadsby PJ (2005) Topiramate inhibits cortical spreading depression in rat and cat: impact in migraine aura. *Neuroreport* 16, 1383–7.

68. Storer RJ, Goadsby PJ (2004) Topiramate inhibits trigeminovascular neurons in the cat. *Cephalalgia* 24, 1049–56.

69. Akerman S, Goadsby PJ (2005) Topiramate inhibits trigeminovascular activation: an intravital microscopy study. *Br J Pharmacol* 146, 7–14.

70. White HS (2005) Molecular pharmacology of topiramate: managing seizures and preventing migraine. *Headache* 45 (Suppl. 1), S48–56.

71. Olesen J (1990) Calcium antagonists in migraine and vertigo. Possible mechanisms of action and review of clinical trials. *Eur Neurol* 30 (Suppl. 2), 31–4; Discussion 39–41.

72. Vahedi K, Taupin P, Djomby R, El-Amrani M, Lutz G, Filipetti V, Landais P, Massiou H, Bousser MG; DIAMIG investigators (2002) Efficacy and tolerability of acetazolamide in migraine prophylaxis: a randomised placebo-controlled trial. *J Neurol* 249, 206–11.

73. Gibbs JW 3rd, Sombati S, DeLorenzo RJ, Coulter DA (2000) Cellular actions of topiramate: blockade of kainate-evoked inward currents in cultured hippocampal neurons. *Epilepsia* 41 (Suppl. 1), S10–16.

74. Gryder DS, Rogawski MA (2003) Selective antagonism of GluR5 kainate-receptor-mediated synaptic currents by topiramate in rat basolateral amygdala neurons. *J Neurosci* 23, 7069–74.

75. Li P, Wilding TJ, Kim SJ, Calejesan AA, Huettner JE, Zhuo M (1999) Kainate-receptor-mediated sensory synaptic transmission in mammalian spinal cord. *Nature* 397, 161–4.

76. Xu H, Wu LJ, Zhao MG, Toyoda H, Vadakkan KI, Jia Y, Pinaud R, Zhuo M (2006) Presynaptic regulation of the inhibitory transmission by GluR5-containing kainate receptors in spinal substantia gelatinosa. *Mol Pain* 2, 29.

77. Sahara Y, Noro N, Iida Y, Soma K, Nakamura Y (1997) Glutamate receptor subunits GluR5 and KA-2 are coexpressed in rat trigeminal ganglion neurons. *J Neurosci* 17, 6611–20.

78. Filla SA, Winter MA, Johnson KW, Bleakman D, Bell MG, Bleisch TJ, Castano AM, Clemens-Smith A, del Prado M, Dieckman DK, Dominguez E, Escribano A, Ho KH, Hudziak KJ, Katofiasc MA, Martinez-Perez JA, Mateo A, Mathes BM, Mattiuz EL, Ogden AM, Phebus LA, Stack DR, Stratford RE, Ornstein PL (2002) Ethyl (3S,4aR,6S,8aR)-6-(4-ethoxycarbonylimidazol-1-ylmethyl)decahydroiso-quinoline-3-carboxylic ester: a prodrug of a GluR5 kainate receptor antagonist active in two animal models of acute migraine. *J Med Chem* 45, 4383–6.

79. Weiss B, Alt A, Ogden AM, Gates M, Dieckman DK, Clemens-Smith A, Ho KH, Jarvie K, Rizkalla G, Wright RA, Calligaro DO, Schoepp D, Mattiuz EL, Stratford RE, Johnson B, Salhoff C, Katofiasc M, Phebus LA, Schenck K, Cohen M, Filla SA, Ornstein PL, Johnson KW, Bleakman D (2006) Pharmacological characterization of the competitive GLUK5 receptor antagonist decahydroisoquinoline LY466195 in vitro and in vivo. *J Pharmacol Exp Ther* 318, 772–81.

80. Sang CN, Ramadan NM, Wallihan RG, Chappell AS, Freitag FG, Smith TR, Silberstein SD, Johnson KW, Phebus LA, Bleakman D, Ornstein PL, Arnold B, Tepper SJ, Vandenhende F (2004) LY293558, a novel AMPA/GluR5 antagonist, is efficacious and well-tolerated in acute migraine. *Cephalalgia* 24, 596–602.

81. Sang CN, Hostetter MP, Gracely RH, Chappell AS, Schoepp DD, Lee G, Whitcup S, Caruso R, Max MB (1998) AMPA/kainate antagonist LY293558 reduces capsaicin-evoked hyperalgesia but not pain in normal skin in humans. *Anesthesiology* 89, 1060–7.

82. Angehagen M, Ronnback L, Hansson E, Ben-Menachem E (2005) Topiramate reduces AMPA-induced Ca^{2+} transients and inhibits GluR1 subunit phosphorylation in astrocytes from primary cultures. *J Neurochem* 94, 1124–30.

83. Kaminski RM, Banerjee M, Rogawski MA (2004) Topiramate selectively protects against seizures induced by ATPA, a GluR5 kainate receptor agonist. *Neuropharmacology* 46, 1097–104.

84. Suman-Chauhan N, Webdale L, Hill DR, Woodruff GN (1993) Characterisation of [^{3}H]gabapentin binding to a novel site in rat brain: homogenate binding studies. *Eur J Pharmacol* 244, 293–301.

85. Dooley DJ, Taylor CP, Donevan S, Feltner D (2007) Ca^{2+} channel $\alpha2\delta$ ligands: novel modulators of neurotransmission. *Trends Pharmacol Sci* 28, 75–82.

86. Field MJ, Hughes J, Singh L (2000) Further evidence for the role of the $\alpha2\delta$ subunit of voltage dependent calcium channels in models of neuropathic pain. *Br J Pharmacol* 131, 282–6.

87. Field MJ, Cox PJ, Stott E, Melrose H, Offord J, Su TZ, Bramwell S, Corradini L, England S, Winks J, Kinloch RA, Hendrich J, Dolphin AC, Webb T, Williams D (2006) Identification of the $\alpha2\text{-}\delta\text{-}1$ subunit of voltage-dependent calcium channels as a molecular target for pain mediating the analgesic actions of pregabalin. *Proc Natl Acad Sci USA* 103, 17537–42.

88. Rogawski MA, Taylor CP (2006) Calcium channel $\alpha2\text{-}\delta$ subunit, a new antiepileptic drug target. In: Löscher W, Schmidt D (eds). New horizons in the development of antiepileptic drugs: innovative strategies. *Epilepsy Res* 69, 183–272.

89. Marais E, Klugbauer N, Hofmann F (2001) Calcium channel $\alpha2\delta$ subunits-structure and Gabapentin binding. *Mol Pharmacol* 59, 1243–8.

90. Davies A, Hendrich J, Van Minh AT, Wratten J, Douglas L, Dolphin AC (2007) Functional biology of the $\alpha2\delta$ subunits of voltage-gated calcium channels. *Trends Pharmacol Sci* 28, 220–8.

91. Dooley DJ, Mieske CA, Borosky SA (2000) Inhibition of K^+-evoked glutamate release from rat neocortical and hippocampal slices by gabapentin. *Neurosci Lett* 280, 107–10.

92. Patel MK, Gonzalez MI, Bramwell S, Pinnock RD, Lee K (2000) Gabapentin inhibits excitatory synaptic transmission in the hyperalgesic spinal cord. *Br J Pharmacol* 130, 1731–4.

93. Fehrenbacher JC, Taylor CP, Vasko MR (2003) Pregabalin and gabapentin reduce release of substance P and CGRP from rat spinal tissues only after inflammation or activation of protein kinase C. *Pain* 105, 133–41.

94. Cunningham MO, Woodhall GL, Thompson SE, Dooley DJ, Jones RS (2004) Dual effects of gabapentin and pregabalin on glutamate release at rat entorhinal synapses in vitro. *Eur J Neurosci* 20, 1566–76.

95. Hendrich J, Van Minh AT, Heblich F, Nieto-Rostro M, Watschinger K, Striessnig J, Wratten J, Davies A, Dolphin AC (2008) Pharmacological disruption of calcium channel trafficking by the $\alpha2\delta$ ligand gabapentin. *Proc Natl Acad Sci USA* 105, 3628–33.

96. Su TZ, Feng MR, Weber ML (2005) Mediation of highly concentrative uptake of pregabalin by L-type amino acid transport in Chinese hamster ovary and Caco-2 cells. *J Pharmacol Exp Ther* 313, 1406–15.

97. Belliotti TR, Capiris T, Ekhato IV, Kinsora JJ, Field MJ, Heffner TG, Meltzer LT, Schwarz JB, Taylor CP, Thorpe AJ, Vartanian MG, Wise LD, Zhi-Su T, Weber ML, Wustrow DJ (2005) Structure-activity relationships of pregabalin and analogues that target the $\alpha2\text{-}\delta$ protein. *J Med Chem* 48, 2294–307.

98. Cundy KC, Branch R, Chernov-Rogan T, Dias T, Estrada T, Hold K, Koller K, Liu X, Mann A, Panuwat M, Raillard SP, Upadhyay S, Wu QQ, Xiang JN, Yan H, Zerangue N, Zhou CX, Barrett RW, Gallop MA (2004) XP13512 [(±)-1-([(α-isobutanoyloxyethoxy)carbonyl] aminomethyl)-

1-cyclohexane acetic acid], a novel gabapentin prodrug: I. Design, synthesis, enzymatic conversion to gabapentin, and transport by intestinal solute transporters. *J Pharmacol Exp Ther* 311, 315–23.

99. Smith TR (2001) Treatment of refractory chronic daily headache with zonisamide: a case series. *Cephalalgia* 21, 482.

100. Krusz JC (2001) Zonisamide in the treatment of headache disorders. *Cephalalgia* 21, 374–5.

101. Bigal ME, Rapoport AM, Sheftell FD, Tepper SJ (2002) New migraine preventive options: an update with pathophysiological considerations. *Rev Hosp Clin Fac Med Sao Paulo* 57, 293–8.

102. Ashkenazi A, Benlifer A, Korenblit J, Silberstein SD (2006) Zonisamide for migraine prophylaxis in refractory patients. *Cephalalgia* 26, 1199–202.

103. Nishimori I, Vullo D, Innocenti A, Scozzafava A, Mastrolorenzo A, Supuran CT (2005) Carbonic anhydrase inhibitors: inhibition of the transmembrane isozyme XIV with sulfonamides. *Bioorg Med Chem Lett* 15, 3828–33.

104. Rogawski MA (2002) Principles of antiepileptic drug action. In: Levy RH, Mattson RH, Meldrum BS, Perucca E (eds) *Antiepileptic Drugs*, 5th edn, pp. 3–22. Lippincott Williams & Wilkins, Philadelphia, PA.

105. Drake ME, Greathouse NI, Armentbright AD, Renner JB (2001) Levetiracetam for preventive treatment of migraine. *Cephalalgia* 21, 373.

106. Krusz JC (2001) Levetiracetam as prophylaxis for resistant headaches. *Cephalalgia* 21, 373.

107. Cochran JW (2004) Levetiracetam as migraine prophylaxis. *Clin J Pain* 20, 198–9.

108. Miller GS (2004) Efficacy and safety of levetiracetam in pediatric migraine. *Headache* 44, 238–43.

109. Rapoport AM, Sheftell FD, Tepper SJ, Bigal ME (2005) Levetiracetam in the preventive treatment of transformed migraine. *Curr Ther Res* 66, 212–21.

110. Vaisleb I, Neft R, Schor N (2005) Role of Levetiracetam in prophylaxis of migraine headaches in childhood. *Neurology* 64, 343.

111. Lynch BA, Lambeng N, Nocka K, Kensel-Hammes P, Bajjalieh SM, Matagne A, Fuks B (2004) The synaptic vesicle protein SV2A is the binding site for the antiepileptic drug levetiracetam. *Proc Natl Acad Sci USA* 101, 9861–6.

112. Custer KL, Austin NS, Sullivan JM, Bajjalieh SM (2006) Synaptic vesicle protein 2 enhances release probability at quiescent synapses. *J Neurosci* 26, 1303-13.

113. Janz R, Goda Y, Geppert M, Missler M, Sudhof TC (1999) SV2A and SV2B function as redundant Ca^{2+} regulators in neurotransmitter release. *Neuron* 24, 1003–16.

114. Duncan S (2007) Teratogenesis of sodium valproate. *Curr Opin Neurol* 20, 175–80.

115. Rogawski MA (2006) Diverse mechanisms of antiepileptic drugs in the development pipeline. *Epilepsy Res* 69, 273–94.

116. Bialer M (2006) New antiepileptic drugs that are second generation to existing antiepileptic drugs. *Expert Opin Investig Drugs* 15, 637–47.

117. Winkler I, Blotnik S, Shimshoni J, Yagen B, Devor M, Bialer M (2005) Efficacy of antiepileptic isomers of valproic acid and valpromide in a rat model of neuropathic pain. *Br J Pharmacol* 146, 198–208.

118. Winkler I, Sobol E, Yagen B, Steinman A, Devor M, Bialer M (2005) Efficacy of antiepileptic tetramethylcyclopropyl analogues of valproic acid amides in a rat model of neuropathic pain. *Neuropharmacology* 49, 1110–20.

119. Isoherranen N, Woodhead JH, White HS, Bialer M (2001) Anticonvulsant profile of valrocemide (TV1901): a new antiepileptic drug. *Epilepsia* 42, 831–6.

120. Isoherranen N, White HS, Klein BD, Roeder M, Woodhead JH, Schurig V, Yagen B, Bialer M (2003) Pharmacokinetic-pharmacodynamic relationships of (2S,3S)-valnoctamide and its stereoisomer (2R,3S)-valnoctamide in rodent models of epilepsy. *Pharm Res* 20, 1293–301.

121. Radatz M, Ehlers K, Yagen B, Bialer M, Nau H (1998) Valnoctamide, valpromide and valnoctic acid are much less teratogenic in mice than valproic acid. *Epilepsy Res* 30, 41–8.

122. Spiegelstein O, Bialer M, Radatz M, Nau H, Yagen B (1999) Enantioselective synthesis and teratogenicity of propylisopropyl acetamide, a CNS-active chiral amide analogue of valproic acid. *Chirality* 11, 645–50.

123. Spiegelstein O, Yagen B, Levy RH, Finnell RH, Bennett GD, Roeder M, Schurig V, Bialer M (1999) Stereoselective pharmacokinetics and pharmacodynamics of propylisopropyl acetamide, a CNS-active chiral amide analog of valproic acid. *Pharm Res* 16, 1582–8.

124. Isoherranen N, Yagen B, Woodhead JH, Spiegelstein O, Blotnik S, Wilcox KS, Finnell RH, Bennett GD, White HS, Bialer M (2003) Characterization of the anticonvulsant profile and enantioselective pharmacokinetics of the chiral valproylamide propylisopropyl acetamide in rodents. *Br J Pharmacol* 138, 602–13.

125. Bialer M, Johannessen SI, Kupferberg HJ, Levy RH, Loiseau P, Perucca E (2001) Progress report on new antiepileptic drugs: a summary of the Fifth Eilat Conference (EILAT V) *Epilepsy Res* 43, 11–58.

126. Wu Y-J, Dworetzky SI (2005) Recent developments on KCNQ potassium channel openers. *Curr Med Chem* 12, 453–60.

127. Tober C, Rostock A, Rundfeldt C, Bartsch R (1996) D-23129: a potent anticonvulsant in the amygdala kindling model of complex partial seizures. *Eur J Pharmacol* 303, 163–9.

128. Rostock A, Tober C, Rundfeldt C, Bartsch R, Engel J, Polymeropoulos EE, Kutscher B, Loscher W, Honack D, White HS, Wolf HH (1996) D-23129: a new anticonvulsant with a broad spectrum activity in animal models of epileptic seizures. *Epilepsy Res* 23, 211–23.

129. Blackburn-Munro G, Dalby-Brown W, Mirza NR, Mikkelsen JD, Blackburn-Munro RE (2005) Retigabine: chemical synthesis to clinical application. *CNS Drug Rev* 11, 1–20.

130. Porter RJ, Partiot A, Sachdeo R, Nohria V, Alves WM; 205 Study Group (2007) Randomized, multicenter, dose-ranging trial of retigabine for partial-onset seizures. *Neurology* 68, 1197–204.

131. Rundfeldt C, Netzer R (2000) The novel anticonvulsant retigabine activates M-currents in Chinese hamster ovary-cells tranfected with human KCNQ2/3 subunits. *Neurosci Lett* 282, 73–6.

132. Main MJ, Cryan JE, Dupere JR, Cox B, Clare JJ, Burbidge SA (2000) Modulation of KCNQ2/3 potassium channels by the novel anticonvulsant retigabine. *Mol Pharmacol* 58, 253–62.

133. Wickenden AD, Zou A, Wagoner PK, Jegla T (2001) Characterization of KCNQ5/Q3 potassium channels expressed in mammalian cells. *Br J Pharmacol* 132, 381–4.

134. Tatulian L, Delmas P, Abogadie FC, Brown DA (2001) Activation of expressed KCNQ potassium currents and native neuronal M-type potassium currents by the anti-convulsant drug retigabine. *J Neurosci* 21, 5535–45.

135. Tatulian L, Brown DA (2003) Effect of the KCNQ potassium channel opener retigabine on single KCNQ2/3 channels expressed in CHO cells. *J Physiol* 549 (Pt 1), 57–63.

136. Passmore GM, Selyanko AA, Mistry M, Al-Qatari M, Marsh SJ, Matthews EA, Dickenson AH, Brown TA, Burbidge SA, Main M, Brown DA (2003) KCNQ/M currents in sensory neurons: significance for pain therapy. *J Neurosci* 23, 7227–36.

137. van Rijn CM, Willems-van Bree E (2003) Synergy between retigabine and GABA in modulating the convulsant site of the GABA$_A$ receptor complex. *Eur J Pharmacol* 464, 95–100.

138. Rundfeldt C, Netzer R (2000) Investigations into the mechanism of action of the new anticonvulsant retigabine. Interaction with GABAergic and glutamatergic neurotransmission and with voltage gated ion channels. *Arzneimittelforschung* 50, 1063–70.

139. Otto JF, Kimball MM, Wilcox KS (2002) Effects of the anticonvulsant retigabine on cultured cortical neurons: changes in electroresponsive properties and synaptic transmission. *Mol Pharmacol* 61, 921–7.

140. Wickenden AD, McNaughton-Smith G, Roeloffs R, London B, Clark S, Wilson WA, Rigdon GC, Wagoner PK (2005) ICA-27243: A novel, potent, and selective KCNQ2/Q3 potassium channel activator. *Soc Neurosci Abst*, Prog No. 153.13.

141. Wu Y-J, Boissard CG, Greco C, Gribkoff VK, Harden DG, He H, L'Heureux A, Kang SH, Kinney GG, Knox RJ, Natale J, Newton AE, Lehtinen-Oboma S, Sinz MW, Sivarao DV, Starrett JE Jr, Sun LQ, Tertyshnikova S, Thompson MW, Weaver D, Wong HS, Zhang L, Dworetzky SI (2003) (S)-N-[1-(3-morpholin-4-ylphenyl)ethyl]-3-phenylacrylamide: an orally bioavailable KCNQ2 opener with significant activity in a cortical spreading depression model of migraine. *J Med Chem* 46, 3197–200.

142. Wu Y-J, Davis CD, Dworetzky S, Fitzpatrick WC, Harden D, He H, Knox RJ, Newton AE, Philip T, Polson C, Sivarao DV, Sun LQ, Tertyshnikova S, Weaver D, Yeola S, Zoeckler M, Sinz MW (2003) Fluorine substitution can block CYP3A4 metabolism-dependent inhibition: identification of (S)-N-[1-(4-fluoro-3-morpholin-4-ylphenyl)ethyl]-3-(4-fluorophenyl)acrylamide as an orally bioavailable KCNQ2 opener devoid of CYP3A4 metabolism-dependent inhibition. *J Med Chem* 46, 3778–81.

143. Wu Y-J, He H, Sun LQ, L'Heureux A, Chen J, Dextraze P, Starrett JE Jr, Boissard CG, Gribkoff VK, Natale J, Dworetzky SI (2004) Synthesis and structure-activity relationship of acrylamides as KCNQ2 potassium channel openers. *J Med Chem* 47, 2887–96.

144. L'Heureux A, Martel A, He H, Chen J, Sun LQ, Starrett JE, Natale J, Dworetzky SI, Knox RJ, Harden DG, Weaver D, Thompson MW, Wu Y-J (2005) (S,E)-N-[1-(3-heteroarylphenyl)ethyl]-3-(2-fluorophenyl)acrylamides: synthesis and KCNQ2 potassium channel opener activity. *Bioorg Med Chem Lett* 15, 363–6.

145. Beyreuther BK, Freitag J, Heers C, Krebsfanger N, Scharfenecker U, Stöhr T (2007) Lacosamide: a review of preclinical properties. *CNS Drug Rev* 13, 21–42.

146. Stöhr T, Krause E, Selve N (2005) Lacosamide displays potent antinociceptive effects in animal models for inflammatory pain. *Eur J Pain* 10, 241–9.

147. Smith MI, Read SJ, Chan WN, Thompson M, Hunter AJ, Upton N, Parsons AA (2000) Repetitive cortical spreading depression in a gyrencephalic feline brain: inhibition by the novel benzoylamino-benzopyran SB-220453. *Cephalalgia* 20, 546–53.

148. Read SJ, Hirst WD, Upton N, Parsons AA (2001) Cortical spreading depression produces increased cGMP levels in cortex and brain stem that is inhibited by tonabersat (SB-220453) but not sumatriptan. *Brain Res* 891, 69–77.

149. Bradley DP, Smith MI, Netsiri C, Smith JM, Bockhorst KH, Hall LD, Huang CL, Leslie RA, Parsons AA, James MF (2001) Diffusion-weighted MRI used to detect in vivo modulation of cortical spreading depression: comparison of sumatriptan and tonabersat. *Exp Neurol* 172, 342–53.

150. Theis M, Sohl G, Eiberger J, Willecke K (2005) Emerging complexities in identity and function of glial connexins. *Trends Neurosci* 28, 188–95.

151. Világi I, Klapka N, Luhmann HJ (2001) Optical recording of spreading depression in rat neocortical slices. *Brain Res* 898, 288–96.

152. Peters O, Schipke CG, Hashimoto Y, Kettenmann H (2003) Different mechanisms promote astrocyte Ca^{2+} waves and spreading depression in the mouse neocortex. *J Neurosci* 23, 9888–96.

153. Frediani F (2004) Anticonvulsant drugs in primary headaches prophylaxis. *Neurol Sci* 25 (Suppl. 3), S161–6.

154. Novak GP, Kelley M, Zannikos P, Klein B (2007) Carisbamate (RWJ-333369). *Neurotherapeutics* 4, 106–9.

155. Carter RB, Wood PL, Wieland S, Hawkinson JE, Belelli D, Lambert JJ, White HS, Wolf HH, Mirsadeghi S, Tahir SH, Bolger MB, Lan NC, Gee KW (1997) Characterization of the anticonvulsant properties of ganaxolone (CCD 1042; 3α-hydroxy-3β-methyl-5α-pregnan-20-one), a selective, high-affinity, steroid modulator of the gamma-aminobutyric acid$_A$ receptor. *J Pharmacol Exp Ther* 280, 1284–95.

156. Hosie AM, Wilkins ME, Smart TG (2007) Neurosteroid binding sites on GABA$_A$ receptors. *Pharmacol Ther* 116, 7–19.

157. Reddy DS, Rogawski MA (2000) Chronic treatment with the neuroactive steroid ganaxolone in the rat induces anticonvulsant tolerance to diazepam but not to itself. *J Pharmacol Exp Ther* 295, 1241–8.

158. Nohria V, Giller E (2007) Ganaxolone. *Neurotherapeutics* 4, 102–5.

159. Monaghan EP, McAuley JW, Data JL (1999) Ganaxolone: a novel positive allosteric modulator of the GABA$_A$ receptor complex for the treatment of epilepsy. *Expert Opin Investig Drugs* 8, 1663–71.

160. Reddy DS, Rogawski MA (2000) Enhanced anticonvulsant activity of ganaxolone after neurosteroid withdrawal in a rat model of catamenial epilepsy. *J Pharmacol Exp Ther* 294, 909–15.

161. Rogawski MA (2008) Common pathophysiological mechanisms in migraine and epilepsy. *Arch Neurol*, 65, 709–14.

21

Discussion summary: Ion channel modulators and antiepileptics

Pramod R. Saxena

Ion channel strategies for migraine drug targets

Dr Arn van den Maagdenberg pointed out that the pathogenesis of the aura and headache phases of migraine is reasonably well understood, but the trigger mechanisms of migraine attacks are poorly delineated. However, the identification of gene mutations in patients with familial hemiplegic migraine (FHM), namely CACNA1A encoding the α1-subunit of voltage-gated neuronal P/Q-type calcium channels,[1] ATP1A2 encoding the α2-subunit of glial cell Na+,K+ pump,[2] and SCN1A encoding the α1-subunit of voltage-gated neuronal sodium channels,[3] suggests that the threshold for migraine trigger, probably cortical spreading depression (CSD), is genetically determined.[4] In support, findings in animal experiments show that CSD is: (1) able to activate the trigeminal-vascular system;[5] (2) more easily evoked in females than in males;[6] and (3) dose-dependently suppressed by some widely prescribed prophylactic antimigraine drugs.[7] Hence, Van den Maagdenberg proposed that knock in mice carrying these ion channel mutations can be useful in unravelling the triggering mechanisms for migraine attacks and in identifying novel migraine prophylactic targets and therapies. Indeed, the mutated mice exhibit some of the behavioural, electrophysiological, and neurobiological characteristics of migraine, including a lower threshold for CSD.[4] It is with expectation that one awaits further validation of these migraine models, for example, by showing effectiveness of current or prospective antimigraine drugs.

K_{ATP} channels and migraine

It is well known that K_{ATP} channel openers cause headache as a side-effect in many healthy subjects suggesting a role of these channels in migraine pathogenesis. When elaborating on this aspect, Dr Inger Jansen-Olesen reported that in rats: (1) dural and pial arteries relax in response to pinacidil and levcromakalim and this effect is attenuated by the K_{ATP} channel blocker glibenclamide;[8] (2) dural arteries are more sensitive than pial arteries to K_{ATP} channel openers and constrict following glibenclamide administration;[8] (3) glibenclamide also attenuates vasodilatation elicited by exogenous as well as endogenous calcitonin gene-related peptide released by perivascular electrical stimulation (Poster IHRS 2007); and (4) basilar and middle cerebral arteries have Kir6.1/SUR2B as major subunits in K_{ATP} channels. Thus, it would seem that K_{ATP} channel blockers with selective affinity for Kir6.1/SUR2B subunits would be particularly interesting as putative novel antimigraine agents. However, one would need to perform similar experiments in human cerebral vessels. Moreover, it is worth investigating if patients co-morbid with migraine and diabetes show a decrease in the frequency of migraine attacks when on treatment with glibenclamide for their diabetes. Similarly, it was raised whether ketogenic diet, that may close K_{ATP} channels by increasing mitochondrial and cellular energetics,[9] is known to decrease migraine frequency. In any case, it may be worthwhile trying such a diet in patients with intractable migraine.

Novel antiepileptic drugs and migraine

Growing understanding of the pathophysiology of epilepsy and the structure and function of ion channels furnish opportunities for improved epilepsy therapy.[10] As both epilepsy and migraine are episodic, paroxysmal disorders involving pathology of voltage-gated ion channels, Dr Mike Rogawski suggested that antiepileptic drug targets may also provide a basis for novel drug development in the migraine field. Indeed, several drugs effective in epilepsy (valproate, topiramate, gabapentin) are employed in migraine therapy and some glutamate receptor antagonists are being explored in migraine.[11] Moreover, the CSD in migraine may be due to neocortical hyperexcitability involving excessive excitatory transmitter release resulting from alterations in Ca^{2+} channel function, as occurs in familial hemiplegic migraine.[12] However, it may be pointed out that there is so far little evidence of such ion channel mutations in other forms of migraine.

References

1. Ophoff RA, Terwindt GM, Vergouwe MN, *et al.* (2006) Familial hemiplegic migraine and episodic ataxia type-2 are caused by mutations in the Ca^{2+} channel gene CACNL1A4. *Cell* 87, 543–52.
2. De Fusco M, Marconi R, Silvestri L, *et al.* (2003) Haploinsufficiency of ATP1A2 encoding the Na^+/K^+ pump alpha2 subunit associated with familial hemiplegic migraine type 2. *Nat Genet* 33, 192–6.
3. Dichgans M, Freilinger T, Eckstein G, *et al.* (2005) Mutation in the neuronal voltage-gated sodium channel SCN1A in familial hemiplegic migraine. *Lancet* 366, 371–7.
4. Van de Ven RCG, Kaja S, Plomp JJ, Frants RR, Van den Maagdenberg AMJM, Ferrari MD (2007) Genetic models of migraine. *Arch Neurol* 64, 643–6.
5. Moskowitz MA, Bolay H, Dalkara T (2004) Deciphering migraine mechanisms: clues from familial hemiplegic migraine genotypes. *Ann Neurol* 55, 276–80.
6. Brennan KC, Romero Reyes M, López Valdés HE, Arnold AP, Charles AC (2007) Reduced threshold for cortical spreading depression in female mice. *Ann Neurol* 61, 603–6.
7. Ayata C, Jin C, Kudo C, Dalkara T, Moskowitz MA (2006) Suppression of cortical spreading depression in migraine prophylaxis. *Ann Neurol* 59, 652–61.
8. Gozalov A, Petersen KA, Mortensen C, Jansen-Olesen I, Klaerke D, Olesen J (2005) Role of K_{ATP} channels in the regulation of rat dural and pial artery diameter. *Cephalalgia* 25, 249–60.
9. Gasior M, Rogawski MA, Hartman AL (2006) Neuroprotective and disease-modifying effects of the ketogenic diet. *Behav Pharmacol* 17, 431–9.

10. Meldrum BS, Rogawski MA (2007) Molecular targets for antiepileptic drug development. *Neurotherapeutics* 4, 18–61.

11. Weiss B, Alt A, Ogden AM, *et al.* (2006) Pharmacological characterization of the competitive GLU$_{K5}$ receptor antagonist decahydroisoquinoline LY466195 *in vitro* and *in vivo*. *J Pharmacol Exp Ther* 318, 772–81.

12. Rogawski MA, Löscher W (2004) The neurobiology of antiepileptic drugs for the treatment of nonepileptic conditions. *Nat Med* 7, 685–92.

Other future targets for headache therapy

22

Innovative drug development for headache disorders: glutamate

Kirk W. Johnson, Eric S. Nisenbaum, Michael P. Johnson, Donna K. Dieckman, Amy Clemens-Smith, Edward R. Siuda, Colin P. Dell, Veronique Dehlinger, Kevin J. Hudziak, Sandra A. Filla, Paul L. Ornstein, Nabih M. Ramadan, and David Bleakman

Glutamate is the major excitatory neurotransmitter in the mammalian central nervous system. Glutamate induces its effects primarily through a family of ionotropic (ligand-gated cation channels) and metabotropic (G-protein coupled) receptors. Experimental evidence collected at the bench and in the clinic indicates a significant role for glutamate in migraine. The emergence of selective pharmacological tools that allow activation or blockade of glutamate receptors have provided further insight into the role of glutamate in migraine, and potential therapies.

Ionotropic glutamate receptors

The three major types of ionotropic glutamate receptors are named after the agonists that were originally used to characterize their pharmacology. This family of receptors includes N-methyl-D-aspartate (NMDA), α-amino-3-hydroxy-5-methyl-4-isoazolepropionic acid (AMPA), and 2-carboxy-3-carboxymethyl-4-isopropenylpyrrolidine (kainate, KA). The ionotropic glutamate receptors primarily function to mediate fast receptor transmission and use-dependent plasticity. The NMDA receptor has seven known subunits (NR1, NR2A, NR2B, NR2C, NR2D, NR3A, and NR3B, although the new nomenclature is Glu_{N1}, Glu_{N2A}, Glu_{N2B}, Glu_{N2C}, Glu_{N2D}, Glu_{N3A}, and Glu_{N3B}, respectively), while the AMPA receptor has four known subunits (iGluR1, iGluR2, iGluR3, and iGluR4 now known as Glu_{A1}, Glu_{A2}, Glu_{A3}, and Glu_{A4}) and KA has five subunits (traditionally named iGluR5, iGluR6, iGluR7, KA-1, and KA-2, but more recently GLU_{K5}, GLU_{K6}, GLU_{K7}, GLU_{K1}, and GLU_{K2}).[1] As the name implies, ionotropic glutamate receptors are ligand-gated ion channels.

Metabotropic glutamate receptors

The metabotropic family of glutamate receptors is divided into three groups according to sequence homology, second messenger coupling, and pharmacology. Group I includes mGlu1 and mGlu5 receptors, which are excitatory and couple through G_q to phospholipase C. Both group II (mGlu2 and mGlu3) and group III (mGlu4, mGlu6, mGlu7, and mGlu8) receptors are inhibitory and couple through G_i/G_o to inhibit adenylate cyclase activity. Metabotropic receptors function primarily to modulate glutamate release and modify postsynaptic glutamate excitability.[2]

Glutamate receptors and migraine

Ionotropic and metabotropic glutamate receptor protein or message has been localized to various sites involved in the transduction of painful migraine signals. For instance, NMDA receptor messenger RNA was found in the trigeminal ganglion of mice,[3] while mGlu1 receptor protein was found in the trigeminal ganglion of rats.[4] Both iGluR5 and KA-2 were coexpressed in rat trigeminal ganglion neurons.[5] Also, high densities of NMDA, AMPA, KA, and mGlu binding sites were found in lamina I and II of rat trigeminal nucleus caudalis (TNC).[6] Kondo et al.[7] found that iGluR1, iGluR2/3, and $GABA_A$ receptors were present in the rat TNC, while primarily the $GABA_A$ receptor-containing neurons projected to the thalamus, not the AMPA receptor-containing neurons. Both mGlu2 and mGlu3 receptors have been found in the trigeminal ganglia and dura of rats, while mGlu3 receptors have also been found in the VPM nucleus of the thalamus.[8,9] Additional characterization has revealed mGlu1, mGlu2/3, mGlu4, mGlu5, and mGlu7 receptors expressed in leptomeninges and/or meningeal microvasculature from adult rats.[9] Ma[10] has shown that the majority of $5-HT_{1B}$, $5-HT_{1D}$, and $5-HT_{1F}$ receptor positive neurons in the trigeminal ganglia of rats were also positive for glutamate, perhaps suggesting the clinical efficacy of the $5-HT_1$ agonists is via the presynaptic inhibition of glutamate release. Goadsby et al.[11] have shown that triptan-sensitive ($5-HT_1$) receptors also exist on postsynaptic central trigeminal neurons. Iontophoresed sumatriptan blocked the increase in the baseline-firing rate of units linked to the superior sagittal sinus, induced by iontophoresis of NMDA receptor agonists into the trigeminocervical complex of anaesthetized cats.[11]

Glutamate and migraine

Pharmacological studies have also been utilized to suggest a role for glutamate in migraine. Hill and Salt[12] found the iontophoretic application of glutamate excited neurons in the rat TNC. Likewise, injection of mustard oil into the temperomandibular joint of rats induced pain and increased extracellular glutamate levels in the TNC.[13] A more recent paper has shown that application of an inflammatory soup to the dura of rats induced a significant increase in extracellular glutamate levels measured in the TNC via microdialysis, as well as caused sensitization of the face as indicated by electrophysiological recordings of secondary sensory neurons in the TNC.[14]

Numerous studies have measured glutamate in various samples taken from migraineurs, both ictal and interictal, with inconsistent results. For instance, Ferrari et al.[15] and Alam et al.[16] have both shown that plasma glutamate levels are significantly higher in migraineurs outside of an attack, and especially during an attack. Other reports have found that plasma glutamate levels may or may not change during an attack, based on the presence of aura. An excellent summary of glutamate levels in migraineurs and controls has been compiled.[17] More recently, a study has shown that both plasma concentrations of glutamate and release of glutamate from platelets were increased in migraineurs with and without aura compared with healthy controls, although more markedly in the group with aura. However, platelet glutamate uptake was increased in migraineurs with aura but decreased in migraineurs without aura, perhaps suggesting unique pathophysiological differences between the two types of migraine.[18]

NMDA antagonists

In preclinical studies, the NMDA receptor antagonist MK-801 has been shown to reduce c-*fos* expression in the TNC induced by either superior sagittal sinus stimulation in cats[19] or intracisternal capsaicin in rats.[20] In addition, competitive and non-competitive NMDA antagonists can block cortical spreading depression in laboratory animals.[21] A recent open-label clinical study found that intranasal ketamine reduced the severity and duration of the neurological effects associated with aura in five of 11 patients with familial hemiplegic migraine. However, only two patients reported a decrease in pain severity.[22] These studies could suggest that migraine pain cannot be effectively treated by an acute therapy that blocks cortical spreading depression and aura.

AMPA and kainate antagonists

The AMPA/KA receptor antagonist, tezampanel (LY293558), has previously been shown to have efficacy in preclinical[23] and clinical models of pain.[24] In addition, LY293558 was efficacious in the rat dural plasma protein extravasation model and shown to inhibit c-*fos* expression in the trigeminal nucleus caudalis following electrical stimulation of the trigeminal ganglion.[25] Evaluation of LY293558 in the preclinical models of pain and migraine required either intravenous or subcutaneous injection of the compound due to low oral bioavailability. In addition, LY293558 did not contract the rabbit saphenous vein *in vitro*, unlike the current 'triptan' therapies.[25]

The efficacy and safety of LY293558 were evaluated in one completed phase IIa acute migraine trial.[26] A randomized, triple-blind, double-dummy trial compared 1.2 mg/kg intravenous LY293558, 6 mg subcutaneous sumatriptan, and placebo when administered to migraineurs experiencing a moderate or severe migraine. The dose of LY293558 was based on the maximally tolerated dose determined from a healthy volunteer study in which hazy vision and sedation were reported at the maximally tolerated dose.[24] Response rates evaluated 2 h post-dose were 69% for LY293558, 86% for sumatriptan, and 25% for placebo. Pain-free rates were 54% for LY293558, 60% for sumatriptan, and 6% for placebo 2 h after dosing. Adverse events were reported by 15% (two of 13) of patients in the LY293558 group, 31% (five of 16) of patients in the placebo group, and 53% (eight of 15) of patients in the sumatriptan group. Dizziness and sedation/drowsiness were the most commonly reported adverse events in the LY293558 and placebo groups. No patients in the LY293558 treatment group reported chest/throat symptoms or heaviness/tingling effects. This study suggests that an AMPA/KA antagonist could represent a novel migraine therapy without vasoconstrictive liabilities.

LY293558 (tezampanel), given subcutaneously, is currently being developed by TorreyPines Therapeutics, Inc., California. The compound is currently in a phase IIb clinical trial for the treatment of acute migraine. TorreyPines' follow-on compound, NGX426, an oral prodrug of tezampanel, is currently undergoing phase I testing.

In order to further dissect the contribution of AMPA and kainate (iGluR5) receptor antagonism to the clinical efficacy and side-effects observed with LY293558, the selective, competitive iGluR5 antagonist, LY466195 (Table 22.1), was characterized in preclinical models[27] and in the clinic. LY466195 was efficacious in the rat dural plasma protein extravassation(PPE) model following intravenous doses of 10 and 100 µg/kg. The orally bioavailable prodrug of LY466195 (LY494582) was also efficacious in the PPE model when evaluated 1 h post-oral administration of 10 and 100 µg/kg doses. LY466195 also decreased c-*fos* expression in the TNC induced by electrical stimulation of the trigeminal ganglion at the same doses found to be active in the PPE model. The prodrug LY494582 was able to block c-*fos* expression at doses of 0.1, 1, and 10 mg/kg following oral administration. The 1 mg/kg dose of LY494582 retained significant efficacy in the c-*fos* assay when evaluated 16 h post-dose. In addition, the selective AMPA antagonist LY300168 was not efficacious in the rat PPE model. These data suggest the efficacy of both LY293558 and LY466195 in the PPE and c-*fos* models is due to antagonism of iGluR5 receptors. LY466915 did not contract the rabbit saphenous vein *in vitro*, differing itself from the triptans.

Table 22.1 *In vitro* characterization of LY466195 binding affinity and functional activity at ionotropic glutamate receptors, in addition to binding affinity at metabotropic glutamate receptors and biogenic amine receptors, including noradrenaline, dopamine, serotonin, histamine, and acetyl choline receptor subtypes. For methods see reference 27.

	LY466195
Assay	K_i (µM)
iGlu5 [3H]ATPA	0.128
iGlu5 [3H]KA	0.052
iGlu1 [3H]AMPA	75
iGlu2 [3H]AMPA	269
iGlu3 [3H]AMPA	312
iGlu4 [3H]AMPA	432
iGlu6 [3H]KA	>100
iGlu7 [3H]KA	8.9
Biogenic amines	>10
mGluR2/3/6/7/8	>12.5
	EC_{50} (µM)
iGlu5 rat DRG (KA)	0.045
NMDA (rat hippocampus)	2.5
AMPA (rat hippocampus)	95
Voltage-gated Ca^{2+} channel (rat hippocampus)	>100

The efficacy and safety of LY466195 were evaluated in acute migraine trials. A randomized, triple-blind, double-dummy trial compared two doses of intravenous LY466195 (1 and 3 mg), 6 mg subcutaneous sumatriptan, and placebo when administered to migraineurs experiencing a moderate or severe migraine. Response rates evaluated 2 h post-dose were 35% for LY466195 (1 mg), 50% for LY466195 (3 mg), 74% for sumatriptan, and 39% for placebo. Pain-free rates were 4% for LY466195 (1 mg), 29% for LY466195 (3 mg), 43% for sumatriptan, and 0% for placebo 2 h after dosing (Figure 22.1). The visual effects reported for LY293558 were also observed in 4% and 21% of patients dosed with the 1 and 3 mg doses of LY466195, respectively. The LY466195 doses selected for this trial were an attempt to establish clinical efficacy for the treatment of acute migraine, while minimizing the occurrence of severity of the visual effects. It is probable this study has not established the ultimate degree of efficacy for this mechanism of action. *In toto*, these data suggest the clinical efficacy, and perhaps visual side-effects, observed with both LY293558 and LY466195 could be due to antagonism of iGluR5 receptors.

Group II metabotropic glutamate receptor agonists, allosteric potentiators, and antagonists

Both mGlu2 and mGlu3 receptors have been found in the trigeminal ganglia and dura of rats, while mGlu3 receptors have also been found in the VPM of the thalamus.[8] In order to investigate the presynaptic, inhibitory effect of mGlu2 receptor activation on glutamate release and potentially migraine, we evaluated the role of group II metabotropic glutamate receptors in the rat dural PPE model.[28] The prototypical mGlu2/3 agonist LY354740 was found to be efficacious in an earlier version of the PPE model. Likewise, the selective mGlu2 allosteric potentiator LY487379 was active in the PPE model following intravenous dosing. The efficacious doses of LY487379 were approximately 300 times

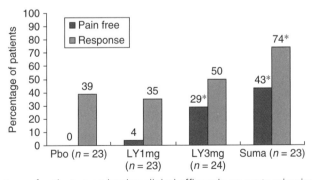

Fig. 22.1 Percentage of patients experiencing clinical efficacy in an acute migraine trial 2 h post-dose of LY466195 (1 mg, iv), LY466195 (3 mg, iv), sumatriptan (Suma) (6 mg, sc), or placebo (Pbo) utilizing a double-dummy design. The response value is the percentage of patients whose headache improved from severe or moderate to mild or none within 2 h post-dose. The pain-free value is the percentage of patients whose headache improved from severe or moderate to none within 2 h post-dose. *$P < 0.05$ (versus placebo).

lower than efficacious doses of LY354740. The inhibitory effects of LY487379 in the PPE model were blocked following pretreatment with the mGlu2/3 antagonist, LY341495. LY341495, when administered alone, actually increased the amount of PPE observed in the dura due to electrical stimulation of the trigeminal ganglion suggesting either mGlu2 or mGlu3 antagonism, or both, exacerbated the PPE.

Recent studies have utilized small, implantable biosensors that continuously measured extracellular glutamate levels in the brains of anaesthetized or conscious rats. These studies indicated that the mGlu2/3 agonist LY379268 could significantly decrease the potassium-evoked release of glutamate in the brains of anaesthetized rats.[29] The same technology was used to show that LY379268 also decreased baseline, resting extracellular glutamate levels in the brains of conscious, freely moving rats. In contrast, LY341495 increased resting glutamate levels in the conscious rats. These data confirm the role of presynaptic mGlu2 receptors in modulating glutamate release. The data also suggest the inhibitory and enhancing effects of mGlu2 agonists/potentiators and antagonists on PPE in the dura could be due to decreased and increased extracellular glutamate levels, respectively.

Evidence suggesting that mGlu3 receptors may be a target for antinociceptive responses in migraine initially has come from studies demonstrating that mGlu3 receptors are prominently expressed in neurons comprising peripheral and central nociceptive pathways for the head and face and may be present within the dura.[8,9] Functionally, mGlu3 receptor activation has been shown to suppress inhibitory inputs to nociceptive relay neurons in the sensory thalamus and these inputs are postulated to 'gate' the transmission of painful stimuli from relay neurons to the somatosensory cortex.[30] As such, antagonism of mGlu3 receptors may enhance the gating action of these inhibitory afferents and reduce pain. In fact, a correlation between compounds' potency for functional inhibition of human mGlu3 receptors and potency in an electrophysiological model quantifying the gating activity in the VPM of the thalamus has been established. In addition, the mGlu2/3 agonist LY354740 was shown to inhibit the inhibitory postsynaptic potentials in the ventral basal thalamus. This disinhibition was absent when the studies were performed in brain slices from mGlu3 knockout mice (E. Nisenbaum, pers. comm.).

LY2171158 is a potent and selective antagonist at mGlu3 receptors (Table 22.2). As such, this compound has been evaluated in the rat dural PPE model. LY2171158 significantly inhibited plasma protein extravasation in the dura following oral doses of 1,

Table 22.2 *In vitro* characterization of LY2171158 in AV12/RGT cells expressing human cloned metabotropic glutamate receptors. The compound was evaluated in three different modes: agonist, antagonist, and potentiator generating EC_{50}, IC_{50}, and EC_{50} values, respectively.

Mode	mGlu1	mGlu2	mGlu3	mGlu4	mGlu5	mGlu8
Agonist (EC_{50}, μM)	>25	>25	>25	>25	>25	>25
Antagonist (IC_{50}, μM)	>12.5	>12.5	0.102	>12.5	>12.5	>12.5
Potentiator (EC_{50}, μM)	>12.5	>12.5	>12.5	>12.5	>12.5	>12.5

10, and 100 µg/kg (Figure 22.2). This compound also had a long duration of effect in the PPE model (>18 h).

Several mGlu2/3 agonists, mGlu2 potentiators, and mGlu3 antagonists were evaluated in the *in vitro* rabbit saphenous vein contraction assay. None of the compounds evaluated significantly contracted the rabbit saphenous vein. As such, these data suggest mGlu2 agonists, mGlu2 allosteric potentiators, and mGlu3 antagonists could represent novel, non-vasoconstrictive antimigraine therapies.

Eli Lilly and Company in Indianapolis has recently announced that an mGlu3 antagonist has been advanced into clinical efficacy trials for the treatment of acute migraine.

Other metabotropic glutamate receptor targets for migraine

Group I metabotropic glutamate receptors are present in the TNC, meninges, hippocampus, and cortex. Metabotropic Glu1 receptor antagonists are efficacious in traditional preclinical models of pain,[31] but no publications exist evaluating their role in migraine pain. Conversely, in 2006 Addex Pharmaceuticals announced the start of the phase II development programme of ADX10059, its selective, negative allosteric modulator of mGlu5 receptors (Addex Pharmaceuticals, unpublished data). This announcement

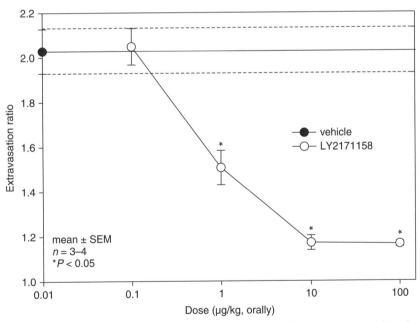

Fig. 22.2 Trigeminal stimulation-induced plasma protein extravasation in the dura of fasted Harlan–Sprague Dawley rats 1 h following oral pretreatment with LY2171158 or vehicle. The extravasation ratio is the average fluorescence intensity of the dura collected from the hemisphere ipsilateral to the stimulation divided by the average fluorescence intensity of the dura collected from the hemisphere contralateral to the stimulation. A ratio of approximately one would indicate a complete inhibition of plasma protein extravasation.

follows the successful completion of three phase I trials, in over 100 healthy subjects, which demonstrated good tolerability of the compound across a broad dose range. The first phase II study, which has started in Germany, evaluates the use of ADX10059 for the acute treatment of migraine.

Glutamate modulation by botulinum toxin type A (Botox)

Recent clinical studies have provided evidence to support botulinum toxin type A (Botox) as an efficacious preventative therapy for migraine.[32] The pharmacological effects of Botox were originally believed to be due to the inhibition of acetylcholine release at the neuromuscular junction, although the reduction of pain often occurred before the reduction of muscular activity. Aoki[33] has shown that Botox can reduce the nociceptive effects of formalin injection into the hindpaw of rats. He also showed that pretreatment with Botox 5 days prior to formalin injection into the paw could prevent the increase in glutamate release and reduce the formalin-mediated increased electrophysiological activity observed in wide dynamic range neurons of the dorsal horn. These data suggest Botox could be working, at least partially, by preventing the release of glutamate from sensory afferents.

Conclusions

There is evidence to support a role for glutamate in migraine as indicated by glutamate levels in migraineurs and the localization of both ionotropic and glutamate receptors in sites on the trigeminal pain pathway. The clinical efficacy of LY293558 and LY466195 also support a role for glutamate, and specifically iGluR5 receptors, in the pathophysiology of migraine. Emerging pharmacological agents, such as mGlu2 allosteric potentiators or mGlu3 antagonists that either modulate the release of glutamate or its postsynaptic effects, could represent additional novel therapies for the treatment of migraine. It is also possible that the definitive mechanism of action for many of the current acute and preventative migraine therapies involves modulation of glutamate levels at some location in the body.

References

1. Kew JNC, Kemp JA (2005) Ionotropic and metabotropic glutamate receptor structure and pharmacology. *Psychopharmacology* 179, 4–29.
2. Swanson CJ, Bures M, Johnson MP, Linden AM, Monn JA, Schoepp DD (2005) Metabotropic glutamate receptors as novel targets for anxiety and stress disorders. *Nat Rev Drug Disc* 4, 131–44.
3. Watanabe M, Mishina M, Inoue Y (1994) Distinct gene expression of the N-methyl-D-aspartate receptor channel subunit in the peripheral neurons of the mouse sensory ganglia and adrenal gland. *Neurosci Lett* 165(1–2), 183–6.
4. Araki T, Kenimer JG, Nishimune A, Sugiyama H, Yoshimura R, Kiyama H (1993) Identification of the metabotropic glutamate receptor-1 protein in the rat trigeminal ganglion. *Brain Res* 627(2), 341–4.
5. Sahara Y, Noro N, Iida Y, Soma K, Nakamura Y (1997) Glutamate receptor subunits GluR5 and KA-2 are coexpressed in rat trigeminal ganglion neurons. *J Neurosci* 17(17), 6611–20.

6. Tallaksen-Greene SJ, Young AB, Penney JB, Beitz AJ (1992) Excitatory amino acid binding sites in the trigeminal principal sensory and spinal trigeminal nuclei of the rat. *Neurosci Lett* 141, 79–83.

7. Kondo E, Kiyama H, Yamano M, Shida T, Ueda Y, Tohyama M (1995) Expression of glutamate (AMPA type) and γ-aminobutyric acid $(GABA)_A$ receptors in the rat caudal trigeminal spinal nucleus. *Neurosci Lett* 186, 169–72.

8. Tamura T, Nomura S, Mizuno N, Shigemoto R (2001) Distribution of metabotropic glutamate receptor mGluR3 in the mouse CNS: differential location relative to pre- and postsynaptic sites. *Neurosci* 106(3), 481–503.

9. Gillard SE, Tzaferis J, Tsui HT, Kingston AE (2003) Expression of metabotropic glutamate receptors in rat meningeal and brain microvasculature and choroid plexus. *J Comp Neurol* 461, 317–32.

10. Ma QP (2001) Co-localization of $5\text{-HT}_{1B/1D/1F}$ receptors and glutamate in trigeminal ganglia in rats. *Neuroreport* 12(8), 1589–91.

11. Goadsby PJ, Akerman S, Storer RJ (2001) Evidence for postfunctional serotonin (5-HT1) receptors in the trigeminocervical complex. *Ann Neurol* 50(6), 804–7.

12. Hill RG, Salt TE (1982) An ionophoretic study of the responses of rat caudal trigeminal nucleus neurons to non-noxious mechanical sensory stimuli. *J Physiol* 327, 65–78.

13. Bereiter DA, Benetti AP (1996) Excitatory amino acid release within spinal trigeminal nucleus after mustard oil injection into the temporamandibular joint region of the rat. *Pain* 67, 451–9.

14. Oshinsky ML, Luo J (2006) Neurochemistry of trigeminal activation in an animal model of migraine. *Headache* 46 (Suppl. 1), S39–44.

15. Ferrari MD, Odink J, Bos KD, Malessy MJ, Bruyn GW (1990) Neuroexcitatory plasma amino acids are elevated in migraine. *Neurology* 40, 1582–6.

16. Alam Z, Coombes N, Waring RH, Williams AC, Steventon GB (1998) Plasma levels of neuroexcitatory amino acids in patients with migraine or tension headache. *J Neurol Sci* 156, 102–6.

17. Ramadan NM (2003) The link between glutamate and migraine. *CNS Spectr* 8(6), 446–9.

18. Vaccaro M, Riva C, Tremolizzao L, *et al.* (2007) Platelet glutamate uptake and release in migraine with and without aura. *Cephalalgia* 27, 35–40.

19. Classey JD, Knight YE, Goadsby PJ (2001) The NMDA receptor antagonist MK-801 reduces Fos-like immunoreactivity within the trigeminocervical complex following superior sagittal sinus stimulation in the cat. *Brain Res* 907(1–2), 117–24.

20. Mitsikostas DD, Sanchez del Rio M, Waeber C, Moskowitz MA, Cutrer FM (1998) The NMDa receptor antagonist MK-801 reduces capsaicin-induced c-*fos* expression within rat trigeminal nucleus caudalis. *Pain* 76, 239–48.

21. Obrenovitch TP, Zilkha E (1996) Inhibition of cortical spreading depression by L-701,324, a novel antagonist at the glycine site of the N-methyl-D-aspartate receptor complex. *Br J Pharmacol* 117(5), 931–7.

22. Kaube H, Herzog J, Kaufer T, Dichgans M, Diener HC (2000) Aura in some patients with familial hemiplegic migraine can be stopped by intranasal ketamine. *Neurology* 55, 139–41.

23. Simmons RM, Li DL, Hoo KH, Deverill M, Ornstein PL, Iyengar S (1998) Kainate GluR5 receptor subtype mediates the nociceptive response to formalin in the rat. *Neuropharmacology* 37, 25–36.

24. Sang CN, Hostetter MP, Gracely RH, *et al.* (1998) AMPA/kainate LY293558 reduces capsaicin-evoked hyperalgesia but not pain in normal skin in humans. *Anesthesiology* 89, 1060–7.

25. Johnson KW, Dieckman DK, Phebus LA, *et al.* (2001) GluR5 antagonists as novel migraine therapies. *Cephalalgia* 21, 268.

26. Sang CN, Ramadan NM, Wallihan RG, *et al.* (2004) LY293558, a novel AMPA/GluR5 antagonist, is efficacious and well-tolerated in acute migraine. *Cephalalgia* 24, 596–602.

27. Weiss B, Alt A, Ogden AM, *et al.* (2006) Pharmacological characterization of the competitive GLUK5 receptor antagonist decahydroisoquinoline LY466195 in vitro and in vivo. *J Pharmacol Exp Ther* 318(2), 772–81.

28. Dieckman DK, Johnson MP, Britton TC, *et al.* (2003) Selective, non-amino acid allosteric mGlu2 receptor potentiators inhibit dural plasma protein extravasation: a potential role in the treatment of migraine. *Headache* 43(5), 582.

29. Huettl P, Quintero JE, Rutherford E, Pomerleau F, Johnson KW, Schoepp DD, Gerhardt GA (2007) Pharmacological studies of mGlu2/3 drugs on glutamate release utilizing ceramic-based microelectrode arrays. 40th Winter Conference on Brain Research, Snowmass Village, CO, January 27–February 2, 2007.

30. Turner JP, Salt TE (2003) Group II and III metabotropic glutamate receptors and the control of NRT input to rat thalamocortical neurons in vitro. *Soc Neurosci Abstr* 26(1–2), abstract 56.11.

31. Fundytus ME (2001) Glutamate receptors and nociception: implications for the drug treatment of pain. *CNS Drugs* 15, 29–58.

32. Blumenfeld A, Chippendale TJ (2006) Botulinum toxin type A compared with divalproex sodium for the prophylactic treatment of migraine: a randomized, evaluator-masked trial. *Neurology* 66(5), A377–8.

33. Aoki KR (2003) Evidence for antinociceptive activity of botulinum toxin type A in pain management. *Headache* 43 (Suppl. 1), S9–15.

23

The modulation of TRPV1 channels by cannabinoid₁ receptors

Beatriz Fioravanti and Todd W. Vanderah

The capsaicin receptor termed transient receptor potential vanilloid 1 (TRPV1) is a non-selective cation channel found on nociceptive afferent fibres and transduces various stimuli such as noxious heat, protons, lipoxygenase, and other lipid products, as well as capsaicin.[1–3] The TRPV1 channel has been extensively studied in the development of novel analgesics.[4,5] Many recent studies over the past 6 years have focused on the functional characteristics of the TRPV1 receptor and its role in acute and chronic pain. Studies have focused on identifying substances that act directly or indirectly in modulating the TRPV1 channel, hence altering the perception of pain. Non-vanilloid endogenous ligands include protons,[2] lipoxygenase products,[6] anandamide,[3,7] and related compounds such as *N*-arachidonoyldopamine.[8] The activation of several G-protein coupled receptors (GPCRs), including galanin GalR2 receptors,[9] somatostatin SSTR2a receptors,[10] bradykinin B₂ receptors,[11,12] cannabinoid CB₁ receptors,[13,14] and tyrosine kinase receptors such as TrkA[12] have been identified as modulating TRPV1 function. Chimeric and site-directed mutation studies of the TRPV1 channel have identified unique amino acid sites within the TRPV1 structure that may modulate the function of TRPV1[1–3,6,12,15–22]. Six different phosphorylation sites have been identified on the TRPV1 channel. The phosphorylation of unique sites on the TRPV1 results in a sensitized channel in the presence of agonists such as capsaicin,[16–19,22] yet the phosphorylation in the absence of the agonist has little effect on the channel. Endogenous TRPV1 ligands include the cannabinoid agonist anandamide and 2-arachidonoyl-glycerol. Recently these endogenous cannabinoid ligands, along with a family of structurally similar lipids, have been referred to as endovanilloids.[23,24] Furthermore, cannabinoid receptors and TRPV1 channels have been shown to be co-localized on nociceptive fibres in cultured rat DRG cells.[25–28] The cannabinoid₁ (CB₁) receptor is a GPCR that has constitutive activity both *in vitro* and *in vivo*.[29–33] SR141716A (Rimonabant), an inverse agonist at the CB₁ receptor with no affinity for the TRPV1 channel, reduced the vasodilatation effects induced by capsaicin.[3] Furthermore, Rimonabant had pharmacological effects in humans in a clinical trial for weight loss and produced a reduction in low-density lipoproteins, suggesting a significant constitutive activity at CB₁ receptors that when attenuated results in a physiological response.[34] These data along with several other studies[29–33] demonstrate a tonic, constitutive activity elicited via CB₁ receptors maintaining an endogenous intracellular level of second messengers that can be altered by inverse agonism.

We have established that the tonic activity of the CB_1 receptor maintains sensitization of the TRPV1 channel. The lack of a pH (Figure 23.1), capsaicin (Figure 23.2A) or 1% formalin response (Figure 23.2B) in the CB_1KO mice compared with a CB_1WT or control ICR mice support the idea that the CB_1 receptors must be present to maintain the activity of the TRPV1 channel.

Although one explanation for the lack of a capsaicin or formalin flinch response may be the loss of TRPV1 in the genetic design of the CB_1KO, using Western blot analysis of tissue from CB_1KO mice identified that the TRPV1 channel in CB_1KO mice is present in a quantity similar to CB_1WT mice. Further support for a role for CB_1 receptors and their modulation of TRPV1 was demonstrated using ICR mice and a CB_1 receptor inverse agonist. Capsaicin's effect was attenuated in a dose-related fashion in wild type or ICR mice pre treated with CB_1 inverse agonists. Several studies have demonstrated that phosphorylation of TRPV1 or removal of PIP_2 result in enhanced capsaicin-induced calcium influx via the TRPV1 channel.[3,6,12,16–22]

We investigated whether intraplantar capsaicin (10 μg/5 μl) would produce neurogenic inflammation in CB_1KO mice. Animals received an intravenous injection of Evans Blue dye in the tail, followed by capsaicin administration in the left paw and vehicle (100% ethanol) injection in the right paw. CB_1KO mice tissue did not display a significant change in the amount of dye extravasated in the left paw when compared with the left paw of control CB_1WT (Figure 23.3) and ICR mice. In all animals, Evans Blue extravasation was not evident in the control paw (right) (Figure 23.3).

The hypothesis that the TRPV1 channel is present but in a desensitized state in the CB_1KO mouse is further supported by pretreating CB_1KO mice with compounds such as galanin and bradykinin that are known to sensitize the TRPV1 channel then applying capsaicin to test for a behavioural response. The 10–15-min pretreatment of CB_1KO mice with either galanin or bradykinin resulted in a capsaicin response similar to wild-type mice. Furthermore, these same CB_1KO mice, when tested 24 or 48 h after gal/cap or BK/cap, no longer responded to the highest dose of capsaicin suggesting the animals had returned to a desensitized state, whereas 24- and 48-h post-testing of CB_1WT or ICR mice resulted in a full capsaicin response.

Studies have demonstrated that TRPV1 function is sensitive to endogenous levels of PIP_2. Capsaicin-induced calcium influx was enhanced by the administration of either bradykinin or NGF, which both act to stimulate phospholipase C (PLC) activity and decrease PIP_2 levels.[12] This enhanced activity via the TRPV1 channel was mimicked using an antibody that sequesters PIP_2. The enhanced capsaicin effect in the presence of PIP_2 antibody was blocked by capsazepine.[12] Similar results were found using rat DRG neurons.[12] Applying PLC to the inside-out patch of the TRPV1 resulted in enhanced activity and could be blocked using an antibody that binds and inhibits PLC activity. These data suggest that PLC activity plays a significant part in the modulation of TRPV1 function. We have demonstrated that the pre-administration of the PLC inhibitor

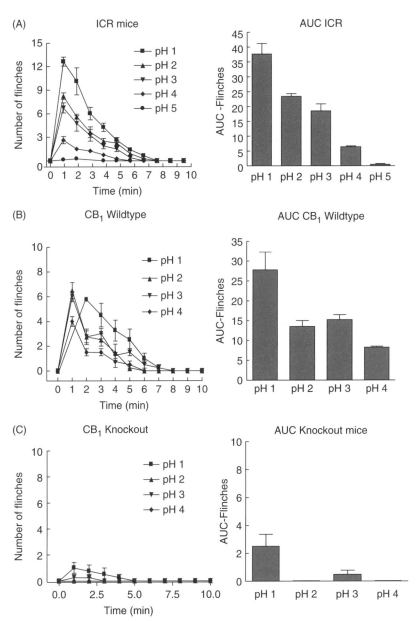

Fig. 23.1 Proton-induced paw flinches in ICR, CB₁WT, or CB₁KO mice. A solution of HCl at pH 4, 3, 2, or 1 increased flinches in ICR mice (A) and in CB₁WT mice (B) over a 10-min period but did not result in a significant number of paw induced flinches in the CB₁KO mice (c).

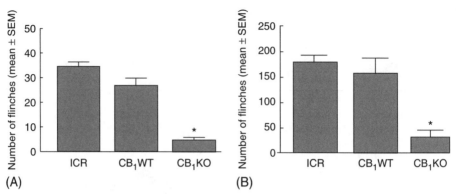

Fig. 23.2 Noxious chemical induced paw flinching in ICR, CB₁WT, or CB₁KO mice.
(A) Capsaicin at a dose of 10 g/5 l was administered directly into the plantar surface of the
hind paw and the number of flinches counted over a 5-min period. Capsaicin-induced flinching
was significantly reduced in CB₁KO mice compared with CB₁WT or ICR mice. (B) A concentration
of 1% formalin (20:l) was administered directly into the plantar surface of the hind paw and the
number of flinches counted over a 30-min period. Formalin-induced flinching was significantly
reduced in CB₁KO mice as compared with CB₁WT or ICR mice.

U73122 at a dose shown to be active *in vivo* significantly reduces a behavioural capsaicin
response in ICR mice, similar to behaviour in animals pretreated with a CB₁ inverse
agonist or CB₁KO mice (Figure 23.4).

The administration of an agonist such as bradykinin, somatostatin, or galanin that
activates the PLC pathway results in capsaicin-induced sensitization.[9,10,12] Here we show
that the pre-administration of bradykinin or galanin restored the capsaicin response in
CB₁KO mice. This supports the idea that the TRPV1 is present in the CB₁KO mice but in
a desensitized state until the intracellular mileu promotes a decrease in PIP₂ by activating

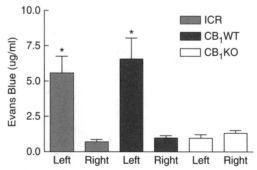

Fig. 23.3 Capsaicin-induced plasma extravasation in the left hind paw of ICR, CB₁WT,
or CB₁KO mice. Evans Blue (100 mg/kg) was injected into the tail vein of mice 15 min after
capsaicin (10 μg/5 μl) administration in the left hind paw. Plasma extravasation into the skin was
measured by spectrophotometry and compared with the right paw, which served as a control.
Capsaicin induced plasma extravasation in the ICR and CB₁WT mice but not in the CB₁KO mice.

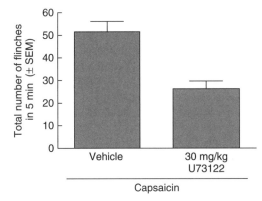

Fig. 23.4 Capsaicin-induced paw flinching is inhibited by pretreatment with the PLC inhibitor U73122. The 30 mg/kg, 30-min pretreatment results in the inhibition of capsaicin-induced paw flinching similar to that in the CB₁KO mice.

PLC and/or activating kinases such as protein kinase C and Cam kinase II restoring the sensitized state of the TRPV1 channel.

The CB₁KO mice had no significant change in their thermal latency when tested in the radiant heat paw flick test, similar to the findings reported by Zimmer et al.[36] These results can be explained by the presence of other heat sensitive channels, including TRPV2 through TRPV4. More importantly, capsaicin, unlike heat, has been shown to be selective for the TRPV1 channel.[1,15] These findings do not apply to all G_{ai} knockout GPCRs present in the nociceptive fibres as we did not see a reduced capsaicin response in mu opioid receptor knockout mice (unpublished observation).

The concept that GPCRs may couple to several different families of G-proteins has gained strength and has moved dual acting compounds into clinical trials (Oxytrex). CB₁ receptors have been shown to couple to G_{ai} and inhibit voltage-gated calcium channels and activate inward rectifying potassium channels to hyperpolarize nociceptors, ultimately inhibiting the release of pain neurotransmitters. However, studies in transfected COS7 cells and *Xenopus* oocytes demonstrated that CB₁ receptors couple to PLC and stimulate the production of inositol 1,4,5-triphosphate and diacylglycerol via $G\alpha14$, $G\alpha15$, and $G\alpha16$.[37,38] It has also been shown that the βγ portion of G-proteins can activate selective PLC isoforms[39,40] suggesting that CB₁ receptors may constitutively activate PLC via the βγ portion of the G-protein resulting in a decrease in PIP_2 and an increase in protein kinase C and Ca^{2+} induced kinases. Hence, the tonic activity of CB₁ and intracellular mileu of lipids and kinases results in a sensitized TRPV1 channel. An increase in cAMP/PKA, an event that occurs in the presence of the inverse agonist SR141716A, results in the inhibition of PLC activity.[17,39,41] Recent studies have shown that CB₁ receptors directly couple to G_{aq} and activate PLC in the presence of a cannabinoid agonist.[42] Although the CB₁ receptor has traditionally been classified as a G_{ai}-protein coupled receptor, several studies demonstrate CB₁ coupling to multiple G-protein subunits and its influence on several signal pathways, including PLC.

Jordt et al.[43] described how a TRPV1-like channel termed ANKTM1 in primary cultured trigeminal rat neurons and transfected HEK cells is activated by mustard oil. The cannabinoid agonists tetra hydro cannabinol (THC) and cannabinol enhanced calcium influx via the ANKTM1 channel. The cotransfection of the ANKTM1 with Muscarinic1 receptor (which activates PLC) increased the influx of intracellular calcium in the presence of mustard oil. They concluded this was due to an increase in protein kinase C activity, but ignored the decrease in possible inhibitory effects of PIP_2 on TRPV1 function.[43] They showed that the chelation of extracellular and intracellular calcium had no effect on THC and mustard oil effects on the ANKTM1 channel and was hence not calcium dependent.

Using Westerns and pharmacological studies we have shown that the neuroblastoma F-11 cell line has both the CB_1 and TRPV1 functional receptors. The administration of capsaicin results in the dose-dependent influx of calcium and can be reversed using the TRPV1 antagonist capsazepine. The pre-administration of the inverse agonist SR141716A or AM251 results in a dose-dependent inhibition of capsaicin-dependent calcium influx in the F-11 cells, suggesting that the pretreatment of F-11 cells with an inverse agonist can change the tonic activity of the CB_1 receptor. Changes of constitutive activity in the CB_1 receptor modulate intracellular transduction signals that decrease capsaicin-induced calcium influx via the TRPV1 channel.

GPCRs are known to produce their biological effect, in part, by modulating ion channels. The TRPV1 ion channel proves to be a very promiscuous channel with multiple intracellular messengers and surface receptors modulating its function. Thus far, the CB_1 receptor's propensity to be constitutively activated by inverse agonists such as rimonabant makes plausible its maintenance of an intracellular environment that results in a capsaicin sensitized TRPV1 channel.

References

1. Caterina MJ, Schumacher MA, Tominaga M, Rosen TA, Levine JD, Julius D (1997) The capsaicin receptor, a heat-activated ion channel in the pain pathway. *Nature* 389, 816–24.

2. Tominaga M, Caterina MJ, Malmberg AB, Rosen TA, Gilbert H, Skinner K, Raumann BE, Basbaum AI, Julius D (1998) The cloned capsaicin receptor integrates multiple pain-producing stimuli. *Neuron* 21, 531–43.

3. Zygmunt PM, Petersson J, Andersson DA, Chuang H, Sorgard M, Di Marzo V, Julius D, Hogestatt ED (1999) Vanilloid receptors on sensory nerves mediate the vasodilator action of anandamide. *Nature* 400, 452–7.

4. Gavva NR, Tamir R, Qu Y, Klionsky L, Zhang TJ, Immke D, Wang J, Zhu D, Vanderah TW, Porreca F, Doherty EM, Norman MH, Wild KD, Bannon AW, Louis JC, Treanor JJ (2005) AMG 9810 [(E)-3-(4-t-butylphenyl)-N-(2,3-dihydrobenzo[b][1,4] dioxin-6-yl)acrylamide], a novel vanilloid receptor 1 (TRPV1) antagonist with antihyperalgesic properties. *J Pharmacol Exp Ther* 313, 474–84.

5. Culshaw AJ, Bevan S, Christiansen M, Copp P, Davis A, Davis C, Dyson A, Dziadulewicz EK, Edwards L, Eggelte H, Fox A, Gentry C, Groarke A, Hallett A, Hart TW, Hughes GA, Knights S,. Kotsonis P, Lee W, Lyothier I, McBryde A, McIntyre P, Paloumbis G, Panesar M, Patel S, Seiler MP, Yaqoob M, Zimmermann K (2006) Identification and biological characterization of 6-aryl-7-isopropylquinazolinones as novel TRPV1 antagonists that are effective in models of chronic pain. *J Med Chem* 49(2), 471–4.

6. Hwang SW, Cho H, Kwak J, Lee SY, Kang CJ, Jung J, Cho S, Min KH, Suh YG, Kim D, Oh U (2000) Direct activation of capsaicin receptors by products of lipoxygenases, endogenous capsaicin-like substances. *Proc Natl Acad Sci USA* 97(11), 6155–60.

7. Smart D, Gunthorpe MJ, Jerman JC, Nasir S, Gray J, Muir AI, Chambers JK, Randall AD, Davis JB (2000) The endogenous lipid anandamide is a full agonist at the human vanilloid receptor (hVR1). *Br J Pharmacol* 129(2), 227–30.

8. Huang SM, Bisogno T, Trevisani M, Al-Hayani A, De Petrocellis L, Fezza F, Tognetto M, Petros TJ, Krey JF, Chu CJ, Miller JD, Davies SN, Geppetti P, Walker JM, Di Marzo V (2002) An endogenous capsaicin-like substance with high potency at recombinant and native vanilloid VR1 receptors. *Proc Natl Acad Sci USA* 99(12), 8400–5.

9. Jimenez-Andrade JM, Zhou S, Du J, Yamani A, Grady JJ, Castañeda-Hernandez G, Carlton SM (2004) Pro-nociceptive role of peripheral galanin in inflammatory pain. *Pain* 110(1–2), 10–21.

10. Carlton SM, Zhou S, Du J, Hargett GL, Ji G, Coggeshall RE (2004) Somatostatin modulates the transient receptor potential vanilloid 1 (TRPV1) ion channel. *Pain* 110(3), 616–27.

11. Cesare P, McNaughton P (1996) A novel heat-activated current in nociceptive neurons and its sensitization by bradykinin. *Proc Natl Acad Sci USA* 93(26), 15435–9.

12. Chuang HH, Prescott ED, Kong H, Shields S, Jordt SE, Basbaum AI, Chao NV, Julius D (2001) Bradykinin and nerve growth factor release the capsaicin receptor from PtdIns(4,5)P2-mediated inhibition. *Nature* 411, 957–62.

13. Jeske NA, Patwardhan AM, Gamper N, Price TJ, Akopian AN, Hargreaves KM (2006) Cannabinoid WIN 55,212-2 regulates TRPV1 phosphorylation in sensory neurons. *J Biol Chem* 281(43), 32879–90.

14. Patwardhan AM, Jeske NA, Price TJ, Gamper N, Akopian AN, Hargreaves KM (2006) The cannabinoid WIN 55,212-2 inhibits transient receptor potential vanilloid 1 (TRPV1) and evokes peripheral antihyperalgesia via calcineurin. *Proc Natl Acad Sci USA* 103(30), 11393–8.

15. Caterina MJ, Julius D (2001) The vanilloid receptor, a molecular gateway to the pain pathway. *Annu Rev Neurosci* 24, 487–517.

16. De Petrocellis L, Harrison S, Bisogno T, Tognetto M, Brandi I, Smith GD, Creminon C, Davis JB, Geppetti P, Di Marzo V (2001) The vanilloid receptor (VR1)-mediated effects of anandamide are potently enhanced by the cAMP-dependent protein kinase. *J Neurochem* 77(6), 1660–3.

17. Bhave G, Zhu W, Wang H, Brasier DJ, Oxford GS, Gereau RW 4th (2002) cAMP-dependent protein kinase regulates desensitization of the capsaicin receptor (VR1) by direct phosphorylation. *Neuron* 35(4), 721–31.

18. Bhave G, Hu HJ, Glauner KS, Zhu W, Wang H, Brasier DJ, Oxford GS, Gereau RW 4th (2003) Protein kinase C phosphorylation sensitizes but does not activate the capsaicin receptor transient receptor potential vanilloid 1 (TRPV1). *Proc Natl Acad Sci USA* 100(21), 12480–5.

19. Rathee PK, Distler C, Obreja O, Neuhuber W, Wang GK, Wang SY, Nau C, Kress M (2002) PKA/AKAP/VR-1 module: a common link of Gs-mediated signaling to thermal hyperalgesia. *J Neurosci* 22(11), 4740–5.

20. Ahern GP (2003) Activation of TRPV1 by the satiety factor oleoylethanolamide. *J Biol Chem* 278, 30429–34.

21. Jung J, Shin JS, Lee SY, Hwang SW, Koo J, Cho H, Oh U (2004) Phosphorylation of vanilloid receptor 1 by Ca2+/calmodulin-dependent kinase II regulates its vanilloid binding. *J Biol Chem* 279(8), 7048–54.

22. Jin X, Morsy N, Winston J, Pasricha PJ, Garrett K, Akbarali HI (2004) Modulation of TRPV1 by nonreceptor tyrosine kinase, c-Src kinase. *Am J Physiol* 287(2), 558–63.

23. Di Marzo V, Blumberg PM, Szallasi A (2002) Endovanilloid signalling in pain. *Curr Opin Neurobiol* 12, 372–9.

24. van der Stelt M, Di Marzo V (2004) Endovanilloids. Putative endogenous ligands of transient receptor potential vanilloid 1 channels. *Eur J Biochem* 271, 1827–34.

25. Ahluwalia J, Urban L, Capogna M, Bevan S, Nagy I (2000) Cannabinoid 1 receptors are expressed in nociceptive primary sensory neurons. *Neuroscience* 100(4), 685–8.

26. Ahluwalia J, Urban L, Bevan S, Capogna MO, Nagy I (2002) Cannabinoid 1 receptors are expressed by nerve growth factor- and glial cell-derived neurotrophic factor-responsive primary sensory neurones. *Neuroscience* 110(4), 747–53.

27. Mitrirattanakul S, Ramakul N, Guerrero AV, Matsuka Y, Ono T, Iwase H, Mackie K, Faull KF, Spigelman I (2006) Site-specific increases in peripheral cannabinoid receptors and their endogenous ligands in a model of neuropathic pain. *Pain* 126(1–3), 102–14.

28. Binzen U, Greffrath W, Hennessy S, Bausen M, Saaler-Reinhardt S, Treede RD (2006) Co-expression of the voltage-gated potassium channel Kv1.4 with transient receptor potential channels (TRPV1 and TRPV2) and the cannabinoid receptor CB1 in rat dorsal root ganglion neurons. *Neuroscience* 142(2), 527–39.

29. Gifford AN, Ashby CR Jr (1996) Electrically evoked acetylcholine release from hippocampal slices is inhibited by the cannabinoid receptor agonist, WIN 55212-2, and is potentiated by the cannabinoid antagonist, SR 141716A. *J Pharmacol Exp Ther* 277(3), 1431–6.

30. Bouaboula M, Perrachon S, Milligan L, Canat X, Rinaldi-Carmona M, Portier M, Barth F, Calandra B, Pecceu F, Lupker J, Maffrand JP, Le Fur G, Casellas P (1997) A selective inverse agonist for central cannabinoid receptor inhibits mitogen-activated protein kinase activation stimulated by insulin or insulin-like growth factor 1. Evidence for a new model of receptor/ligand interactions. *J Biol Chem* 272, 22330–9.

31. Meschler JP, Kraichely DM, Wilken GH, Howlett AC (2000) Inverse agonist properties of N-(piperidin-1-yl)-5-(4-chlorophenyl)-1-(2,4-dichlorophenyl)-4-methyl-1H-pyrazole-3-carbox-amide HCl (SR141716A) and 1-(2-chlorophenyl)-4-cyano-5-(4-methoxyphenyl)-1H-pyrazole-3-carboxylic acid phenylamide (CP-272871) for the CB(1) cannabinoid receptor. *Biochem Pharmacol* 60(9), 1315–23.

32. Shearman LP, Rosko KM, Fleischer R, Wang J, Xu S, Tong XS, Rocha BA (2003) Antidepressant-like and anorectic effects of the cannabinoid CB1 receptor inverse agonist AM251 in mice. *Behavioral Pharmacol* 14, 573–82.

33. Zhou D, Shearman LP (2004) Voluntary exercise augments acute effects of CB1-receptor inverse agonist on body weight loss in obese and lean mice. *Pharmacol Biochem Behav* 77, 117–25.

34. Despres JP, Golay A, Sjostrom L (2005) Rimonabant in Obesity-Lipids Study Group. Effects of rimonabant on metabolic risk factors in overweight patients with dyslipidemia. *N Engl J Med* 353(20), 2121–34.

35. Sim-Selley LJ, Brunk LK, Selley DE (2001) Inhibitory effects of SR141716A on G-protein activation in rat brain. *Eur J Pharmacol* 414, 135–43.

36. Zimmer A, Zimmer AM, Hohmann AG, Herkenham M, Bonner TI (1999) Increased mortality, hypoactivity, and hypoalgesia in cannabinoid CB1 receptor knockout mice. *Proc Natl Acad Sci USA* 96, 5780–5.

37. Ho BY, Current L, Drewett JG (2002) Role of intracellular loops of cannabinoid CB(1) receptor in functional interaction with G(alpha16). *FEBS Lett* 522(1–3), 130–4.

38. Ho BY, Uezono Y, Takada S, Takase I, Izumi F (1999) Coupling of the expressed cannabinoid CB1 and CB2 receptors to phospholipase C and G protein-coupled inwardly rectifying K+ channels. *Receptors Channels* 6(5), 363–74.

39. Liu M, Simon MI (1996) Regulation by cAMP-dependent protein kinease of a G-protein-mediated phospholipase C. *Nature* 382, 83–7.

40. Huang C-L, Feng S, Hilgemann DW (1998) Direct activation of inward rectifier potassium channels by PIP2 and its stabilization by Gβγ. *Nature* 391, 803–6.

41. Wen Y, Anwer K, Singh SP, Sanborn BM (2005) Protein kinase-A inhibits phospholipase-C activity and alters protein phosphorylation in rat myometrial plasma membranes. *Endocrinology* 131(3), 1377–82.

42. Lauckner JE, Hille B, Mackie K (2005) The cannabinoid agonist WIN55,212-2 increases intracellular calcium via CB1 receptor coupling to Gq/11 G proteins. *Proc Natl Acad Sci USA* 102(52), 19144–9.

43. Jordt SE, Bautista DM, Chuang HH, McKemy DD, Zygmunt PM, Högestätt ED, Meng ID, Julius D (2004) Mustard oils and cannabinoids excite sensory nerve fibres through the TRP channel ANKTM1. *Nature* 427(6971), 260–5.

24

Future targets for headache therapy: prostanoids

Christian Waeber

Aspirin is the best-known and most widely used medicine to treat headaches and many other minor illnesses. It is estimated that 100 billion tablets are swallowed in the world every year. Aspirin's active ingredient, acetyl salicylic acid, is a synthetic derivative of salicin, which occurs naturally in plants, notably the willow tree and the perennial herb meadowsweet. As early as 400 BC, Hippocrates recommended a brew made from willow leaves to treat labour pains.[1] In the middle of the nineteenth century, 1853, French scientists made salicylic acid from salicin. Gastric irritation and the unpleasant taste of salicylic acid were, however, problematic side-effects. In 1897, the German chemist Felix Hoffmann developed and patented a process for synthesizing an altered version of salicin, which caused less irritation to the lining of the mouth and stomach than salicylic acid. The trade name 'Aspirin' was registered in 1899 ('A' for acetyl and 'spir' from the first part of *Spirea ulmania*, the Latin name for meadowsweet).

The mechanism of action of aspirin was only elucidated in the 1970s by Sir John Vane (who was awarded the Nobel Prize in 1982 for this work). The transformation of arachidonic acid to prostaglandin H_2 (PGH_2) is a step that commits arachidonic acid down the path of prostaglandin–thromboxane synthesis. This transformation is catalysed by cytosolic cyclooxygenase (COX, also known as prostaglandin G/H synthase), which is inhibited by aspirin. Prostaglandin H_2 is an unstable intermediate and is further converted to one of many prostanoids, such as prostacyclin (PGI_2) and thromboxane A_2 (TXA_2), by tissue-specific isomerases.

At the beginning of the twenty-first century, aspirin remains a cornerstone of pain therapy, based upon its more than 100-year track record of efficacy, its cost-effectiveness, and relative safety. Non-aspirin 'non-steroidal anti-inflammatory drugs' (NSAIDs) have enjoyed a much shorter history than aspirin. Ibuprofen, the first of the non-aspirin NSAIDs, was identified in the early 1950s, and by the 1970s it was being widely prescribed for the treatment of painful musculoskeletal anti-inflammatory conditions. Over the following years, new classes of NSAIDs were identified and a series of novel agents was brought to market. These drugs are now among the most widely prescribed of all therapeutic agents, but also have a significant history of toxicity and adverse effects. Indeed, chronic use of aspirin and other NSAIDs gives rise to serious iatrogenic effects in the gastrointestinal (GI) tract. These include the development of haemorrhage and ulcers in a significant proportion of the patient population. Over 100 000 hospitalizations and

16 500 deaths result every year from NSAID-induced serious adverse events in the USA alone.[2] Even low doses of aspirin can have detrimental effects on the gastric mucosa: a meta-analysis of 24 randomized trials involving over 66 000 patients reported a twofold increase in the risk of GI bleeding for those taking chronic low-dose aspirin compared with those not taking aspirin.[3] Various formulation improvements (e.g. coating, buffering) only slightly decrease the incidence of these adverse reactions.[4] A possible explanation is that systemic effects (e.g. on platelets, and prostaglandin synthesis), which are unlikely to differ according to the aspirin preparation used, are at least as harmful as local effects on the gastric or duodenal mucosa. In addition, many NSAIDs cause GI damage when administered parenterally. A better understanding of the mechanism underlying GI injury has led to significant pharmacological advances. These newer approaches have predominantly concerned the development of selective inhibitors of the inducible isoform of the enzyme COX, known as the COX-2 inhibitors or coxibs[5] (see below) and of agents that offer protection mechanisms to the gut against potential injury, such as those that contain or are combined with prostanoid analogues or nitric oxide (NO)-releasing moieties. These latter agents are known as the NO NSAIDs[6] and more recently as CINODS (COX-inhibiting NO donating drugs).[7]

Development of cyclooxygenase-2 selective agents

It was evident from early studies that there were different COX isoforms formed at the inflammatory sites and in the gastric mucosa. The contribution of any pharmacokinetic disposition to the site selectivity of the agents studied was not known, and whether it reflected uptake or selectivity of action of the agents by the inflammatory cells themselves was also not found. However, the findings did indicate the potential for site-selective COX inhibitors to yield anti-inflammatory agents with less GI toxicity.[8] The biochemical rationale for the development of COX-2 selective drugs arose 10 years later from an understanding of the molecular biology of COX, with the identification of two distinct isoforms.[9–11]

The COX-1 isoform present in the GI mucosa, renal systems, and platelets was identified as a constitutive enzyme. The prostanoids synthesized by this COX-1 enzyme are involved in the control of many physiological functions including microvascular blood flow, platelet aggregation, renal tubular functions, and the regulation of gastric acid production and mucosal integrity. The second isoform, COX-2, was found to be inducible, and expressed within 4–24 h in a number of cell systems following challenge with inflammatory mediators such as interleukin-1, lipopolysaccharide, and various mitogens.[9–12] COX-2 is considered to be the primary source of the proinflammatory prostanoids, making it an appropriate target for drug development,[13–16] leading to the new drug class of anti-inflammatory agents, the coxibs. Preclinical evaluation of the coxibs has clearly demonstrated that, in contrast to the classical NSAIDs, they do not provoke gastric mucosal injury under a number of experimental settings.[14,15] Two large clinical studies confirmed the superiority of coxibs' GI profile over that of conventional NSAIDs.[17,18] For one of these trials, however,[17] the GI superiority of celecoxib observed in the 6-month data failed to manifest in the 12-month data.[19] This may have been related to the fact that COX-2 is expressed constitutively in some tissues under physiological situations, and may also play a defensive role in the gut and kidney.[20] In the gastric mucosa, COX-2 inhibitors can aggravate the damage provoked by ischaemia–reperfusion,[21] and can attenuate the protective response elicited by mild irritants to subsequent more severe challenge.[22] Moreover, COX-2 may have a functional role in the healing of mucosal ulcers.[23]

Subsequent trials were designed to show the efficacy of coxibs for novel indications. One such trial[24] was prematurely terminated after investigators found an increased cardiovascular risk among patients taking the drug. Several studies have shown that TXA_2, a vasoconstrictor and promoter of platelet aggregation, is largely COX-1-derived, whereas the synthesis of the vasodilator and potent inhibitor of platelet aggregation, PGI_2, is linked to COX-2 induction.[25,26] Specifically, COX-2 upregulation (e.g. by interleukin-1β) shifts arachidonic acid metabolism from TXA_2 synthesis to the preferential production of PGI_2.[27] Furthermore, although non-selective COX inhibitors, such as aspirin and ibuprofen, suppress TXA_2 production in platelets, selective COX-2 inhibitors do not.[25,26] Taken together, these data suggest that COX-2 inhibition can tip vascular homeostasis into a prothrombotic state.

Cyclooxygenase inhibition and migraine

The previous section would suggest that COX inhibitors are old non-specific drugs, ridden with numerous side-effects. Why, then, consider them in a scientific session centred on future targets for headache therapy? The following sections will deal with four possible answers to this question: (1) the fact that clinical trials support the efficacy of COX inhibition in migraine therapy; (2) that inflammatory mechanisms are known to be involved in migraine pathophysiology; (3) recent data implicate specific prostaglandin receptor subtypes in inflammatory and nociceptive mechanisms; and, therefore (4) current or future subtype selective agents might specifically target migraine pain, without affecting other physiological functions such as microvascular blood flow, platelet aggregation, renal tubular functions, gastric acid production, and mucosal integrity.

The established efficacy of NSAIDs in migraine therapy has been summarized extensively elsewhere (see for instance reference 28) and a full review is beyond the scope of this paper. It has been shown for instance that intravenous administration of the COX inhibitor aspirin is effective in treating acute migraine.[29] Furthermore, NSAIDs such as paracetamol, ibuprofen, ketoprofen, and diclofenac, have been shown to be two- to threefold more effective than placebo in treating migraine and tension headache.[30–33] Finally, it is important to mention that rofecoxib, a long-acting (about 17-hour half-life) selective COX-2 inhibitor has also been shown to be superior to placebo in a large parallel-groups trial.[34]

Migraine and inflammation

Although inflammation and pain usually go hand in hand, migraine has not classically been considered an inflammatory disease, possibly because it is not obviously associated with heat, redness, and swelling. Instead, a vascular aetiology was proposed, and for most of the twentieth century, the prevailing theory of migraine held that pain results from an abnormal dilatation of intracranial blood vessels, leading to mechanical excitation of sensory fibres that innervate these vessels. In recent years, accumulating evidence has shifted the emphasis away from vascular smooth muscle and toward mechanisms related to inflammation within cephalic tissue, with concomitant activation of meningeal afferents, release of neuropeptides, vasodilatation, and extravasation of plasma proteins.[35] According to this 'neurogenic inflammation' theory, ions and inflammatory agents are released in the vicinity of sensory fibres innervating the meninges, where they activate and sensitize peripheral nociceptors. Exposure of perivascular fibres to chemical agents alters their sensitivity to subsequent stimuli and leads to the sensation of head pain. The cause of the initial release of these chemicals has not been established but may arise from brain, blood, or meningeal tissues. Exogenous agents such as NO donors cause migraine or migraine-like attacks,[36] and it is possible that other precipitants found in air, food, or drugs activate similar pathways in susceptible individuals.[37] In addition, several lines of evidence suggest that perivascular fibres are also activated by endogenous factors released during cortical spreading depression-like phenomena.[38]

Neurogenic inflammation occurs in many organs.[39] Although it often appears to be a beneficial and protective response, neurogenic inflammation can also be maladaptive and destructive, and may be involved in the pathophysiology of diseases such as arthritis, multiple sclerosis, and asthma. In dura mater, activation of meningeal nociceptors causes sensory fibres to release neuropeptides, including substance P and calcitonin gene-related peptide (CGRP).[35] This initiates a process of neurogenic inflammation, leading to a further secretion of inflammatory agents (such as bradykinin and prostanoids). In rats, after application of a cocktail containing these inflammatory mediators to the dural sinuses, meningeal primary afferent neurons rapidly become mechanically hypersensitive (i.e. neurons that showed no or minimal response to a small dural indentation before the chemical irritation show a strong response minutes after application of these inflammatory mediators).[40] Similarly, this cocktail causes central trigeminal neurons receiving convergent input from the dura and the skin to lower their thresholds to mechanical dural stimulation and to mechanical and thermal stimulation of the skin. Lidocaine application to the dura abolishes the response to dural stimulation, but has minimal effect on the increased response to cutaneous stimulation, suggesting involvement of a central mechanism in maintaining the sensitized state, which can last up to 10 h.[41] Based on these studies, Burstein has proposed that: (1) sensitization of both peripheral and central trigeminovascular neurons accounts for the intracranial hypersensitivity observed in migraineurs; (2) sensitization of central but not peripheral trigeminal neurons is responsible for the extracranial hypersensitivity (extracranial tenderness and cutaneous allodynia) often seen in these patients.[42]

Prostanoids and migraine

Various lines of clinical evidence implicate prostanoids in the pathogenesis of migraine headache. Levels of PGE_2 are elevated in the plasma, saliva, or venous blood of migraineurs during migraine attacks.[43–45] In addition, migraine-like symptoms can be induced in migraineurs by the exogenous administration of prostaglandins of the E series.[46,47] Finally, a major side-effect of the IP receptor agonist iloprost is headache.[48,49] Taken together, these observations suggest that not only inhibiting prostanoid synthesis, but also blocking prostanoid receptors would be an effective approach to treat migraine headache.

Potential drug targets

Arachidonic acid metabolites play a pivotal role in both inflammation and pain. These metabolites include both enzymatically generated products (thromboxanes, prostaglandins, leucotrienes, lipoxins, and epoxyeicosatrienoic acids) and non-enzymatically produced substances (isoprostanes and cyclopentenone prostaglandins). In response to cell stimulation, prostanoids are synthesized by the COX pathway from arachidonic acid released from membrane phospholipids by the actions of phospholipases (Figure 24.1). Prostanoids, once formed, are quickly released. Owing to their chemical and metabolic instability, they probably only act in the vicinity of their sites of production. Thus, they are 'short-range hormones', maintaining local homeostasis in a variety of tissues and cells. While some prostaglandins have anti-inflammatory effects (they decrease inflammation, increase oxygen flow, prevent cell aggregation, and decrease pain), others are known to have proinflammatory effects.

The actions of the five naturally occurring prostanoid metabolites of arachidonic acid (PGD_2, PGE_2, PGF_2, PGI_2, and TXA_2) are mediated via interaction with specific plasma membrane G protein-coupled receptors. Five major subdivisions of the prostanoid receptor family, termed DP, EP, FP, IP, and TP, have been defined on the basis of their pharmacological sensitivity and molecular identity[50,51] (Table 24.1). In smooth muscle,

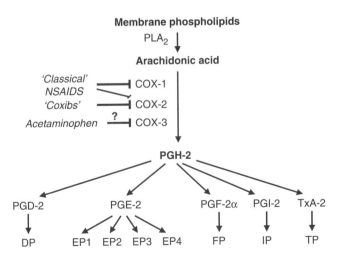

Fig. 24.1 Summary of biosynthetic routes to the major prostaglandins and thromboxane A_2.

Table 24.1 Properties of prostanoid receptor subtypes.

Subtype	Potency order	G protein	Signalling	Alternative splicing
DP	D>>E>F>I,T	Gs	cAMP increase	None
EP				
EP$_1$	E>F,I>D,T	Gq/11	Ca^{2+} increase	2 (rat)
EP$_2$	E>F,I>D,T	Gs	cAMP increase	None
EP$_3$	E>F,I>D,T	Gq/11, Gi/o, Gs	cAMP increase	3 (mouse)
			Ca^{2+} increase	4 (rat)
			cAMP decrease	8 (human)
EP$_4$	E>F,I>D,T	Gs	cAMP increase	None
FP	F>D>E>I,T	Gq/11	Ca^{2+} increase	2 (cow)
IP	I>>D,E,F>T	Gs, Gq/11	cAMP increase	None
			Ca^{2+} increase	
TP	T,H>>D,E,F,I	Gq/11, Gi/o, Gs	cAMP increase	2 (human)
			Ca^{2+} increase	
			cAMP decrease	

D: PGD$_2$; E: PGE$_2$; F: PGF$_{2\alpha}$; H: PGH$_2$; I: prostacyclin or PGI$_2$; T: thromboxane.

FP and TP receptors are functionally associated with contractile responses, while DP and IP receptors mediate relaxation. Electrical or inflammatory mediated stimulation of rat trigeminal ganglia *in vitro* has been demonstrated to cause a delayed synthesis and release of PGE$_2$ from dura mater.[52,53] This, in turn, can lead to the activation of pain-stimulating trigeminovascular afferents that innervate and cause vasodilatation of the cranial and cerebral vasculature.[54]

PGE$_2$ has received the most attention among prostaglandins because of its contribution to nociception and inflammation. PGE$_2$ stereospecifically exerts potent (within the nanomolar to micromolar range) tissue- and cell type-selective actions. PGE$_2$ is not only thought to play a key role in nociception (e.g. intradermal PGE$_2$ is largely responsible for hyperalgesia in the peripheral nervous system) but also appears to be involved in a wide variety of other functions, including altered microvascular permeability, and febrile responses.[55,56] PGE$_2$ induces different cellular responses via interaction with specific receptors (EP$_1$–EP$_4$), with restricted patterns of expression and receptor-specific actions.[57] The most widely accepted explanation for the effects of prostaglandins on nociception relates to the activation of the adenyl cyclase/cAMP/protein kinase A pathway following PGE$_2$ binding to EP$_2$ receptors, which leads to enhanced, tetrodotoxin-resistant sodium currents (probably via phosphorylation of Na$_v$1.8), inhibition of voltage-dependent potassium currents, and increased voltage-dependent calcium influx in nociceptive afferent fibres.[58] These changes in ion influx result in decreased firing thresholds, increased firing rates, and the release of excitatory amino acids, substance P, CGRP, and NO. Additionally, protein kinase A activated following PGE$_2$ binding to EP$_2$ receptors may selectively block inhibitory (strychnine-sensitive) glycinergic neurotransmission on to superficial dorsal horn neurons.[59] This PGE$_2$-induced 'disinhibition' may facilitate transmission of nociceptive input to higher areas of the central nervous system.

A complex interplay of receptor subtypes may be involved in various hypersensitivity states, and different subtypes could be activated depending upon the amount of agonist present. Utilizing EP$_1$ and EP$_3$ receptor knockout mice, Minami *et al.*[60] demonstrated that spinal EP$_1$ receptors contribute to PGE$_2$-induced allodynia (apparently upstream from N-methyl-D-aspartate receptor activation and resultant NO generation). At low doses of PGE$_2$, however, it appears that spinal EP$_3$ receptors may play a key role in PGE$_2$-induced hyperalgesia.[60] Nanomolar concentrations of PGE$_2$ reduce the responsiveness of postsynaptic inhibitory glycine receptors in the superficial layers of the spinal cord dorsal horn[59] and may also directly depolarize deep dorsal horn neurons.

cAMP-coupled, functional EP prostanoid receptors have recently been observed on cultured rat trigeminal neurons, where stimulation mediates Ca^{2+}-dependent CGRP release.[61] A recent study showed that EP$_4$ receptors mediate PGE$_2$-induced vasodilatation of human middle cerebral artery, in addition to IP receptors mediating relaxation and TP receptors mediating contraction.[62] In this context, it is worth mentioning that considerable species differences have been reported regarding the effects of prostanoids on isolated cerebral blood vessels. PGE$_2$ has been demonstrated to weakly relax 5-hydroxytryptamine pre-contracted feline basilar and middle cerebral arteries,[63] but to contract canine, rabbit, and human basilar arteries.[64,65] Because endogenously produced prostaglandins, most notably PGE$_2$, seem to play a direct role in the pathophysiology of migraine by stimulating CGRP release from trigeminal afferents, selective EP$_4$ antagonists may be therapeutically beneficial.

Although PGE$_2$ seems to be the key prostaglandin involved in nociceptive processes, PGI$_2$ may contribute to hyperalgesia under certain circumstances. PGI$_2$ levels are elevated in the central nervous system during the early phase of carrageenan-induced paw oedema, and PGI$_2$ is thought to contribute to pain and inflammation because IP knockout mice show a reduction in pain and oedema.[66] IP and EP$_3$ receptors seem to mediate the enhanced acetic acid-induced writhing response in mice previously exposed to lipopolysaccharide.[67] Bradykinin-evoked increases in isolated nodose ganglion neuron excitability demonstrate the dependence on PGI$_2$ in the neuronal membrane, as inhibitors of PGI$_2$ synthesis block the effect of bradykinin.[68] PGD$_2$ may lead to hyperalgia via DP effects on substance P release, with subsequent binding to neurokinin-1 receptors on small-diameter primary afferent fibres.[58] DP effects have also been implicated in antagonizing PGE$_2$-induced allodynia.[58]

Alternative strategies

COX inhibitors act relatively high up on the arachidonid acid-prostanoid signalling cascade (Figure 24.1). This proximal molecular site of action may underlie their effectiveness in pain, and, more specifically, migraine therapy, but it is also inherently non-specific, which may cause untoward side-effects. The goal of the previous section was to identify potentially more specific receptor targets for migraine therapy. This approach may be valid because 45% of the known drug targets are receptors,[69] and the existence of multiple receptor subtypes might enable medicinal chemists to design highly specific agents. However, this strategy may fail if prostanoid receptors act in a significantly redundant manner. If this is the case, antimigraine drug design might have to use the older strategy (i.e. act high up in the prostanoid signalling cascade). The following paragraph highlights a potential target of this kind.

Bradykinin is a known stimulator of sensory neurons[70] and activates pathways known to be implicated in pain transmission during migraine headache. Bradykinin stimulates primary afferent neurons and also increases the firing rate of second-order neurons of the trigeminal nucleus caudalis.[71] In addition, bradykinin has also been shown to enhance CGRP release from cultured dorsal root and trigeminal ganglion neurons.[61,72] Bradykinin exerts its effects through the activation of seven transmembrane G-protein coupled receptors (B_1 or B_2 receptors). B_1 receptors are upregulated in response to inflammation and tissue damage, whereas bradykinin B_2 receptors exhibit a more widespread constitutive distribution pattern.[73] Both receptors are constitutively expressed in both dorsal root and trigeminal ganglia.[74,75] Chemical stimulation of the trigeminal ganglion with an 'inflammatory soup' containing bradykinin induces PGE_2 release from rat dura mater.[71] When tested on its own, bradykinin induces PGE_2 release via B_2 receptors, protein kinase C and mitogen-activated protein kinase-dependent activation of phospholipase A_2 and consequent stimulation of COXs.[76] Taken together, these results suggest bradykinin receptor antagonists may provide additional therapeutic approaches to the treatment of migraine.

Conclusions

Although therapeutic inhibition of the COX pathway has been used for millennia, most of the potential targets in this cascade have currently not been 'drugged'. Substantial data from animal pain models, taken together with the results of studies specifically focused on the trigeminal/meningeal system, strongly suggest that blocking one or several of the prostaglandin receptor subtypes may be useful in migraine therapy. Only clinical trials will be able to demonstrate whether the efficacy of current COX inhibitors will be retained in these more specific agents, and whether the side-effect profiles of these drugs will be significantly improved.

Arachidonic acid is generated from membrane phospholipids via the action of two types of phospholipase A_2 (a secreted 14 kDa form, and the type IV cytosolic 85 kDa isoform[77]). Arachidonic acid is then converted to the prostaglandin endoperoxides PGG_2 (not shown) and PGH_2 by two enzymes, COX-1 and COX-2. A COX-1 splice variant, named COX-3, has been cloned and found to be abundantly expressed in mature brain and spinal cord.[78] It was initially suggested to account for the therapeutic efficacy of acetaminophen. In humans however, an acetaminophen sensitive COX-3 protein is not expressed because the retention of intron-1 adds 94 nucleotides to the COX-3 mRNA, resulting in a frameshift in the mRNA and the production of a truncated protein lacking acetaminophen sensitivity. PGH_2 spontaneously decomposes in aqueous solution to form a mixture of PGD_2, PGE_2, and PGF_2. However, distinct enzymes catalyse the formation of each of these prostaglandins, as well as TXA_2 and PGI_2. The cellular expression pattern of each of these enzymes may influence the type of prostaglandin produced by a particular cell. Prostaglandins are liberated from cells and bind to a family of G-protein coupled receptors (see Table 24.1).

References

1. Jones R (2001) Nonsteroidal anti-inflammatory drug prescribing: past, present, and future. *Am J Med* 110(1A), 4–7S.

2. Wolfe MM, Lichtenstein DR, Singh G (1999) Gastrointestinal toxicity of nonsteroidal antiinflammatory drugs. *N Engl J Med* 340(24), 1888–99.

3. Derry S, Loke YK (2000) Risk of gastrointestinal haemorrhage with long term use of aspirin: meta-analysis. *BMJ* 321(7270), 1183–7.

4. Kelly JP, Kaufman DW, Jurgelon JM, Sheehan J, Koff RS, Shapiro S (1996) Risk of aspirin-associated major upper-gastrointestinal bleeding with enteric-coated or buffered product. *Lancet* 348(9039), 1413–16.

5. Hawkey CJ (1999) COX-2 inhibitors. *Lancet* 353(9149), 307–14.

6. Wallace JL, Reuter B, Cicala C, McKnight W, Grisham MB, Cirino G (1994) Novel nonsteroidal anti-inflammatory drug derivatives with markedly reduced ulcerogenic properties in the rat. *Gastroenterology* 107, 173–9.

7. Fagerholm U, Bjornsson MA (2005) Clinical pharmacokinetics of the cyclooxygenase inhibiting nitric oxide donor (CINOD) AZD3582. *J Pharm Pharmacol* 57(12), 1539–54.

8. Whittle BJ, Higgs GA, Eakins KE, Moncada S, Vane JR (1980) Selective inhibition of prostaglandin production in inflammatory exudates and gastric mucosa. *Nature* 284(5753), 271–3.

9. Fu JY, Masferrer JL, Seibert K, Raz A, Needleman P (1990) The induction and suppression of prostaglandin H2 synthase (cyclooxygenase) in human monocytes. *J Biol Chem* 265(28), 16737–40.

10. Xie WL, Chipman JG, Robertson DL, Erikson RL, Simmons DL (1991) Expression of a mitogen-responsive gene encoding prostaglandin synthase is regulated by mRNA splicing. *Proc Natl Acad Sci USA* 88(7), 2692–6.

11. O'Banion MK, Sadowski HB, Winn V, Young DA (1991) A serum- and glucocorticoid-regulated 4-kilobase mRNA encodes a cyclooxygenase-related protein. *J Biol Chem* 266(34), 23261–7.

12. Mitchell JA, Warner TD (1999) Cyclo-oxygenase-2: pharmacology, physiology, biochemistry and relevance to NSAID therapy. *Br J Pharmacol* 128(6), 1121–32.

13. FitzGerald GA, Patrono C (2001) The coxibs, selective inhibitors of cyclooxygenase-2. *N Engl J Med* 345(6), 433–42.

14. Masferrer JL, Zweifel BS, Manning PT, *et al.* (1994) Selective inhibition of inducible cyclooxygenase 2 in vivo is antiinflammatory and nonulcerogenic. *Proc Natl Acad Sci USA* 91(8), 3228–32.

15. Chan CC, Boyce S, Brideau C, *et al.* (1999) Rofecoxib [Vioxx, MK-0966; 4-(4'-methylsulfonylphenyl)-3-phenyl-2-(5H)-furanone]: a potent and orally active cyclooxygenase-2 inhibitor. Pharmacological and biochemical profiles. *J Pharmacol Exp Ther* 290(2), 551–60.

16. Warner TD, Giuliano F, Vojnovic I, Bukasa A, Mitchell JA, Vane JR (1999) Nonsteroid drug selectivities for cyclo-oxygenase-1 rather than cyclo-oxygenase-2 are associated with human gastrointestinal toxicity: a full in vitro analysis. *Proc Natl Acad Sci USA* 96(13), 7563–8.

17. Silverstein FE, Faich G, Goldstein JL, *et al.* (2000) Gastrointestinal toxicity with celecoxib vs nonsteroidal anti-inflammatory drugs for osteoarthritis and rheumatoid arthritis: the CLASS study: A randomized controlled trial. Celecoxib Long-term Arthritis Safety Study. *JAMA* 284(10), 1247–55.

18. Bombardier C, Laine L, Reicin A, *et al.* (2000) Comparison of upper gastrointestinal toxicity of rofecoxib and naproxen in patients with rheumatoid arthritis. VIGOR Study Group. *N Engl J Med* 343(21), 1520–82.

19. Drazen JM (2005) COX-2 inhibitors–a lesson in unexpected problems. *N Engl J Med* 352(11), 1131–2.

20. Kishimoto Y, Wada K, Nakamoto K, Kawasaki H, Hasegawa J (1998) Levels of cyclooxygenase-1 and -2 mRNA expression at various stages of acute gastric injury induced by ischemia-reperfusion in rats. *Arch Biochem Biophys* 352(1), 153–7.

21. Maricic N, Ehrlich K, Gretzer B, Schuligoi R, Respondek M, Peskar BM (1999) Selective cyclo-oxygenase-2 inhibitors aggravate ischaemia-reperfusion injury in the rat stomach. *Br J Pharmacol* 128(8), 1659–66.

22. Schmassmann A, Peskar BM, Stettler C, *et al.* (1998) Effects of inhibition of prostaglandin endoperoxide synthase-2 in chronic gastro-intestinal ulcer models in rats. *Br J Pharmacol* 123(5), 795–804.

23. Halter F, Tarnawski AS, Schmassmann A, Peskar BM (2001) Cyclooxygenase 2-implications on maintenance of gastric mucosal integrity and ulcer healing: controversial issues and perspectives. *Gut* 49(3), 443–53.

24. Bresalier RS, Sandler RS, Quan H, *et al.* (2005) Cardiovascular events associated with rofecoxib in a colorectal adenoma chemoprevention trial. *N Engl J Med* 352(11), 1092–102.

25. Cullen L, Kelly L, Connor SO, Fitzgerald DJ (1998) Selective cyclooxygenase-2 inhibition by nimesulide in man. *J Pharmacol Exp Ther* 287(2), 578–82.

26. McAdam BF, Catella-Lawson F, Mardini IA, Kapoor S, Lawson JA, FitzGerald GA (1999) Systemic biosynthesis of prostacyclin by cyclooxygenase (COX)-2: the human pharmacology of a selective inhibitor of COX-2. *Proc Natl Acad Sci USA* 96, 272–7.

27. Caughey GE, Cleland LG, Penglis PS, Gamble JR, James MJ (2001) Roles of cyclooxygenase (COX)-1 and COX-2 in prostanoid production by human endothelial cells: selective up-regulation of prostacyclin synthesis by COX-2. *J Immunol* 167(5), 2831–8.

28. Tfelt-Hansen P, Rolan P (2006) Nonsteroidal anti-inflammatory drugs in the acute treatment of migraines. In: Olesen J, Goadsby PJ, Ramadan N, Tfelt-Hansen P, Welch K (eds) *The Headaches*, 3rd edn, pp. 449–57. Lippincott Williams & Wilkins, Philadelphia, PA.

29. Diener HC (1999) Efficacy and safety of intravenous acetylsalicylic acid lysinate compared to subcutaneous sumatriptan and parenteral placebo in the acute treatment of migraine. A double-blind, double-dummy, randomized, multicenter, parallel group study. The ASASUMAMIG Study Group. *Cephalalgia* 19(6), 581–8; discussion 42.

30. Kellstein DE, Lipton RB, Geetha R, *et al.* (2000) Evaluation of a novel solubilized formulation of ibuprofen in the treatment of migraine headache: a randomized, double-blind, placebo-controlled, dose-ranging study. *Cephalalgia* 20(4), 233–43.

31. Codispoti JR, Prior MJ, Fu M, Harte CM, Nelson EB (2001) Efficacy of nonprescription doses of ibuprofen for treating migraine headache: a randomized controlled trial. *Headache* 41(7), 665–79.

32. Dib M, Massiou H, Weber M, Henry P, Garcia-Acosta S, Bousser MG (2002) Efficacy of oral ketoprofen in acute migraine: a double-blind randomized clinical trial. *Neurology* 58(11), 1660–5.

33. Prior MJ, Cooper KM, May LG, Bowen DL (2002) Efficacy and safety of acetaminophen and naproxen in the treatment of tension-type headache. A randomized, double-blind, placebo-controlled trial. *Cephalalgia* 22(9), 740–8.

34. Silberstein S, Tepper S, Brandes J, *et al.* (2004) Randomized, placebo-controlled trial of rofecoxib in the acute treatment of migraine. *Neurology* 62(9), 1552–7.

35. Moskowitz MA (1992) Neurogenic versus vascular mechanisms of sumatriptan and ergot alkaloids in migraine. *Trends Pharmacol Sci* 13(8), 307–11.

36. Olesen J, Iversen HK, Thomsen LL (1993) Nitric oxide supersensitivity: a possible molecular mechanism of migraine pain. *Neuroreport* 4(8), 1027–30.

37. Reuter U, Bolay H, Jansen-Olesen I, *et al.* (2001) Delayed inflammation in rat meninges: implications for migraine pathophysiology. *Brain* 124(Pt 12), 2490–502.

38. Bolay H, Reuter U, Dunn AK, Huang Z, Boas DA, Moskowitz MA (2002) Intrinsic brain activity triggers trigeminal meningeal afferents in a migraine model. *Nat Med* 8(2), 136–42.

39. Barnes PJ, Belvisi MG, Rogers DF (1990) Modulation of neurogenic inflammation: novel approaches to inflammatory disease. *Trends Pharmacol Sci* 11(5), 185–9.

40. Strassman AM, Raymond SA, Burstein R (1996) Sensitization of meningeal sensory neurons and the origin of headaches. *Nature* 384(6609), 560–4.

41. Burstein R, Yamamura H, Malick A, Strassman AM (1998) Chemical stimulation of the intracranial dura induces enhanced responses to facial stimulation in brain stem trigeminal neurons. *J Neurophysiol* 79(2), 964–82.

42. Burstein R (2001) Deconstructing migraine headache into peripheral and central sensitization. *Pain* 89(2–3), 107–10.

43. Nattero G, Allais G, De Lorenzo C, *et al.* (1989) Relevance of prostaglandins in true menstrual migraine. *Headache* 29(4), 233–8.

44. Tuca JO, Planas JM, Parellada PP (1989) Increase in PGE2 and TXA_2 in the saliva of common migraine patients. Action of calcium channel blockers. *Headache* 29(8), 498–501.

45. Sarchielli P, Alberti A, Codini M, Floridi A, Gallai V (2000) Nitric oxide metabolites, prostaglandins and trigeminal vasoactive peptides in internal jugular vein blood during spontaneous migraine attacks. *Cephalalgia* 20(10), 907–18.

46. Carlson LA, Ekelund LG, Oro L (1968) Clinical and metabolic effects of different doses of prostaglandin E1 in man. Prostaglandin and related factors. *Acta Med Scand* 183(5), 423–30.

47. Peatfield RC, Gawel MJ, Rose FC (1981) The effect of infused prostacyclin in migraine and cluster headache. *Headache* 21(5), 190–5.

48. Hildebrand M (1997) Pharmacokinetics and tolerability of oral iloprost in thromboangiitis obliterans patients. *Eur J Clin Pharmacol* 53, 51–6.

49. Gao IK, Scholz P, Boehme MW, Norden C, Lemmel EM (2002) A 7-day oral treatment of patients with active rheumatoid arthritis using the prostacyclin analog iloprost: cytokine modulation, safety, and clinical effects. *Rheumatol Int* 22(2), 45–51.

50. Coleman RA, Smith WL, Narumiya S (1994) International Union of Pharmacology classification of prostanoid receptors: properties, distribution, and structure of the receptors and their subtypes. *Pharmacol Rev* 46(2), 205–29.

51. Tsuboi K, Sugimoto Y, Ichikawa A (2002) Prostanoid receptor subtypes. *Prostaglandins Other Lipid Mediat* 68–69, 535–56.

52. Rich G, Yoder EJ, Moore SA (1998) Regulation of prostaglandin H synthase-2 expression in cerebromicrovascular smooth muscle by serum and epidermal growth factor. *J Cell Physiol* 176(3), 495–505.

53. Ebersberger A, Averbeck B, Messlinger K, Reeh PW (1999) Release of substance P, calcitonin gene-related peptide and prostaglandin E2 from rat dura mater encephali following electrical and chemical stimulation in vitro. *Neuroscience* 89(3), 901–7.

54. Williamson DJ, Hargreaves RJ, Hill RG, Shepheard SL (1997) Sumatriptan inhibits neurogenic vasodilation of dural blood vessels in the anaesthetized rat–intravital microscope studies. *Cephalalgia* 17(4), 525–31.

55. Williams TJ, Peck MJ (1977) Role of prostaglandin-mediated vasodilatation in inflammation. *Nature* 270(5637), 530–2.

56. Raud J, Dahlen SE, Sydbom A, Lindbom L, Hedqvist P (1988) Enhancement of acute allergic inflammation by indomethacin is reversed by prostaglandin E2: apparent correlation with in vivo modulation of mediator release. *Proc Natl Acad Sci USA* 85(7), 2315–19.

57. Narumiya S, FitzGerald GA (2001) Genetic and pharmacological analysis of prostanoid receptor function. *J Clin Invest* 108, 25–30.

58. Vanegas H, Schaible HG (2001) Prostaglandins and cyclooxygenases in the spinal cord. *Prog Neurobiol* 64(4), 327–63.

59. Ahmadi S, Lippross S, Neuhuber WL, Zeilhofer HU (2002) PGE(2) selectively blocks inhibitory glycinergic neurotransmission onto rat superficial dorsal horn neurons. *Nat Neurosci* 5, 34–40.

60. Minami T, Nakano H, Kobayashi T, *et al.* (2001) Characterization of EP receptor subtypes responsible for prostaglandin E2-induced pain responses by use of EP1 and EP3 receptor knockout mice. *Br J Pharmacol* 133(3), 438–44.

61. Jenkins DW, Feniuk W, Humphrey PP (2001) Characterization of the prostanoid receptor types involved in mediating calcitonin gene-related peptide release from cultured rat trigeminal neurones. *Br J Pharmacol* 134(6), 1296–302.

62. Davis RJ, Murdoch CE, Ali M, *et al.* (2004) EP4 prostanoid receptor-mediated vasodilatation of human middle cerebral arteries. *Br J Pharmacol* 141(4), 580–5.

63. Whalley ET, Schilling L, Wahl M (1989) Cerebrovascular effects of prostanoids: in-vitro studies in feline middle cerebral and basilar artery. *Prostaglandins* 38(6), 625–34.

64. Nakagomi T, Kassell NF, Sasaki T, *et al.* (1988) Effect of removal of the endothelium on vasocontraction in canine and rabbit basilar arteries. *J Neurosurg* 68(5), 757–66.

65. Parsons AA, Whalley ET (1989) Effects of prostanoids on human and rabbit basilar arteries precontracted in vitro. *Cephalalgia* 9(3), 165–71.

66. Murata T, Ushikubi F, Matsuoka T, *et al.* (1997) Altered pain perception and inflammatory response in mice lacking prostacyclin receptor. *Nature* 388(6643), 678–82.

67. Ueno A, Matsumoto H, Naraba H, *et al.* (2001) Major roles of prostanoid receptors IP and EP(3) in endotoxin-induced enhancement of pain perception. *Biochem Pharmacol* 62(2), 157–60.

68. Weinreich D, Koschorke GM, Undem BJ, Taylor GE (1995) Prevention of the excitatory actions of bradykinin by inhibition of PGI_2 formation in nodose neurones of the guinea-pig. *J Physiol* 483 (Pt 3), 735–46.

69. Drews J (2000) Drug discovery: a historical perspective. *Science* 287(5460), 1960–4.

70. Calixto JB, Cabrini DA, Ferreira J, Campos MM (2000) Kinins in pain and inflammation. *Pain* 87(1), 1–5.

71. Ebersberger A, Ringkamp M, Reeh PW, Handwerker HO (1997) Recordings from brain stem neurons responding to chemical stimulation of the subarachnoid space. *J Neurophysiol* 77(6), 3122–33.

72. Vasko MR, Campbell WB, Waite KJ (1994) Prostaglandin E2 enhances bradykinin-stimulated release of neuropeptides from rat sensory neurons in culture. *J Neurosci* 14(8), 4987–97.

73. Marceau F, Hess JF, Bachvarov DR (1998) The B1 receptors for kinins. *Pharmacol Rev* 50(3), 357–86.

74. Ma QP, Hill R, Sirinathsinghji D (2000) Basal expression of bradykinin B1 receptor in peripheral sensory ganglia in the rat. *Neuroreport* 11(18), 4003–5.

75. Seabrook GR, Bowery BJ, Heavens R, *et al.* (1997) Expression of B1 and B2 bradykinin receptor mRNA and their functional roles in sympathetic ganglia and sensory dorsal root ganglia neurones from wild-type and B2 receptor knockout mice. *Neuropharmacology* 36(7), 1009–17.

76. Jenkins DW, Sellers LA, Feniuk W, Humphrey PP (2003) Characterization of bradykinin-induced prostaglandin E2 release from cultured rat trigeminal ganglion neurones. *Eur J Pharmacol* 469(1–3), 29–36.

77. Bingham CO 3rd, Murakami M, Fujishima H, Hunt JE, Austen KF, Arm JP (1996) A heparin-sensitive phospholipase A2 and prostaglandin endoperoxide synthase-2 are functionally linked in the delayed phase of prostaglandin D2 generation in mouse bone marrow-derived mast cells. *J Biol Chem* 271(42), 25936–44.

78. Chandrasekharan NV, Dai H, Roos KL, *et al.* (2002) COX-3, a cyclooxygenase-1 variant inhibited by acetaminophen and other analgesic/antipyretic drugs: cloning, structure, and expression. *Proc Natl Acad Sci USA* 99(21), 13926–31.

25

Role of anandamide in the modulation of nitroglycerin-induced hyperalgesia: a study in the rat

Cristina Tassorelli, Rosaria Greco, Armando Perrotta, Simona Buscone, Giorgio Sandrini, and Giuseppe Nappi

Introduction

Alterations of endocannabinoid levels have been found in animal models of pain, neurological and neurodegenerative disorders, and inflammatory conditions. Migraine is a disabling neurological disorder mediated by the activation of the trigeminovascular system. Trigeminal sensory nerve fibres that innervate the cranial vasculature contain calcitonin gene-related peptide, substance P, and neurokinin. It has been proposed that migraine may be caused by cerebral vasodilatation, abnormal neuronal (trigeminal) firing, and neurogenic dural inflammation. The role of the endocannabinoid system in the pathogenesis of headaches has been recently put under scrutiny.

A recent study reported that anandamide (AEA), an endogenous ligand to the cannabinoid receptor, is able to inhibit neurogenic dural vasodilatation, induced by either calcitonin gene-related peptide or nitric oxide.[1] AEA seems to be tonically released to modulate the trigeminovascular system. Systemic nitroglycerin (NTG) is a nitric oxide donor that provokes spontaneous-like migraine attacks in migraine sufferers and induces a condition of hyperalgesia in the rat, 4 h after its administration.[2,3] The NTG-induced hyperalgesic state can be detected as an increase of nociceptive behaviour at the formalin test.

Aims

The aim of this study was to probe the possible role for AEA in the neurochemical mechanisms mediating NTG-induced hyperalgesia.

Materials and methods

Adult male Sprague–Dawley rats, weighing 180–220 g, were used in the present investigation. All animals ($n = 6$ per group) underwent formalin test.

Formalin test

The formalin test is a well-established rat model of persistent somatic pain that was refined by Tjølsen *et al.*[4] Following injection of 100 µl of a 1% solution of formalin into the plantar surface of the right hind paw, animals were placed in a plexiglas observation chamber ($10 \times 20 \times 24$ cm) in which a mirror (angled at 45°) allowed unimpeded observation of the animals' paws. The total number of flinches and shakes per min was counted during the period from 1 to 5 min after injection (phase 1) and, subsequently, for 1-min periods at 5-min intervals during the period from 15 to 60 min (phase 2) after formalin injection. Incomplete formalin injection constituted an exclusion criterion for the study.

Experimental groups

- *AEA:* i.p. injection of AEA (20 mg/kg i.p.) 30 min before the formalin test;
- *Control:* i.p. injection of 4% Tween 80 (vehicle) 30 min before the formalin test;
- *NTG4h :* i.p. injection of NTG (10 mg/kg i.p.) 4 h before the formalin test;
- *Control for NTG4h:* i.p. injection of saline 4 h before the formalin test;
- *AEA + NTG4h:* i.p. injection of NTG (10 mg/kg) (4 h before formalin test) and administration of AEA (20 mg/kg) 30 min before the formalin test.

Statistical evaluation

The total number of flinches and shakes evoked by formalin injection were counted for phases 1 and 2 of the formalin test. Differences between groups were analysed by Student's t test and a probability level of less than 5% was regarded as significant.

Results

In the control group, the injection of formalin resulted in a highly reliable, typical, biphasic pattern of flinches/shakes of the injected paw, being characterized by an initial acute phase of nociception within the first 5 min, followed by a prolonged tonic response from 15 to 60 min after formalin injection.

AEA administration significantly reduced the nociceptive behaviour in both phases of the formalin test (Figure 25.1).

NTG administration significantly increased the total number of flinches + shakes in phase 2 of formalin test (Figure 25.2), therefore confirming previous reports. AEA treatment significantly inhibited the nociceptive behaviour induced by NTG administration during phase 2 of test (Figure 25.3).

Conclusions

Recent clinical studies show that cerebrospinal fluid levels of AEA are significantly lowered in patients with chronic migraine with respect to control subjects.[5] In addition, AEA degradation seems to be increased in platelets of female migraineurs, to suggest an

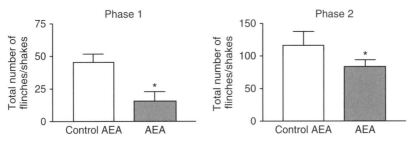

Fig. 25.1 Effect of treatment with anandamide (AEA) upon nociceptive behaviour at the formalin test. The histograms illustrate the total number of flinches and shakes per phase of formalin test. Data are expressed as mean ± SD. Each group was formed by six animals. Student's *t*-test: *$P < 0.05$ versus control group.

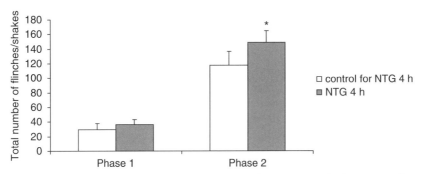

Fig. 25.2 Hyperalgesic effect of nitroglycerin (NTG) at the formalin test. The histograms illustrate the total number of flinches and shakes per phase of formalin test. Data are expressed as mean ± SD. Each group was formed by six animals. Student's *t*-test: *$P < 0.05$ versus control for NTG 4 h group.

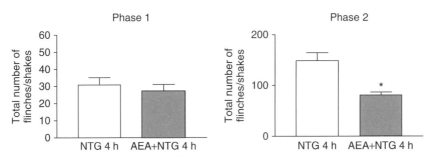

Fig. 25.3 Effect of treatment of anandamide (AEA) upon nitroglycerin (NTG)-induced hyperalgesia at the formalin test. The histograms illustrate the total number of flinches and shakes per phase of formalin test in rats evaluated 4 h after NTG administration. Data are expressed as mean ± SD. Groups were formed by six animals. Student's *t*-test: *$P < 0.05$ versus NTG 4 h group.

intriguing explanation for the prevalence of migraine in women.[6] Activation of the cannabinoid CB_1 receptor by synthetic agonists and pharmacological elevation of endocannabinoid levels suppress hyperalgesia and allodynia in animal models of neuropathic pain.

NTG administration activates specific cerebral nuclei via the intervention of selected neurotransmitters and neuromediators, with a specific time-pattern in brain and spinal areas of the rat. Endocannabinoid receptors have been identified in many of the NTG-activated areas. NTG-induced hyperalgesic condition in rat is mediated by cyclooxygenase induction, NMDA activation, *ex novo* nitric oxide synthesis,[7] and calcitonin gene-related peptide/substance P release. In the present study, we show that AEA administration significantly reduces NTG-induced hyperalgesic state. By combining the present data with the findings available from the literature,[8] we can hypothesize that a dysfunctional endocannabinoid system may contribute to the development of migraine attacks and that endocannabinoids or ligands of the cannabinoid receptor or, again, inhibitors of endocannabinoid-degrading enzymes may represent promising targets for the clinical management of migraine pain.

References

1. Akerman S, Kaube H, Goadsby PJ (2004) Anandamide is able to inhibit trigeminal neurons using an in vivo model of trigeminovascular-mediated nociception. *J Pharmacol Exp Ther* 309, 56–63.
2. Tassorelli C, Greco R, Sandrini G, Nappi G (2003) Central components of the analgesic/antihyperalgesic effect of nimesulide: studies in animal models of pain and hyperalgesia. *Drugs* 63, 9–22.
3. Tassorelli C, Greco R, Wang D, Morelli G, Nappi G (2003) Nitroglycerin induces hyperalgesia in rats: a time-course study. *Eur J Pharmacol* 464, 159–62.
4. Tjølsen Aberge OG, Hunskaar S, Rosland JH, Hole K (1992) The formalin test: an evaluation of the method. *Pain* 51, 5–17.
5. Sarchielli P, Pini LA, Coppola F, Rossi C, Baldi A, Mancini ML, Calabresi P (2007) Endocannabinoids in chronic migraine: CSF findings suggest a system failure. *Neuropsychopharmacology* 32(6), 1384–90.
6. Cupini LM, Bari M, Battista N, Argiro G, Finazzi-Agrò A, Calabresi P, MacCarrone M (2006) Biochemical changes in endocannabinoid system are expressed in platelets of female but not male migrain. *Cephalagia*, 26, 277–81.
7. Tassorelli C, Greco R, Wang D, Sandrini G, Nappi G (2006) Prostaglandins, glutamate and nitric oxide synthase mediate nitroglycerin-induced hyperalgesia in the formalin test. *Eur J Pharmacol* 534, 103–7.
8. Hohmann AG, Suplita RL (2006) Endocannabinoid mechanisms of pain modulation, 2006. *AAPS J* 8, 693–708.

Index

The index entries appear in letter-by-letter alphabetical order. Page references in italics indicate information in figures and tables.